# FINDING HOPE IN DESPAIR

## CLINICAL STUDIES IN INFANT MENTAL HEALTH

Edited by Marian Birch

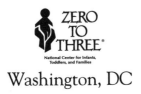

ZERO
TO
THREE®

National Center for Infants,
Toddlers, and Families

Washington, DC

Published by

ZERO TO THREE
2000 M St., NW, Suite 200, Washington, DC 20036–3307
(202) 638–1144
Toll-free orders (800) 899–4301, Fax: (202) 638–0851
Web: http://www.zerotothree.org

The mission of the ZERO TO THREE Press is to publish authoritative research, practical resources, and new ideas for those who work with and care about infants, toddlers, and their families. Books are selected for publication by an independent Editorial Board.

The views contained in this book are those of the authors and do not necessarily reflect those of ZERO TO THREE: National Center for Infants, Toddlers and Families, Inc.

These materials are intended for education and training to help promote a high standard of care by professionals. Use of these materials is voluntary and their use does not confer any professional credentials or qualification to take any registration, certification, board or licensure examination, and neither confers nor infers competency to perform any related professional functions.

The user of these materials is solely responsible for compliance with all local, state or federal rules, regulations or licensing requirements. Despite efforts to ensure that these materials are consistent with acceptable practices, they are not intended to be used as a compliance guide and are not intended to supplant or to be used as a substitute for or in contravention of any applicable local, state or federal rules, regulations or licensing requirements. ZERO TO THREE expressly disclaims any liability arising from use of these materials in contravention of such rules, regulations or licensing requirements.

The views expressed in these materials represent the opinions of the respective authors. Publication of these materials does not constitute an endorsement by ZERO TO THREE of any view expressed herein, and ZERO TO THREE expressly disclaims any liability arising from any inaccuracy or misstatement.

Cover design: K Art and Design, Inc.
Text design and composition: Black Dot Group

Library of Congress cataloging-in-infant-Publication Data
Finding hope in despair: clinical studies in infant mental health/edited by Marian Birch.
    p.;cm.
  Includes bibliographical references.
  ISBN 978-1-934019-25-2
1.  Infant psychiatry–Case studies.  I.  Birch, Marian.
  [DNLM: 1.  Infant–Case Reports.  2.  Mental Disorders–therapy–Case Reports.  3.  Child Psychology–Case  Reports.  4.  Family  Therapy–methods–Case  Reports.  5.  Parent–Child Relations–Case Reports. WS 350 F494 2008]
  RJ502.5.F56 2008
  618.92'89–dc22                                     2008012108

Copyright © 2008 by ZERO TO THREE. All rights reserved.
For permission for academic photocopying (for course packets, study materials, etc.) by copy centers, educators, or university bookstores or libraries, of this and other ZERO TO THREE materials, please contact Copyright Clearance Center, 222 Rosewood Drive, Danvers, MA 01923; phone, (978) 750–8400; fax, (978) 750–4744; or visit its Web site at www.copyright.com.

10 9 8 7 6 5 4 3 2 1
ISBN 0-978-1-934019-25-2
Printed in the United States of America

**Suggested citations:**
Book citation: Birch, M. (Ed.), (2008). *Finding hope in despair: Clinical studies in infant mental health.* Washington, DC: ZERO TO THREE.
Chapter citation: Sklan, S. (2008). How to mother when your mother leaves you again and again. In M. Birch (Ed.), *Finding hope in despair: Clinical studies in infant mental health* (pp. 29–66). Washington, DC: ZERO TO THREE.

# TABLE OF CONTENTS

# ACKNOWLEDGMENTS

This book has two mothers: it was conceived by Jeree Pawl and the late, much-missed Emily Fenichel. These two remarkable women decided that I was the person to write and edit a book to balance the many reports of successful treatment of infants and their families. Until her sudden death in June 2006, Emily Fenichel was a tireless supporter and participant in the project. My debt to Jeree goes further back, as she, Alicia Lieberman, and Graeme Hanson were my teachers and mentors as well as role models as an infant–parent psychotherapist. This trio sponsored me for a ZERO TO THREE fellowship, and offered their wisdom and support unstintingly. Other teachers and supervisors to whom I owe immense gratitude include Nathan Adler, Eleanor Dansky, Lester Eisenstadt, Daniel Greenson, Mary Main, and Elizabeth Lloyd Mayer.

I am grateful to my colleagues on the Olympic Peninsula: Mary Jane Apple, Carolyn Johnston, Heidi Kaas, Dott Kelly, Carol Hathaway, Nita Lynn, Cheryl Mantle, Bill Maier, Maureen Martin, Mary Morgan, Janet Proebstel, Sheri Stutesman, and Quen Zorrah, with all of whom I have discussed many of the ideas in this book. Likewise, my colleagues at the Center for Infant Mental Health and Development, at the University of Washington, Kathryn Barnard, Melissa Hoffman, Rosemary Kelly, Lisa Mennet, Susan Spieker, Joanne Solchany, and Donna Weston contributed to my understanding of the issues addressed here. I am particularly grateful to Lisa Mennet for reading preliminary sections of the book with her brilliant editorial scrutiny.

I cannot overstate how deeply grateful I feel for the wise and courageous work of my fellow authors, Toni Vaughn Heineman, Martin Maldonado-Durán, Richard Ruth, Susan Sklan, and Julie Stone. It has been a great pleasure and honor to work with them. It has truly been a collaborative and healing journey for all of us.

A special word of gratitude is due to the many families in pain who allowed me into their lives and who taught me more than I can ever tell.

Finally, with all love, I thank my husband, Bronson West, a trauma specialist and a child protective services supervisor, whose passion about all the questions in this book is the equal of mine, and whose love and support are immeasurably precious.

# FOREWORD

My very first young child case was a 3-year-old boy with a big, twinkling smile who would come to his sessions in whatever outfit suited his fancy that afternoon: pajamas, bathing trunks (in winter), snow pants (in summer), and everything in between. His long and very curly hair stuck straight up and out in masses of knots and tangles. He had three first names (two were Spanish and one was African) and a hyphenated last name; his mother called him by one of his Spanish first names, and his father by his African name. He referred to himself as either. His mother, depressed, overwhelmed, and morbidly obese, had already given birth to a second child, who was—at 1 year old—significantly delayed. Coping with her infant daughter's disabilities sapped her limited emotional and financial resources, leaving my little patient to make his own choices and to sort out the confusion and chaos of his daily life on his own. I never met the father, whose vaguely malevolent presence cast a long shadow over the treatment. I saw this family nearly 30 years ago, and they haunt me still. I could have done more, I could have helped more, I should have made the unbearable bearable and saved that sweet little boy from his own demons and the demons that surrounded him.

This case is one of the "heartbreaking failures" that are at the heart of Marian Birch and her colleagues' discussion of limits and limitations of infant–parent psychotherapy. This was the case that introduced me to the dark side of the hope with which we approach so many challenging cases—the hope that with our sensitivity, attunement, and robust capacity to mentalize, we will help the parent hold the child in mind, such that they can weather the storms of adversity, regardless of its strength or breadth. But as we quickly learn, the dark side of hope is, of course, despair, confusion, and all of the other nasty messes of anger, resentment, guilt, and fear that plague us when we confront the limits of our work and our capabilities.

So little of our professional literature—and by professional literature I mean not only the literature of infant–parent psychotherapy but the larger literature on psychotherapy and psychoanalytically informed treatment of both children and adults—concerns itself with the dark side of the therapeutic process. And yet most of us confront it regularly. Every therapist knows the familiar, sinking, and increasingly desperate feeling that sets in when we realize that we are losing a grip on a case. Usually these failures occur despite our best efforts, when we are working with families whose risk factors often seem beyond counting, and whose strengths have been all but obliterated by external circumstance and entrenched, generations-deep psychopathology. They occur when we have put more than our "all" into a case, when–in the case, for example, of impoverished families whose humanity is being eroded by systems out of their control—we have tried to move mountains and oceans both. There are other times when we actually *haven't* made our best efforts, but have instead given in to complacency or routine, and retreated into a kind of comfortable denial. In either instance, "losing" a case almost always engenders intense feelings, among them grief, sadness, guilt, anger, and worry for the future. We tell ourselves that we should have done better, we should have done more.

To date, discussions of treatment failures have been enormously limited. For the most part, failures are seen as just that, *failures*: failures of imagination, of compassion, of technique, of good ideas, of analyzing the transference, the countertransference, and so forth. Most therapists believe that when a case turns out badly, *they* have failed. Indeed, professional discussion of derailed treatments often carry the implicit message that were the therapist only more imaginative, compassionate, technically savvy, and so forth, (as the critic no doubt would have been!), the case would have had a more successful outcome. The roots for this self-blame are pervasive in our history. Psychoanalysis was conceived in an atmosphere that privileged understanding as an agent of change; even now, over 100 years later, we often see our failures as failures of understanding, as if understanding could somehow work miracles. Psychoanalysis was also conceived in an atmosphere that privileged *neutrality*. Even worse than failing to understand is *letting our own feelings get in the way*, the scourge of countertransference. Freud long ago implicated the therapist's neuroses in many aspects of treatment failure, especially when his or her strong feelings were aroused in the course of the work. It is hard to imagine how Freud's notions would have changed were he to have worked with vulnerable mothers and their infants.

In a way, treatment failures have been the field's "dirty little secret." For experienced therapists, the secret of one's derailed cases becomes an old, private, and unwelcome friend, ready to provoke shame and guilt at the slightest provocation. To the trainee, however, the first failures are never secret, but are there for the trainee, supervisor, and others to examine in painful detail. But because there is little open discussion of the reality and multidimensional aspects of treatment ruptures, they are often perceived by trainees as a *personal and unique failure,* and as such a source of burning shame and self-criticism. For all therapists, there is also a sense of loss and of lost opportunities that softens only with time.

Marian Birch and her colleagues—Susan Sklan, Richard Ruth, Julie Stone, Martin Maldonado-Durán, and Toni Heineman—have bravely initiated a remarkably lucid, honest, and probing examination of the treatment ruptures that inevitably occur even *and especially* within the context of "good enough" and even very good care. Using a series of beautifully documented and considered case presentations to organize their conversation, the authors begin to develop what has been so sorely missing in our field: a language for the limitations and limits of the work we do. Together, their diverse voices offer unusual insight into the internal processes of experienced and deeply thoughtful clinicians as they grapple with the disappointment, frustration, and heartbreak that is so much a part of what we do.

One of the themes that organizes the volume is hate. Within the strengths-based, relational model that is at the heart of infant–parent psychotherapy, we so often think of ourselves as helping parents become more attuned, sensitive, and reflective by modeling these capacities in our relationships with both mother and baby. But how do we think about mothers whose hatred of their babies and unrelenting aggression seems impermeable and immutable?

Sometimes the hatred is in the room, palpable and devastating, sometimes it is in the child, left behind by an abusive or abandoning parent whose absence is a forceful presence. How can we hold the rage—the child's, the parent's, the foster or adoptive parent's—without disrupting fragile structures and tenuous alliances? Linked to addressing bare and raw aggression is the issue of parental psychopathology. The benign or hopeful model of infant–parent psychotherapy has generally minimized the impact of severe parental (or, for that matter, child) psychopathology, and yet all infant–parent psychotherapists confront this reality on a regular basis. How can these factors be addressed within the framework of a model in which the infant–parent psychotherapist—who may or may not be trained in adult psychotherapy or evaluation—is often the *only* therapist allowed access to a vulnerable, suspicious, and beleaguered family?

Related to these crucial questions is the issue of our own fear and dread. As Birch notes, "What is it, in work with infants, that makes us so partial to being supportive and makes it so difficult to tolerate, metabolize, and use therapeutically the intense countertransference feelings that are evoked when we see children suffering and cannot stop it? Is there a special kind of 'parental countertransference' that such cases evoke?" (p. 256). On the one hand, this countertransference makes it difficult for the infant–parent psychotherapist to sit with the child or parent's unbearable pain or rage. It also makes it difficult to confront the complexities and ambiguities inherent in the fact that their availability to families is supported (financially and otherwise) by and embedded within a suspect and often distinctly unresponsive social service system. And, in some instances, it provokes enactments that may have long-term consequences for both patient and therapist.

The seeds for such ruptures are, suggest Birch and her colleagues, many, and include unresolved chronic trauma; the absence of "angels" in the form of family, social, or community supports; issues of race, class, and gender; lack of peer contact and supervision for the therapist, and the vagaries of working with enormously disorganized families and family systems in which consistency and regularity are all but impossible; and forced, abrupt terminations that are the rule rather than the exception.

This book makes abundantly clear how much we have needed—as a field—a full and honest discussion of the factors that underlie our "heartbreaking failures." It is the only way to put them in context. And it is the only way to begin to develop a language for understanding the limits of the infant–parent psychotherapy model, the limits of our own capacities as therapists and human beings, and the limits of what we can reasonably expect to change. I hope that this work will serve as a model for trainees, who often begin their work without a language for its inevitable ruptures. And I hope that this will make our good work better, but at the same time allow us to forgive ourselves and the families we work with when things go wrong. Maybe we'll be able to see the obstacles before we have flattened ourselves against them and maybe we can even navigate around them once in awhile. This is the radical hope of this volume.

Arietta Slade, PhD

The City College and Graduate Center
The City University of New York
*and*
Yale Child Study Center

CHAPTER 1

# THE REASON FOR SUCH A BOOK

*Marian Birch*

Psychotherapeutic work with the families of very young children offers some of the most rewarding experiences in the career of a psychotherapist. The opportunity to intervene preventively, when both infant and parent are in a developmental state that is uniquely and intrinsically receptive and open to change, is exciting and prognostically hopeful (Fonagy, 1998). The preponderance of evidence indicates that such intervention does lead, in a significant majority of cases, to improved developmental and psychiatric outcomes for high-risk infants and their families (Balbernie, 2006).

Many of us in the new and exciting field of infant mental health have been career-long advocates, even missionaries, for this model of intervention. We have believed that if only all young parents had access to the help we can offer, there would eventually be far less repair work for the therapists of adults, adolescents, and older children. Infant mental health is a wonderful specialty for those of us who believe in miracles and who like to midwife them. The results of our work with young parents and their infants are often profoundly positive in a way that is deeply satisfying. Just as there are few experiences that touch the human heart with the immediate intensity of a baby's trusting smile, there are few professional satisfactions as deeply felt as those that derive from successfully helping a baby and her parents find one another emotionally.

As the field of infant mental health enters its fourth decade, if we date its birth with the publication of *Ghosts in the Nursery* (Fraiberg, Adelson, &

I

Shapiro) in 1975, such miracles have been amply documented in what is by now an extensive archive of brilliant case histories, beginning with those of Selma Fraiberg (Fraiberg, 1980; Fraiberg et al., 1975), and subsequently those of many other gifted therapists, including some of the contributors to this volume (Birch, 1997, 1998, 2000; Birch, Mennet, & Zorrah, 2005; Heineman, 1998, 2000; Maldonado-Durán, 1997; Maldonado-Durán & Lartigue, 2002; Stone, 2007).

In this inspiring clinical archive, typically, a desperately unhappy family engages with a marvelously sensitive, insightful, and patient therapist who helps the family members attain a new way of relating to their infant. In the words of Fraiberg and her colleagues (1975), such work enables the client family to become unburdened by

> the ghosts of the past. If we can help ensure the bonds between (a mother) and her baby in the first days and weeks of the infant's life, we think the intruding ghosts will depart, as they do in most nurseries, when the child is protected by the magic circle of family. (Fraiberg et al., 1975).

Fraiberg et al. (1975) have described the power of such work, which has been beautifully documented in their own and others' case histories, as "like having God on your side." But believing that God is on your side is a tricky enterprise. Where does it leave us when we come up against our own limitations and those of the model? Those of us who have worked in infant mental health for any length of time have encountered families where, if God is on our side, it is the God of the Book of Job. The predicaments of these families are more likely to make us think about the Devil, evil, and the universal human capacity for hatred, destructiveness, and cruelty. There are families that remind us of the anthropologist Sarah Hrdy's (1999) meticulous documentation of the inevitability and the "naturalness" of abuse, neglect, and cruelty, as well as abandonment of children when parents' own needs are unmet or unmeetable.

The field of infant mental health, focusing as it does on the promise of new beginnings that the infant represents, may have had a tendency to be a bit too hopeful, too trusting in the innate goodness of the human species. This optimism, although it has an immense power to inspire both clinicians and families, risks a certain blindness that can place a heavy burden of expectation on therapists.

We have found that clinical work with infants and their families can also be searingly painful and disappointing. We cannot always find the emotional bridges to connect a baby to the loving and protective aspects of her caregivers. Sometimes the chasms between what is and what ought to be are too vast for our modest tools to span. Our ability to help may be compromised by the sheer number of and intensity of risk factors that compromise the family's potential to nurture and thrive, as well as by a lack of protective factors (Emde, Everhart, & Wise, 2004).

Insurmountable challenges may originate within the child: in severe and intractable sequelae of trauma and neglect, or in sensory processing difficulties, developmental delays, and disabilities. Obstacles to therapeutic success may reside within the caregivers in the form of intractable mental or medical illness, irreversible disability, developmental delays, limited education, or treatment-resistant addictions. Our nemeses may rest as well within the web of social circumstances and resources that is the matrix for the infant and the family: unemployment, cultural dislocation, lack of access to medical or mental health services, poverty, and community violence. At times, we face a veritable "Perfect Storm" of dysfunction that combines all of these.

## QUESTIONS ABOUT INFANT–PARENT INTERVENTION

The seeds for this book are rooted in my experiences as a clinician and a supervisor. This experience heightened my awareness of the impact that these "failures" can have on clinicians.

From 2001 to 2004, I was the clinical coordinator of the certificate program in Infant Mental Health at the University of Washington. This was a new training program, created in the Department of Family and Child Nursing at the University of Washington by Dr. Kathryn Barnard, along with a faculty comprising Dr. Barnard, myself, Melissa Hoffman, Rosemary Kelly, Lisa Mennet, Joanne Solchany, Susan Spieker, and Donna Weston. My position as clinical coordinator involved creating and implementing a program of clinical experiences, supervision, and case conferences, as well as reading for students from a wide range of backgrounds.

During this same period, I was also the clinical director of the Changes Are Relationship Embedded (CARE) Project in Port Angeles, Washington. The CARE Project was a collaboration between the Washington State Department of Child and Family Services, a family support agency, and an infant mental health specialist (myself). The intervention model combined the monitoring of child health and safety by a social worker from protective services, concrete family support services, and in-home, relationship-based, infant–parent psychotherapy. Experienced home visitors and family support specialists provided up to 7 hours per week of services for participating families. The services were offered to families that had extensive histories of repeated referrals to protective services and chronic difficulty engaging with services, families severely affected by chronic neglect who were living in a rural community.

During these years, in my capacity as a teacher and clinical supervisor overseeing 25 clinicians and their work with close to 100 families, my own unbridled optimism about the possibilities of early intervention was tempered and tested by the following observations.

## Working in the Home

Infant–parent psychotherapists working in the home are exposed to greater emotional stress than office-based psychotherapists working with adults or older children. With home visits, therapists are routinely exposed to extremely chaotic, unpredictable, and often terribly painful environments, behavior, emotions, and narratives. They have none of the props that provide a containment function for the office practice. Such protections include, for example, a room with a door and perhaps a sign on the door; the structure provided by charging and collecting fees; or the necessity for the patient to come to the therapist's office, guaranteeing some minimal level of willingness and commitment to our therapeutic work. These added stresses, this absence of standard protective procedures, and the routine use of active outreach make it challenging to maintain a modicum of emotional reserve and objectivity. The emotional responses that we as therapists have, when we are exposed to infants in states of activated attachment need, are rooted in our biology and our personal history. These responses further becloud our capacity for analytic distance and dispassionate assessment.

## Parental Mental Illness

A parent's mental illness is a major factor in many families referred for infant mental health services. There may be real limits to the extent that it is possible to protect an infant from parental psychopathology, for two reasons. First, there is no evidence that such psychopathology (schizophrenia, severe depression, bipolar disorder, severe personality disorder), if it can be treated at all, is treatable within a time frame consistent with an infant's developmental needs. Second, the "job description" of the infant mental health specialist is to treat the relationship between caregiver and infant. The infant–parent therapist often has little or no training in psychotherapeutic work with adults, which is not what is being offered to the family anyway. The goal of helping the parents to "compartmentalize" their psychiatric symptoms and create a relatively protected sphere for the infant–parent relationship is very complex theoretically. On the one hand, the many forms of psychopathology are often thought of as originating within early relationships and then transmitted to the next generation in the parent–infant relationship (Fonagy, 2001; Lyons-Ruth, 1995; Main & Hesse, 1990). On the other hand, we suggest that, in the case of severe parental psychopathology, the relationship-based components of mental illness can somehow be sequestered to permit an uncontaminated space for emotional connectedness between the mentally ill parent and her infant. Even if this were true, there would inevitably be some sacrifice in the depth and richness of a relationship that is founded on excluding part of who the parent really is. To what extent does this require a sensitive infant "not to know what he knows" about his parent (Bowlby, 1988)?

## Severely Impaired Infants

Another challenge to therapeutic effectiveness arises when a child is so severely impaired that she or he cannot and may never be able to offer caregivers the ordinary expectable rewards for caregiving. There are many case reports describing heroically devoted parents who make their child's special needs their lifework. This type of heroism calls, however, not for the ordinary "good-enough mother," but for something more. For the many parents who struggle with their own ghosts and whose infants already serve, to some degree, as posttraumatic triggers for their unresolved early tragedies, the child who cannot "give back" in the ordinary expectable way is a true conundrum.

## Parent–Infant Therapy Without a Parent

We have not established clear guidelines, theoretically or technically, for those cases in which the child and family are caught in the child welfare–foster care system and there is no one who functions as a parent even in the minimal sense of sharing a life with a child and witnessing most of the child's experiences. Invariably, as the therapist works to keep such a child's capacity for love and connection alive, she herself is drawn in as a stand-in for the lost or nonexistent parent, and this feels far more "real" and compelling than the ordinary common garden varieties of transference and countertransference. Adoption of the child in such circumstances by therapists is not rare. The child welfare system has become one of the principal consumers of infant mental health services. Yet in many ways, our model is inadequate to address the concerns of these children.

## Countertransference Pressures

All of these factors compound to create and amplify countertransference pressures within the therapist. The longing to help can feel overwhelming in work with very young children, and failure can be deeply painful. It can feel, in the words of one of my supervisees, "like a crime against humanity."

The basic transference/countertransference paradigm in clinical work with infants is the activation, in the therapeutic relationship with the family, of the attachment systems of all the participants: parent, child, and therapist (Lieberman, Silverman, & Pawl, 2000; Stern, 1995). As our theoretical base increasingly emphasizes the central, mutative role of the therapeutic relationship, and the therapist's "use of self" as a primary intervention technique (Heffron, Ivins, & Weston, 2005), it behooves us to examine carefully the strains and risks entailed in such a relational model when it is applied within such a complex and often chaotic intersubjective field.

Cases in which we are unable to achieve an outcome that puts a child securely on a positive developmental trajectory are exceptionally and sometimes overwhelmingly painful to therapists. It is not uncommon for such cases to lead to fairly extraordinary boundary "failures" and "enactments." These include instances of the therapist's adoption of the child in question. Even with intensive reflective supervision, trainees in infant mental health often speak of being "blindsided" by the intensity of the feelings stirred up in them by the predicaments of their client families. Experienced practitioners speak of the constant struggle to maintain a balance between caring engagement and keeping a clearly professional role.

These challenges require us to reexamine the dominant model of intervention in infant mental health. This model, as described by Fraiberg (1980), Stern (1995), Lieberman et al., (2000), as well as others, assumes that the therapist will be able to dispel the ghosts that interfere with a parent's inherent capacity and motivation to cherish and protect her child. This model also assumes an inherent capacity and motivation on the part of infants to woo and draw their parents into the intense and intimate emotional orbit of attachment. The inclusion of "concrete support" as a component of what the therapist offers the infant–parent dyad in the model rests on the assumption that adequate social services exist to meet the needs of these desperate families, if they can only be helped to access them. These assumptions, unfortunately, are not always true. At times, we find ourselves working with children whom nobody truly wants or even sees, and with parents whose capacities for attachment are mortally wounded, in communities with few if any appropriate services for the families of infants.

## FACING NEW CHALLENGES

When we look at the history of any discipline, including psychotherapy, we see a recurrent cycle. New theories and techniques lead to the observation of phenomena that were previously invisible. These phenomena require new theories and new techniques (Kuhn, 1962). Forty years of experience have shown us things about intervention with infants and their families that were unimaginable before.

In this volume, we explore the limits of the tools of infant–parent psychotherapy and reflect on what can be learned from the sometimes excruciating distress of failures. This is not an exercise in despair, but an effort to grow our field into a new maturity, in which failures and limited outcomes can be acknowledged and endured without despair.

One model I draw on for this book is *Deep Trouble*, by Matt Broze and George Gronseth (1997). *Deep Trouble* is a book for sea kayakers. Each chapter recounts a paddling voyage that went desperately, often fatally, wrong. Yet each narrative does full justice to the beauty and allure of the sea and to the carefully honed skills of the paddlers. Our work with young children and their families brings us, like kayakers, into a privileged yet perilous intimacy with mighty forces—not unlike those of tide, current, sun, and wind—over which we have very modest control.

The "moments of meeting" (Stern et al., 1998), when child and parent find one another through our help, are profoundly inspiring. To do the work well, however, we must open ourselves up to deep, wild places within ourselves. When we cannot help, when a child remains outside of the "magic circle," Fraiberg et al. (1975) invoked, everyone involved, not least we therapists, can be deeply hurt and confused.

Like good paddlers, who study and respect the sea, we need to know and understand the risks we face, so we can make the best possible choices about whether to put on the raingear, whether to attempt a crossing, or whether to leave shore at all.

As training programs in infant mental health proliferate and the field struggles to define "competencies" for infant mental health clinicians, seasoned clinicians have an obligation to tell newcomers the "facts of life." We need to let novices know that there are sometimes ghosts that simply will not go away. We must begin the work of refining our understanding of the *possible* in infant–parent psychotherapy.

## CONTRIBUTORS

This book offers a nonjudgmental and reflective discussion of six puzzling and difficult cases; cases of the kind that can leave the therapist heartbroken and doubting the usefulness of her tools. The clinicians who contributed these cases are all seasoned and experienced veterans. Many have published inspiring accounts of more "successful" clinical endeavors. Each clinician has had the courage and fortitude to offer a case from his or her own practice that left him or her troubled and doubting, questioning the value of the work each had done, and wondering if someone or something else would have been more useful. Such courage is rare—in mental health or elsewhere. Harold F. Searles, a psychiatrist who could be considered a world-class expert on therapeutic hopelessness and futility after spending decades providing psychoanalytic treatment to unmedicated chronic schizophrenic individuals, once said that self-disclosure in psychotherapy is most often limited to disclosure of thoughts, feelings, and acts that make the therapist look thoughtful, sensitive, and generous (heard at a talk sponsored by San Francisco Psychoanalytic Institute in 1992). Our contributors have gone well beyond that.

Susan Sklan (chapter 2) is a clinical social worker with a background in child development. She has years of experience in early intervention and overseeing a program for adolescent parents. She is a graduate of the Infant

Mental Health Fellowship program at Boston Institute for Psychotherapy. Her practice and interests include therapeutic support for the parent–infant and parent–child relationship, home-visit-based psychotherapy, and provision of clinical services to underserved populations. She is currently the clinical director of The Parents Program of the Newton Community Service Center, Newton, Massachusetts, a faculty member of the Infant–Parent Training Institute of Jewish Family and Children's Service of Boston, where she teaches a course in Infant Observation, and a staff clinician at the Rice Center for Children and Families clinic at the Boston Institute for Psychotherapy. She also has a private practice.

Her chapter describes an attempt to provide infant–parent psychotherapy to an adolescent mother who was being abandoned first by her own parent, then again by her foster mother, and then again by the rotating shifts of the staff at the residential shelter where she and her son were placed. Despite Sklan's heroic efforts to preserve the treatment, this was ultimately not possible. Treatment ended with toddler and teen mother in a very precarious situation with few resources to draw upon.

I am a psychologist in private practice in Port Angeles, Washington. I work extensively with infants, toddlers, and their families involved with protective services. I also am a consultant to a family support center, where I provide group treatment for mothers and infants coping with postpartum depression. A ZERO TO THREE Fellow (1983–1985), I was trained at the Infant–Parent Program in San Francisco and have been a consultant, supervisor, and practitioner in infant mental health programs for 25 years. I was clinical coordinator for the Center on Infant Mental Health and Development at the University of Washington from 2001 to 2004, and have written extensively on clinical work with infants and families.

I discuss my work (chapter 4) with a severely traumatized toddler and his adoptive family. This intervention occurred many years ago, and was an inspiration for many of the reflections found in this volume. After an enormously hopeful beginning, the treatment fell apart with the adoption of the child's biological sister. The second adoption precipitated a profound regression in the older brother that both the parents and therapist were unsuccessful in addressing. In this chapter, I examine the unfolding of this failed treatment, and reflect on thoughts about its meaning. I also look at the ghosts that abused and neglected children bring with them into new homes, and examine and critique a therapeutic approach in which "strengths" and "safety" are used—sometimes at the expense of tolerating and containing anguish, terror, and violence.

Richard Ruth is a psychologist/psychoanalyst in Wheaton, Maryland, working with children and families. His affiliation is with the Washington School of Psychiatry. He is on the clinical faculty of the Center for Professional Psychology at George Washington University.

In his chapter (chapter 6), Ruth describes and reflects on his work with a family referred to him by the courts. The mother and several of her five children had been diagnosed as developmentally delayed. Despite an encouraging beginning in which the therapist felt that he had made a positive alliance with the family and that they were receptive to his offer to help them provide a more consistent and nurturing environment for their children, this treatment never seemed to find a "direction." Apparent growth and learning had dissipated or was "forgotten." The theme of "running out"—as in running out of needed daily necessities (e.g., food), as in running out in the street or running away from unmanageable responsibilities, and as in running out of time in the child welfare system—pervades the material presented in these chapters.

Julie Stone (chapter 8) is an infant, child, and family psychiatrist. She has worked within Australia's hospital system and provides consultation and reflective supervision to colleagues practicing within the child protective system. Stone works with children orphaned or made vulnerable by the AIDS pandemic in Africa, helping to ensure that their emotional well-being has not been forgotten. She was also a ZERO TO THREE Fellow (2003–2005).

In her chapter, Stone discusses the aborted treatment of a little boy whose mother needed to see him as damaged and defective. She discusses the potential for professionals to be drawn into unwholesome alliances with distressed and disturbed parents, and examines how children can be in danger of being abused and neglected by the very care systems intended to help and protect them when those working in those systems refuse to, or are unable to, embrace the possibility that parents may have powerful agendas other than the best interests of their child.

Martin Maldonado-Durán is a psychiatrist and psychoanalyst at the Menninger Clinic in Topeka, Kansas. He directs an early intervention program serving both pregnant women and children who are less than 36 months old. Treating these patients involves collaboration with several public health agencies. In this program, therapists research the symptoms presented by the infants and their families, and study the attachment patterns in the child and in the primary caretaker. Maldonado-Durán is interested in further work in primary and secondary prevention of infant mental health problems. He has written extensively on a range of infant mental health topics and is the editor of *Infant and Toddler Mental Health: Models of Clinical Intervention With Infants and Their Families* (2002). Maldonado-Durán works closely with colleagues in Latin America and has coedited two books in Spanish: one on child psychopathology for use by pediatricians and the other on feeding difficulties in infants.

In Maldonado-Durán's chapter (chapter 10), he documents his thwarted efforts as a consulting psychiatrist to engage the family of an out-of-control toddler in an exploration of environmental and emotional factors within the family system that amplify their difficulties with the toddler. His work with the family elicited a paranoid response from them. The grandmother formally complained that the psychiatrist was *causing* rather than relieving the child's problems.

Toni Vaughn Heineman (chapter 12) is a psychotherapist in private practice working with children and adults in San Francisco. She is the executive director of A Home Within, a nationwide organization providing long-term psychotherapy to children in foster care. She is the author/editor of two books on work with abused and neglected children. She was a ZERO TO THREE Fellow (2003–2005).

In her chapter, she examines her work with a little girl enmeshed throughout her childhood in the foster care system. Infant–parent psychotherapy is based on the assumption that young children in emotional distress come to us in the company of a caregiver. However, this is too often not the case for young children in foster care. Heineman questions how we define the role of the therapist if there is no relationship to treat. What is the therapist to do if the infant, rather than being held in the arms of a single person who has primary responsibility for her care, is tossed from one pair of hands to another?

Each of the coauthors of this volume, in addition to writing a case history from his or her own experiences, has contributed a discussion of the case history of another of the book's coauthors. This format, it is hoped, offers more of a "conversation" between us, rather that a series of sad, unconnected stories. It certainly demonstrates how very much kinder seasoned clinicians are about the work of others than they are about their own. Thus, in its form as well as its content, the book demonstrates one of the central tools for sustaining hope and faith in this work—that of sharing the work with others and seeing oneself and one's efforts through experienced but less enmeshed eyes.

The case histories and the discussions address the intense countertransference pressures that can contribute to unrealistic goals, boundary problems, and crushing disappointment. We hope to contribute to a deeper understanding of the therapeutic skills needed to persevere with realistic expectations in our efforts to use psychotherapeutic intervention to diminish the intergenerational transmission of anguish and dysfunction.

## CORE CONCEPTS IN INFANT–PARENT PSYCHOTHERAPY

A brief statement seems in order of what we understand to be the core concepts and techniques of therapeutic intervention with infants and very young children and their families (Greenspan & Wieder, 1987; Lieberman et al., 2000; Stern, 1995). Such a review will provide a context for our reflections on its limits.

From conception through the third year of life, there is, in Winnicott's (1960) pithy phrase, "no such thing as a baby." There is, rather, the dynamic, nonlinear system (Sander, 1975) of the infant-and-caregiving environment.

The caregiving environment is, most immediately, in most cases, the mother; equally critically, it is the web of familial, social, and economic relationships and resources that support the mother so that she is able to find within herself the psychological and physical resources to successfully rear a healthy, happy, and competent child. A mother can no more parent successfully without such environmental support than an infant can thrive and grow without a mother (Hrdy, 1999).

The tasks of the infant–parent psychotherapist include addressing internal obstacles that impede the parent from accessing the support she needs, as well as providing practical assistance in identifying and accessing available resources.

When babies grow up and have their own babies, their capacity to find and accept the help they need from others is directly and strongly correlated with the kind of caregiving they received as infants. In terms of attachment theory, a securely attached infant grows up to become a mother who is able to use relationships with others to meet her need for support. An anxiously attached infant, barring intervening help, becomes a mother who has significant constrictions in her ability to do so. The infant with no organized attachment strategy is likely to become a mother with no organized strategy for obtaining the support she needs, and who, in powerful and automatic ways, perceives others as threatening, not helpful. Similarly, the mother's representation of her infant and her ability to be sensitively responsive to her infant are shaped to a significant degree by her own early experience and the way it is registered in her psyche (Main, Kaplan, & Cassidy, 1985).

Our intention, as infant–parent psychotherapists, is to expand the mother's range of choices in both spheres: in response to her infant, and in meeting her own psychological and practical needs.

When the infant–parent dyad is not working well, it is often because the mother has rigid defenses against being aware of and experiencing what

Tronick (1998) called "a dyadic expansion of consciousness" within the dyad. On the mother's side, this dyadic expansion of consciousness, when accessible, provides her an entrance into a long-forgotten world of primitive nonverbal feeling and experience that permit her, for example, to distinguish a hungry cry from a tired cry, or, in the case of many mothers in developing countries, to unerringly hold the baby out at arms' length at the moment just before he pees.

When a mother cannot tolerate this primitive way of knowing, it is usually because she received inadequate help, when she herself was an infant, in tolerating, managing, and regulating her own primitive preverbal feelings. Thus, in her infancy, she experienced her affects as overwhelming and traumatic, not as reliable signals to herself and her caregivers about needs and wishes. Her infantile distress and arousal met with neglect, abuse, intrusion, projection, and negative attributions. Furthermore, her subsequent experiences may not have afforded her an opportunity to revise her early, infantile ways of coping with these failures of caregiving with more mature and adaptive mechanisms.

This is the help that we come, as infant–parent psychotherapists, at the 11th hour, to offer. Our objective is to exorcise the ghosts in the nursery, which cloud the mother's perception of and ability to respond to her infant. But, of course, these selfsame obstacles are the chief impediment to the mother's accepting any help we have to offer.

We cannot expect the mother to have a "realistic" view of our helpful intentions and purposes in intruding ourselves into her life, any more than she has a realistic view of her baby's motives for occupying so much of the territory formerly known as her life. We do not take her wariness, hostility, and evasive vagueness personally. We do not waste too much breath trying to persuade her that we are different from the others—the parents, teachers, doctors, social workers, and so forth—who have disappointed her in the past. Instead, we try to understand how she experienced those disappointments and how they shaped her, and in our way of doing so we try to offer a different experience of being listened to, understood, and cared about.

This importantly includes acknowledging and perhaps even apologizing for the inevitably intrusive, humiliating, and insufficient aspects of our presence in her life. It also includes acknowledging that our interest, caring, and helpfulness are professional. In the brutally crude terms of one of my clients, we are paid to care. This falls far short of what our clients want, and may need.

It cannot be overemphasized how sensitive, deeply personal, and intimately tied up with self-esteem and her evil stepsisters—self-doubt and self-loathing—is the territory which we presume to enter. Often we come with only a flimsy and awkward excuse for an invitation. "Your CPS [Child Protective Services] worker, or your pediatrician thought you needed help." How special does that make a mother feel?

We, as therapists, do not like to think about this. We have our own self-esteem issues and probably would not be doing this kind of work if we did not have some fairly deeply rooted need to help. To be effective, and to survive as an infant–parent psychotherapist, we have to let go of this need, or at least, loosen its grip.

The current dominant model is that we help parents become more sensitive, responsive, and protective of their babies through the therapeutic relationship itself: We have to become more sensitive, responsive, and protective of the parents. In the words of Jeree Pawl (1995), we "do unto others as we would have others do unto others" (J. Pawl, personal communication, October 30, 2007).

This doing unto mothers what we hope mothers will do for their babies—provide sensitive, attuned, and comforting responses—has been described by Fonagy, Gergely, Jurist, and Target (2002, p. 403) as "the creation of an interpersonal situation where the potential for reflective function could be specifically and safely exercised." We believe that our cumulative interactive exchanges with the mother help her to think about her own and her infant's feelings and experiences as meaningful and understandable by another and by herself. We are trying to provide an attuned, supportive relationship, a holding environment, a container within which the mother can reflect on and resolve some of the obstacles to attunement, mutuality, and growth in her relationship with her infant.

Work with infants and families is tremendously challenging. It requires us to keep a therapeutic focus and balance in the often chaotic, distracting, and disturbing settings in which our clients live. To maintain such balance, it is absolutely essential to have ongoing consultation, supervision, and training. There must be dedicated time for the therapist to think about the system he or she is trying to join—time away from the infant-caregiver system and the multiple and often conflicting demands it makes for her attention and intervention. She also needs help seeing herself in the system, such as the opportunities that individual supervision and clinical case review with peers and consultants can provide.

## THE THERAPEUTIC CHALLENGES WE FACE

In her radical innovation in psychoanalytic practice, what she referred to as "psychotherapy in the kitchen," Selma Fraiberg and her colleagues (1975, p. 394) grafted a set of techniques that had long been central to the practice of nursing and social work onto an essentially classical, ego psychological model of psychotherapy. These techniques were home visiting, case management (including referral and advocacy), and educational guidance.

Furthermore, Fraiberg et al. (1975) defined the patient of infant–parent psychotherapy as the dynamic relationship between an infant and his or her caregiving environment. This was a conceptualization that was far closer to family systems theory (Bateson, Jackson, Haley, & Weakland, 1956) than to the American ego psychoanalysis to which Fraiberg et al. claimed allegiance. Stern (1995) 20 years later likewise defined the patient of infant–parent psychotherapy as the infant–parent relationship.

Fraiberg et al.'s (1975) "parameters," or special modifications of classical psychoanalytic practice, emerged in the '70s and '80s of the last century, in the same historical context as other adaptations (e.g., Heinz Kohut, Kurt Eissler, and Harold Searles) to the classical model of a rigorously "neutral" analyst who facilitated psychological change through interpreting the patient's free associations and, in particular, "resistances" and "defenses" (Mitchell, 1988). The classical model was viewed as effective only for "neurotic" patients—those whose problems stemmed from maladaptive efforts to manage unacceptable impulses. Its practice and its failures had led to increasing awareness of different kinds of emotional problems that required different techniques (Fonagy, 2001). The rehabilitation of John Bowlby and Melanie Klein, both of whom emphasized the central motivational role of relatedness, from the status of psychoanalytic pariahs, which they had endured in the '50s and '60s, also began in this period.

Fraiberg et al. (1975) explained that their parameters, their new techniques—(a) home visits, concrete and emotional support, and developmental guidance; and (b) dyadic relationship as patient—made it possible to offer therapeutic services to families who lacked the inner and outer resources required to come to office appointments. This was initially discussed in terms of the logistical difficulties frequently facing parents with infants. It gradually became clear in practice, however, that the inability to access center-based services often reflected deep-seated distrust and disorganization in relationships. Such techniques were seen as concrete, operational statements of the therapist's implicit and explicit offer to meet the family where and as they were. Again, the goal of this practice was to engage distrustful caregivers in a therapeutic endeavor on behalf of the infant.

The practice of home visiting provided an incredibly rich and immediate access point or "portal of entry" (Stern, 1995) for collecting clinically relevant data. After an hour in a family's home, the therapist often was privy to data that would take years to gather in an office setting—if, in fact, it could ever be gathered there at all.

It has seldom been acknowledged, either in infant mental health or in psychoanalysis, just how much these adaptations changed the therapeutic situation. Let us examine, then, the further implications of these innovations for the therapist's understanding of her role and of what is supposed to be happening in therapy.

In several ways, the dominant model of infant–parent psychotherapy obscures and complicates the issues of informed consent and professional boundaries. The adaptation of home visiting forfeits one of the key features of office-based psychotherapy, namely, the patient indicates his engagement in a therapeutic endeavor by his physical presence (Clarkin, Kernberg, & Yeomans, 2006; Greenson, 1967). In addition, the formal setting of an office—often with signs, diplomas, professional books—conveys implicitly that the therapist is offering specialized skills and services. Home visits and case management services (e.g., helping to locate housing or complete legal paperwork) make it more difficult to communicate clearly that the goal of therapy is to help the caregiver to overcome internal, mental obstacles to growth. The special quality of the patient's transference and the therapist's countertransference feelings and enactments (Bromberg, 1998), as a kind of "play" that occurs in the protective haven of the therapy, is easily obscured when the therapist actively seeks to engage the family in its own setting. The caregivers' wishes that the relationship with the therapist would actually function, on a permanent basis, as a replacement for their own tormented ties to their families of origin are implicitly validated by this active, unconditionally accepting approach. Further complicating matters, our emotional availability to the caregivers is actually far from unconditional: We are motivated by a primary goal of promoting the infant's healthy development, not the optimal future for the caregivers.

A further consequence of working in the home, with a dependent infant present, is that it is much riskier to invite and work with profoundly regressive and intense feelings and states. An office offers the safety of a private, anonymous haven that the patient chooses to come to and that she can leave behind. Likewise, the therapist in an office can be emotionally engaged with the patient's intense and primitive material safe in the knowledge that the hour will end, there are no lethal weapons on site, and the patient is almost always able to pull himself together and leave, or at least sit in the waiting room until he can. In our work with parent–infant dyads, we are always titrating the depth to which our dialogue can go against the ever-present physical and emotional need of the infant, as well as our own sense of safety (Lieberman, 2000).

The hypothesis that the therapist's provision of warm, sensitive, attuned responsiveness leads to the caregiver's enhanced capacity to provide the same to the infant has led to an emphasis on strengths-based, supportive interventions (Fraiberg, 1980; McDonough, 2000; Olds, 2005; Pawl, 1995). This approach is a far cry from the often painful "interpretations of resistance" prescribed by the old classical model (Greenson, 1967). We try to find something positive and growth-promoting to admire and validate in the parent–infant relationship. Although we often observe situations and interactions that profoundly disturb us, we also often feel that we cannot address them directly lest we lose the fragile alliance with the caregiver. Finding the boundary between being supportive versus colluding with subtle forms of neglect and maltreatment can be extraordinarily difficult. If we believe in the unconscious, it is inevitable that our concealed feelings of worry, revulsion, anger, and fear have an impact even though we do not openly express them. We need better ways to think about that (displaced) impact.

Like the public health nurse, and like the social worker, the infant–parent psychotherapist may provide developmental guidance and concrete support. However, rather than being ends in themselves, these activities are understood as ways of establishing the kind of relationship with the infant and its caregivers that, because it is sensitive, nurturing, and warmly positive, facilitates the caregivers' abilities to relate to the infant in similar growth-promoting ways.

This trickle-down effect is beautifully captured in Jeree Pawl's (1995) koan-like "do unto others as you would have others do unto others." It is presumed to work by altering the caregivers' internal working model of relationship, rooted in their own infancy, so that it is more flexible, hopeful, and generous and less rigid, fearful, and withholding (Lyons-Ruth, 1998; Main & Hesse, 1990; Slade, 1999).

This can work beautifully when

- There is a clearly identified parent or caregiver who claims the child.

- This caregiver or parent has a psychological makeup that permits him or her to alter and soften lifelong unconscious strategies for maintaining psychic coherence within the time frame set by the infant's inexorable developmental processes.

- The therapist is able to maintain a balance in her attention to and investment in both caregiver and infant. Therapy must focus on optimizing this relationship as opposed to the oft-wished-for happy ending for one or the other of the dyad (Seligman, 2000).

What happens if one or more of these conditions are not met, as is the case in the situations described in this volume?

Contemporary writing about psychoanalytic work with adults and children has been marked by a very dramatic and rich expansion of the concept of *counter-transference*. Writers such as Stephen Mitchell (1988, 2000), Thomas Ogden (1986), and Philip Bromberg (1998), to name but a few, have vastly enlarged our understanding of the ways that, in Freud's terms, "the analyst turns his unconscious like a receptive organ to the unconscious of the patient" (1912, p. 118), and uses the behaviors, thoughts, affects, images, and impulses that are evoked in him as a rich source of "data" about the clinical situation. With these discoveries has come a profound acknowledgment of the fallible humanity of the analyst; that, in the words of Harry Stack Sullivan (1953), "We are all much more simply human than otherwise" (p. 32). Harold F. Searles, a psychoanalyst renowned for his Herculean efforts to treat schizophrenic patients psychoanalytically, has eloquently complained that the more classical view of the neutral and abstinent analyst requires the analyst to be a person who somehow transcends the ordinary human vulnerability to confusion, envy, destructiveness, and perversity, and is able to listen to extraordinarily painful and disturbing material with the serenity of a Mother Teresa.

With few exceptions, within the field of infant–parent psychotherapy, the therapist is still expected to be superhuman in this way. Yet infant–parent psychotherapy evokes what are arguably the most intense and disturbing countertransference responses imaginable.

Intimate work with an infant in distress is guaranteed to stimulate the therapist's loving and protective feelings. To a lesser extent, the kinds of narcissistic hungers that are assuaged by producing a healthy child, the longings and impulses that Erikson (1952) so graciously called *generative*, are also engaged. When the child is actually in a life-threatening predicament, as may be the case in medical crises or instances of parental or institutional neglect or abuse, these countertransferential feelings take on a terrifying immediacy and power.

In 1999, Arietta Slade wrote the following:

> Therapy concerns itself over and over again with loss, separation, and reunion—both in its consideration of such events in patients' lives, and in the constant separations and reunions that are intrinsic to the therapeutic process. And just as losses, separations and reunions have meaning for patients, so do they have meaning for therapists. Similarly, just as being cared for may be quite evocative for patients, so may the experience of caring be evocative for therapists. Many therapists have suffered early loss and abandonment; naturally, they will vary in the degree to which they have reconciled and come to terms with these experiences. And, regardless of the degree to which a therapist has come to terms with his or her own early experiences, different patients will engage the therapist's attachment dramas in different ways (p. 589).

When a child or infant is dangerously uncared for or maltreated in his family, finding the appropriate therapeutic stance can be very challenging. On the one hand, these situations seem to call for an intense level of therapist activity. The ethics of standing by as a child appears to slip away into physical or psychological death are tricky. On the other hand, activity may be a defense against thinking and feeling, including thinking that, in reality, the therapist's power and influence are often very limited. Sometimes it seems there is no other option other than standing by; at other times, one's most sincere and strenuous efforts are unavailing. There are few things more painful and difficult in life than watching helplessly as a beloved child slips away. The feelings are not just feelings of grief, but inevitably of failure and self-reproach. Adults are supposed to be able to protect and care for children.

Perhaps, given the actual impossibility of the task, we are supposed to have illusions that we can. Anyone whose career has involved him or her for any length of time with high-risk infants and their families has had such comforting illusions remorselessly eroded. Again and again, we have seen children we have grown to care for overwhelmed by circumstances beyond our control, and we see the window of opportunity for growth and healing in a place of safety slam shut. To continue in this work is to find a way to bear this without burning out or shutting down. This is the challenge to which the present volume hopes to make a modest contribution.

The stories in this book are based on the authors' experiences. Some of the cases represent actual people and circumstances. Individuals' names and identifying details have been changed to protect their identities. Other vignettes are composite accounts that do not represent the lives or experiences of specific individuals, and no implications should be inferred.

## REFERENCES

Balbernie, R. (2006). Conference Report: ZERO TO THREE NTI. *The Signal, 14,* 11–13.

Bateson, G., Jackson, D. D., Haley, J., & Weakland, J. (1956). Toward a theory of schizophrenia. *Behavioral Science, 1,* 251–264.

Birch, M. (1997). In the land of counterpane: Travels in the realm of play. *Psychoanalytic Study of the Child, 52,* 57–75.

Birch, M. (1998, August). *Love in the countertransference.* Presentation as part of the Intergeneration Transmission of Trauma panel at the 106th Annual Convention of the American Psychological Association, San Francisco, CA.

Birch, M. (2000). A case of pediatric undernutrition. *Journal of Infant, Child & Adolescent Psychotherapy, 1,* 29–46.

Birch, M., Mennet, L., & Zorrah, Q. (2005). Multiple births: The experience of learning in infant-parent psychotherapy. *Infants and Young Children, 18,* 282–294.

Bowlby, J. (1988). *A secure base: Clinical applications of attachment theory.* London: Routledge.

Bromberg, P. (1998). *Standing in the spaces: Essays on clinical process, trauma and dissociation.* Hillsdale, NJ: Analytic Press.

Broze, M., & Gronseth, G. (1997). *Deep trouble: True stories and their lessons.* Camden, ME: Ragged Edge Press.

Clarkin, J., Kernberg, O., & Yeomans, F. (2006). *Psychotherapy for borderline pathology: Focusing on object relations.* Washington, DC: American Psychiatric Press.

Emde, R., Everhart, K. D., Wise, B. K. (2004). Therapeutic relationships in infant mental health and the concept of leverage. In A. Sameroff, S. C. McDonough, & K. L. Rosenblum (Eds.), *Treating parent–infant relationships: Strategies of intervention* (pp. 267–292). New York: Guilford Press.

Erikson, E. (1952). *Childhood and society.* New York: Norton.

Fonagy, P. (1998). Prevention, the appropriate target of infant psychotherapy. *Infant Mental Health Journal, 19,* 124–150.

Fonagy, P. (2001). *Attachment theory and psychoanalysis.* New York: Other Press.

Fonagy, P., Gergely, G., Jurist, E., & Target, M. (2002). *Affect regulation, mentalization and the development of the self.* New York: Other Press.

Fraiberg, S. (1980). *Clinical studies in infant mental health.* New York: Basic Books.

Fraiberg, S., Adelson, E., & Shapiro, V. (1975). Ghosts in the nursery: A psychoanalytic approach to impaired infant–mother relationships. *Journal of the American Academy of Child Psychiatry, 14,* 387–422.

Freud, S. (1912). Recommendations to physicians practising psychoanalysis. In J. Strachey (Ed. & Trans.), *The standard edition of the complete psychological works of Sigmund Freud* (Vol. 12, pp. 111–120). London: Hogarth Press.

Greenson, R. (1967). *The technique and practice of psychoanalysis*. New York: International Universities Press.

Greenspan, S., & Wieder, S. (1987). *Dimensions and levels of the therapeutic process*. In S. Greenspan (Ed.), *Infants in multirisk families: Case studies in preventive intervention* (Clinical Infant Reports Series of the National Center for Clinical Infant Programs—Number 3). Madison, CT: International Universities Press.

Heffron, M. C., Ivins, B., & Weston, D. R. (2005). Finding an authentic voice-use of self: Essential learning processes for relationship-based work. *Infants and Young Children, 18*, 323–336.

Heineman, T. V. (1998). *The abused child: Psychodynamic understanding and treatment*. New York: Guilford Press.

Heineman, T. V. (2000). Beginning to say goodbye: A two-year-old confronts the death of his father. *Journal of Infant, Child & Adolescent Psychotherapy, 1*, 1–22.

Hrdy, S. B. (1999). *Mother nature: A history of mothers, infants and natural selection*. New York: Pantheon.

Kuhn, T. (1962). *The structure of scientific revolutions*. Chicago: University of Chicago Press.

Lieberman, A. (2000). Modeling an attitude of protectiveness. *Zero to Three, 20*(5), 15–19.

Lieberman, A. F., Silverman, R., & Pawl, J. (2000). Infant–parent psychotherapy: Core concepts and current approaches. In C. H. Zeanah (Ed.), *Handbook of infant mental health* (2nd ed., pp. 472–484). New York: Guilford Press.

Lyons-Ruth, K. (1995). Broadening our conceptual framework: Can we introduce relational strategies and implicit representational systems to the study of psychopathology? *Developmental Psychology, 31*, 432–436.

Lyons-Ruth, K. (1998). Implicit relational knowing: Its role in development and psychoanalytic treatment. *Infant Mental Health Journal, 19,* 282–289.

Main, M., & Hesse, E. (1990). Parents' unresolved traumatic experiences are related to infant disorganized attachment status: Is frightened and/or frightening parental behavior the linking mechanism? In M. Greenberg, D. Cicchetti, & E. M. Cummings (Eds.), *Attachment in the preschool years: Theory, research, and intervention* (pp. 161–182). Chicago: University of Chicago Press.

Main, M., Kaplan, N., & Cassidy, J. (1985). Security in infancy, childhood and adulthood: A move to the level of representation. In I. Bretherton & E. Waters (Eds.), *Growing points of attachment theory and research* (Monographs of the Society for Research in Child Development). Chicago: University of Chicago Press.

Maldonado-Durán, J. M. (1997). Adjustment disorder: Jalil aged 9 months. In A. Lieberman, S. Wieder, & E. Fenichel (Eds.), *DC 0–3 Casebook: A guide to the use of Zero to Three's "Diagnostic Classification of Mental Health and Developmental Disorders of Infancy and Childhood" in assessment and treatment* (pp. 181–194). Washington, DC: ZERO TO THREE.

Maldonado-Durán, J. M., & Lartigue, T. (2002). Multimodal parent-infant psychotherapy. In J. M. Maldonado-Durán (Ed.), *Infant and toddler mental health: Models of clinical intervention with infants and their families* (pp. 129–159). Washington, DC: American Psychiatric Publishing.

McDonough, S. (2000). Interaction guidance: An approach for difficult-to-engage families. In C. H. Zeanah (Ed.), *Handbook of infant mental health* (2nd ed., pp. 485–493). New York: Guilford Press.

Mitchell, S. (1988). *Relational concepts in psychoanalysis.* Cambridge, MA: Harvard University Press.

Mitchell, S. (2000). *Relationality: From attachment to intersubjectivity.* Hillsdale, NJ: Analytic Press.

Ogden, T. (1986). *The matrix of the mind: Object relations and the psychoanalytic dialogue*. Northvale, NJ: Jason Aronson.

Olds, D. (2005). The nurse–family partnership: Foundations in attachment theory and epidemiology. In L. Berlin, Y. Ziv, L. Amaya-Jackson, & M. Greenberg (Eds.), *Enhancing early attachments: Theory, research, and policy* (pp. 217–249). New York: Guilford Press.

Pawl, J. (1995). The therapeutic relationship as human connectedness: Being held in another's mind. *Zero to Three, 15*(4), 1–5.

Sander, L. (1975). Infant and caregiving environment: Investigation and conceptualization of adaptive behavior in a system of increasing complexity. In E. J. Anthony (Ed.), *Explorations in child psychiatry* (pp. 129–166). New York: Plenum Press.

Seligman, S. (2000). Clinical interviews with families of infants. In C. Zeanah (Ed.), *Handbook of infant mental health* (2nd ed., pp. 211–221). New York: Guilford Press.

Slade, A. (1999). Attachment theory and research: Implications for the theory and practice of individual psychotherapy with adults. In J. Cassidy & P. Shaver (Eds.), *Handbook of attachment: Theory, research, and clinical applications* (pp. 575–594). New York: Guilford Press.

Stern, D. (1995). *The motherhood constellation: A unified view of parent–infant psychotherapy*. New York: Basic Books.

Stern, D., Sander, L. W., Nahum, J. P., Harrison, A. M., Lyons-Ruth, K., Morgan, A. C., et al. (1998). Non-interpretive mechanisms in psychoanalytic therapy: The "something more" than interpretation. *International Journal of Psychoanalysis, 79*, 903–921.

Stone, J. (2007). Tom's perfect world: Conversations with an infant facing death. In F. Thomson-Salo & C. Paul (Eds.), *The baby as subject: New directions in infant–parent therapy from the Royal Children's Hospital* (2nd ed., pp. 111–119). Melbourne, Australia: Stonnington Press.

Sullivan, H. S. (1953). *The interpersonal theory of psychiatry*. New York: Norton.

Tronick, E. (1998). Dyadically expanded states of consciousness and the process of therapeutic change. *Infant Mental Health Journal, 19,* 290–299.

Winnicott, D. W. (1960). The theory of the parent-infant relationship. In D. W. Winnicott, *The maturational processes and the facilitating environment* (pp. 37–55). London: Karnac.

# CHAPTER 2

# HOW TO MOTHER WHEN YOUR MOTHER
# LEAVES YOU AGAIN AND AGAIN

*Susan Sklan*

In this chapter, I describe 2 years of parent–infant therapy with an adolescent mother and her son. The young mother and infant were identified as at risk because of concern that the mother's history of trauma, unresolved loss, and conflict with her own parents would have an impact on her attachment relationship with her baby.

## REFERRAL

Julia gave birth to a baby boy a week before her 16th birthday. Julia was born in the Dominican Republic and came to the United States when she was 10 years old. Julia became pregnant while she was in foster care. She chose to return to live with her mother 2 months before the baby was born. Julia knew of the program for parenting teens where I worked. She called when she was 6 months pregnant to request a home visitor to support her with her new baby.

I began seeing Julia weekly in her mother's apartment. I continued to see Julia and her son Miguel over 2 years, as they ricocheted from her mother's home to foster care and then to a specialized shelter for teen parents and their children.

## MOTHER'S HISTORY OF ABUSE AND ABANDONMENT

I learned thirdhand that Julia had a history of sexual abuse. The Child Protective Services (CPS) worker told me that Julia's mother had told her that Julia was sexually assaulted at age 9 in Santiago, before she came to the United States. Julia's parents had immigrated to the United States when she was 5 years old. They sent for her to join them when she was 10 years old. Julia herself told me about her second assault. At 13, her parents sent her and her 5-year-old sister to stay with a favorite aunt, her mother's sister in Atlanta. Julia was raped by the aunt's boyfriend. The family blamed Julia and told her not to tell anyone. Julia was later medically examined. When she was found to be pregnant, the hospital reported the pregnancy of an underage girl to the police for investigation. Julia's aunt drove her in silence to have an abortion. The police arrested the boyfriend, and his DNA matched the fetus. The family, in particular Julia's mother, still blames Julia for causing this trouble. Julia's mother brought the girls back home; Julia was enraged and behaved recklessly. Her parents separated, and her mother could not parent her. As a result CPS placed Julia in foster care. She became involved with a physically abusive 30-year-old boyfriend. He continued to beat her while she was pregnant with Miguel. Julia broke off her relationship with the father of her baby when she learned that he had a number of other women in his life and other children. She then moved back to live with her mother 2 months before she had her baby.

## HOPES AND GOALS

In this chapter, I look at the themes of abandonment and loss that played out for Julia and her infant son. Julia had a complex history of many separations from her parents as a child, as well as abuse and neglect. Julia's own journey as a child immigrant to this country is a backdrop of another separation and loss. Julia's infant son had the instability of his mother's emotional state and multiple caregivers in a series of abrupt transitions and losses as he moved with his young mother from her mother's home to a foster home and then into a shelter.

Questions that informed the treatment included the following:

1. How would Julia's history of multiple traumas and rejection by her parents affect her sense of self, emotional functioning, and parenting abilities?

2. How does an infant mental health practitioner best address the issues raised in the first question and use the therapeutic relationship?

3. How could I make a difference so that the family cycle of violent rejections was not repeated again for the infant Miguel?

4. Would Julia keep her baby at a distance, as her own parents had done to her?

5. What were Julia's expectations of herself as a mother and of her infant?

6. What is Julia's relationship to her own needs? Julia's experience growing up was that if you speak up about your needs, bad things will happen.

Becoming a parent opens up the possibility of new patterns of relationship for a trauma survivor. It may stir sadness for the parent who was not herself treated as tenderly as she treats her infant. The infant–parent psychotherapist invites the parent to consider her own feelings and the feelings of her infant, with compassion for both. I worked to underscore, observe, and verbalize how Miguel was a unique individual, not a reincarnation of a host of negative characters from Julia's past. I carefully listened to uncover the harmful ghosts of Julia's earliest relationships in which she felt helpless and fearful as an infant and child (Fraiberg, Adelson, & Shapiro, 1975). I also worked to elicit the angels who had nurtured and protected her (Lieberman, Padron, Van Horn, & Harris, 2005).

The essence of the work is to develop the mother's capacity for mindfulness and reflective functioning so that she can take in the baby's needs and intentions in order to "keep the baby in mind." This is a key to parental sensitivity and to the development of a strong, positive attachment relationship between parent and child (Fonagy, 2001; Slade, Sadler, & Mayes, 2005). I hoped that this type of attachment-based intervention would be an instrument of therapeutic change and support for Julia, helping her ensure the safety and protection of Miguel and not repeat her own parents' lack of protection for herself. These themes were played out in almost every home visit.

Relationship therapy requires the therapist's authentic presence and the pro-vision of a space to witness the parent's hopes, struggles, and fears. Unhealthy early attachment relationships can leave a permanent vulnerability to anx-ious or depressed states. The art for both therapist and parent is to allow for both dark and light, the full range of human emotions, without being engulfed or terrified.

Amini et al. (1996) saw the focus of psychotherapy with individuals with impaired attachment relationships as regulating affective homeostasis and restructuring attachment-related implicit memory. The patient's implicit memory of early attachment relationships is played out and addressed in the therapeutic relationship. In Amini's terms, my work as a therapist is to engage with Julia and Miguel in an "affective trio." The therapist's job is to enable the music to begin and take up her place in the melody, in order to change the music. The use of the therapeutic relationship provides oppor-tunities to acknowledge the therapist's misattunements or lapses in empathy. The therapist then explores with the parent and infant how to repair this rela-tionship by reestablishing mutual understanding and building trust that they can work it out together (Lieberman, Silverman, & Pawl, 2000; Lieberman & Zeanah, 1999).

This chapter includes process notes of home visits to illustrate how the parent–infant therapist works at the level of the interaction to facilitate moments of connection between parent and child, such that the new, devel-oping relationship patterns are experienced as not merely possible but as achieved. The home visit allows the therapist a context in which to provide "holding" in a multidimensional and sometimes nonverbal way for the parent–infant dyad that parallels the infant's ongoing development and the unfolding parent–infant relationship (Fraiberg et al., 1975; Stern, 1985; Winnicott, 1971). Fraiberg (1987) referred to the importance of nurturing these psychologically undernourished young mothers, and Stern (1995) spoke of the importance to all new parents, both advantaged and disadvan-taged, for the therapist to offer support with positive regard. The therapist provides ongoing witness to the parent as a loving parent who is reliable and trustworthy (McDonough, 2000).

These hopes for Julia and her infant were housed in a home visitation program for adolescent parents. I was guided by the work of Alicia Lieberman, Susan McDonough, and others. Home visiting provides the context for the therapist to earn credibility as consistent and dependable. Case management helps the parent to identify needs and then helps to link the family to appropriate resources for concrete assistance with the problems of daily living (e.g., child care, housing, medical care, and transportation). The therapist mentors the parents to develop confidence and skills in seeking resources and services for themselves and their children (Lieberman & Van Horn, 2005). Case management also offers a metaphor of hopeful change as it addresses emotional, social, and environmental threats to the parent and infant's well-being, while promoting loving connections.

## INTERVENTION: FIRST PHASE AT HER MOTHER'S HOME

I began seeing Julia weekly in her mother's apartment during her pregnancy. Julia's baby boy, Miguel, was born 2 weeks early. She called me from the hospital, and I visited her and Miguel in the hospital. I resumed weekly home visits thereafter.

### Observation of Baby

After his natural delivery and birth, Miguel was monitored at the hospital and then discharged with one visiting nurse visit to the home. Julia breast-fed him for 2 months and faithfully took him to see his pediatrician for follow-up clinic appointments. Miguel fed easily, put on weight, transitioned to sleep easily and slept well. During his first 4 months, Miguel was surrounded by a family circle of caring that included his mother, grandmother, young aunt and uncle, and a child care provider whom he interacted with daily. He had a wider circle of his pediatrician, myself, and family friends. His outer circle included the CPS worker and some extended family. Miguel seemed peaceful and content in the center of these circles as he grew into a responsive 4-month-old, gazing, smiling, vocalizing, and reaching for social and emotional interaction. He would drift asleep or Julia would gently put him to sleep in the midst of family activity, his bassinet being kept in the living room. We all admired Miguel and his great accomplishments of sleeping, feeding, pooping, and growing.

## Observation of Parent

Julia was an engaging, attractive, very personable young woman who appeared older than her years. She was bright and alert to the world and fun to be with in her 16-year-old chatter. Julia's resilience and resourcefulness in finding ways to get her needs met impressed me. Julia was also very mindful of her mother and sister. At one point she fantasized about home schooling for herself and a part-time job. Doing such would allow her to be home in the afternoon for her younger sister so that her own mother would not have to pay for after-school care. She was creative and open to new ideas. Julia's presentation was a good camouflage of someone who lives in a dangerous, chaotic world. When she did share some of her pain, when I asked her how she was feeling, she said, "I don't feel anything. I must move on and not let it get me down." As I got to know more of Julia, I perceived an anger that could erupt anytime, and I was aware of a deep sorrow. She identified the obstacles for her goal to finish high school: bad friends, boys, fear, and love.

Julia returned to school when the baby was 2 months old. Miguel was cared for by a family day care provider while she was in school. To do this, Julia had to navigate the circuitous and unyielding systems of the public schools, CPS, welfare, and child care. Julia's mother worked long hours, mostly at night, and slept during the day. She was depressed and stressed by family disapproval of Julia and pressure to have Miguel adopted. Julia's mother also had a court eviction notice from the landlord and did not know how to afford a move. Julia had been trying to find them an apartment from the newspaper.

### Observation of Parent–Infant Interactions and Intervention

I considered it fortunate to be present right at the beginning of Julia's and Miguel's relationship, having met Julia shortly before he was born. I helped her prepare for the birth, and Julia was able to talk about her imagined baby. She told me that her baby would always love her and not leave her, alerting me to an unsatisfied psychological hunger, a fantasy, and a hope for something better (Fraiberg, 1987). Once he was born, I was there to help Julia and Miguel negotiate the arousal–sleep–wake cycle and feeding. Julia was an attentive and mostly skillful parent in this first 4-month period. I noted that Julia seemed to understand how to support an infant through routine transitions. For example, she gently helped him learn to fall asleep by himself, a challenge for many new parents. I was pleased to see this and did my best to give her positive feedback for her parenting strengths while clarifying Miguel's needs and abilities. We examined Julia's concerns that Miguel was not looking at her eyes. This concern was shared by the pediatrician who had the baby's vision checked by an eye specialist. I was able to show her how Miguel was actively seeking out her gaze. Was Julia afraid that her infant was rejecting her?

I had some concerns that Julia was overfeeding her baby, choosing to feed him when he began to fuss rather than to explore if he wanted to be held or have some other social interaction. Those concerns abated as Julia learned to read Miguel's cues and needs. Miguel now turned to her voice, sought eye contact with her, and smiled and cooed to engage his mother in an exchange whenever I saw them together. He was clearly in love with her, so everything was going well on his part. Julia was able to play and initiate an exchange with him. Truly reciprocal interchanges were well established between Julia and Miguel in his third and fourth months (Sander, 1962). I observed Julia respond to him and reflect back what he was giving her. She also responded in kind with an added feature, thus enlarging Miguel's experience of social interactions. Julia liked to report and show me Miguel's new tricks. "Miguel, you are so cool" she would endearingly tell him. I asked her how she had learned to care for her baby. She replied, "I just know what I didn't have and I want him to have this. I want him to know that I am there for him."

## Mother's Internal World

Julia responded to my regular presence, asking at the end of a visit, "Same time next week?" At first Julia saw me as someone to help her with her baby. I had not known then how to tell her I could offer more. Both her mother and the CPS worker spoke to me about Julia' refusal to be in therapy. Julia herself had told me that she had had bad experiences with counselors, and she did not want to talk with anyone. She thought it was best to keep things inside her. I wanted Julia to choose how she used our time together and told her that, if she wished, she could use our visits to think about how her past affected her now.

At the next home visit, Julia was alone. She had just put Miguel down to sleep. Having set a stage, she sat and poured out her life: her rape at age 13 and then her abusive relationship at age 15 in which she became pregnant with Miguel. I stood rocking the baby who had awoken in the darkened room. I was conscious that Miguel was agitated, a state I had not seen him in before. It seemed as if he had responded to his mother's state as she told her heavy, sad story.

Julia continued talk of her family, its culture, and her past, dropping emotionally charged information into my lap. Each week I could count on another crisis: an eviction, a court date, the baby may be blind, Julia's belief that no one in her family wants her or her baby, CPS wants to have Miguel adopted, her uncle was just shot in front of Julia's grandmother in Santiago.

In December, escalating conflict caused Julia to call the police on her mother while her mother called Julia's CPS worker from a different cell phone, both accusing the other of hitting her. Julia and Miguel were placed together in a foster home, thus solving her mother's predicament about finding an apartment for all of them.

I introduced the idea that this uproar and rejection might be a repeating pattern that had occurred before in Julia's life. I asked her if she would like to think about this idea with me. Another theme I pursued was to give both Miguel and Julia a voice. I wanted to establish that their relationship was one in which they communicated and Miguel was allowed to talk and be heard. So many adults had told Julia to be silent. Julia had picked up on my subtext of giving both her and Miguel a voice. I was pleased that Julia introduced me to her new foster sister as her advocate.

## Pressures Upon the Therapist

In addition to the therapeutic relationship, I had other relationships to develop and maintain as part of the work of supporting this vulnerable parent–infant dyad. During this first phase, I was very conscious of the need for a three-generational approach, which included working with Julia's mother. This was a tricky dance as Julia's relationship with her mother had been repeatedly disrupted and conflictual, and they had just reunited. I saw this recent mother–daughter reunion as a hopeful effort on both their parts to do better together and to do better for the baby's sake. Working in a program for adolescent parents, I was aware of the research and had seen firsthand that an adolescent parent does best when she has the support of her own mother who can provide developmentally supportive assistance to her daughter and mentor the daughter's parenting (Wakschlag & Hans, 2000). Although I had to pay attention to the boundaries, and be there for Julia and her baby, I also was available to Julia's mother when she approached me with their urgent housing needs. I was able to refer her to some affordable housing search resources and legal help with her upcoming eviction. At other times I observed that Julia's mother was mindful of the baby's needs and assisted Julia. It made me hopeful that Julia's mother was supporting Julia as the mother of her own baby. She had not taken over the baby or left Julia to work out infant care and her own baby's needs by herself. I had helped Julia put together child care arrangements, but it was Julia's mother who sometimes helped by driving Miguel to or from child care.

Another key relationship in Julia's life was with her CPS worker. With Julia's permission, I introduced myself to her and explained my work. One day Julia booked us both to visit her at the same time. The CPS worker arrived and saw us both playing on the floor with Miguel. "This is beautiful," the worker acknowledged. The CPS worker did continue to champion for Julia and Miguel to remain together, which I greatly appreciated.

When Julia left her mother's home in the wake of their conflict, I lost contact with her for 2 months. I felt compelled to maintain a thread of continuity for her and Miguel. I was unwilling to let them drop out of sight, especially after such a tumultuous departure from the supportive circles that had surrounded them in Miguel's first months. I eventually found them and continued weekly visits at Julia's new foster mother's house a few towns away. I noted that it was actually Julia's mother who helped me find them as she shared with me her version of their mother–daughter conflict and her own despair. She told me to call CPS. "See what you can do for her," she encouraged me. I gratefully had Julia's mother's blessing.

## INTERVENTION: SECOND PHASE IN FOSTER CARE

To continue my work with Julia and Miguel, I also needed the blessing of Julia's foster mother. First I had to speak with her, explain my work with Julia and her baby, and get her permission to visit Julia in her home. There was a difference between my approach and the foster mother's concerns about how Julia should parent. Out of myriad parenting details, one example is as follows: Julia's foster mother thought Miguel was delayed developmentally because at 6 months he did not hold his own bottle. I, in contrast, was delighted, as it indicated to me that Julia held his bottle as he was fed. I worked to include the foster mother in some of our play with Miguel, to defuse tension and share some developmental knowledge with her. I did not want Julia to be split between us. Later, as I gained the foster mother's trust, she shared her concerns for both Julia and Miguel, and her sensitivity to their immediate needs and entitlements, not all of which the system could meet. On the last day of Julia's stay in foster care, I learned that the foster mother had been unaware of Julia's trauma history. This may have made it difficult for her to respond to Julia's acting out with any understanding. Unknowingly, she had reprimanded her and doled out harsh discipline.

## Observation of Infant in Foster Care

Miguel was a calm baby, who cried very little, loved to be held, and was easily soothed. I noted that he responded to changes in his environment, such as when he first moved to the foster mother's household with a large number of new people in his daily life and the loss of his grandmother and young aunt and uncle. Julia reported to me that he did not feed or sleep well for the month after their move. I observed that Miguel looked dull and withdrawn when I saw him in the foster home. Was he using his infant emotional detector skills and reflecting the emotions of his mother at that moment? He regrouped and seemed to navigate the changes. At Julia's insistence to her CPS caseworker, he continued to go to the same caring and competent family day care provider. Miguel continued to do well overall in his development, and he was very socially responsive with gorgeous smiles. I was pleased to see that Miguel at 8 months preferred to be with his mother, letting us know that she was his primary attachment figure and he was developmentally on target for normal separation anxiety. His child care provider, whom he had known since he was 2 months old, could also soothe him. He had begun to use "ba-ba" to indicate his bottle, so language was beginning. And he was creeping on all fours. He was a very sweet-looking baby, and Julia informed me that he looked just like his father.

## Observation of Mother

During the 4 months that Julia was in foster care it was clear that Julia was under a lot of stress dealing with the impact of becoming a ward of the state after an abrupt abandonment by her mother. Initially, Julia held up valiantly, trying to please and welcome the new cast of characters in her life, while clinging to some who represented some continuity for Miguel and herself. She kept Miguel's pediatrician and day care provider, even though they were some distance from her foster home. She was always there for my scheduled visits, except when there was no van service to collect Miguel. I felt this represented a huge commitment on Julia's part to our sessions.

Her foster mother observed to me that, whatever happened with her own mother, Julia was a well brought up young lady, who was responsible and helped around the house without being asked. She reported that Julia never had to be reminded to feed or change Miguel. When the initial honeymoon period was over, her foster mother expressed concerns about Julia: she was too interested in older men, and she needed "an education while she is rippin' and roaring through her adolescence." Julia began staying out, and her foster mother was not sure what she was up to.

## Process Note of a Home Visit at Foster Home

Smiling, Julia opened the door of her foster mother's home. She ushered me into the living room, which was unusually quiet with no TV or other people's presence. We sat on the couch, and I asked her how she was doing. She told me that she was still angry and each day was different, sometimes she was up and sometimes she was down. "How was today?" I asked her. She told me today was a good day. She had gone out with Miguel to the mall and had met with his godmother, her friend Elsie, who was enjoying her school break. On Tuesday she had even sent Miguel to day care so that she could have some time for herself. I smiled and told her it was good that she was able to take care of herself while taking care of Miguel. Julia jumped up and said she would bring in her little man. She disappeared into the back of the house, soon emerging with Miguel in her arms, riding on her hip. He was smiling. "Miguel will be 6 months old tomorrow," I acknowledged to her. Julia seemed pleased that I remembered this. "Yes, he will be 6 months. Just think all I have gone through," she said. "Yes, you have both gone through a lot of changes," I replied while thinking that I wanted her to recognize Miguel as having these changes, too.

I had brought Miguel a two-handled cup for his 6-month birthday. We examined the cup, and Julia pronounced it cool. "Is he ready for a cup now?" she asked. I explained how she could introduce it gradually so that he could learn how to swallow from the cup as well as from the bottle. Julia discussed his formula with me. She was now giving him a formula without iron, as it did not make him spit up. I asked who had helped her work this out. "Myself," she grinned. "I wonder if he needs the iron?" I inquired. "Maybe you can check when you speak to WIC [the Women, Infants, and Children's Program] this week." "I called my pediatrician, and she said he needed the iron," Julia replied. "She said she was not worried about his spitting up a bit." "Good for you for checking in with his doctor," I praised her. "I see he is growing well, so the amount he spits up is not leaving him hungry." "No," said Julia. "Look how happy he is sitting with you," I commented. She looked at Miguel, and they both grinned at each other.

Julia told me that Miguel was now sleeping by himself in his own room through the night. "How did you both manage this?" I asked. "Well, he was tired, not too tired, but getting ready to go to sleep. I put a vibrator under his mattress and laid him in the bed. I turned off the lights and nearly closed the door. I came back in 10 minutes and he was asleep. He stayed there until about one in the morning. I got up and went in and found him laughing and playing. I left him and he went back to sleep until 6!" "Wow, Julia, he is growing to manage this. You watch him so carefully and you know just when and how he will manage this. I recall you also helped him when he was much younger to fall asleep by himself on the sofa bed." Julia nodded.

"I don't think Miguel is going to crawl. I think he is just going to walk," Julia announced. "Why do you think this? Let us see how he is on the floor," I responded. To myself I wondered if this was Julia's mother's negative voice speaking? Was this something that Julia was afraid that Miguel would miss, would not be quite right? We put a blanket I had brought on the floor, and we sat on it with Miguel on his back. Playing with Miguel was a pleasure. He was into everything, alert and calm as he explored the toys I had brought, rolling around the blanket—grasping, reaching, sucking, blowing raspberries, and indulging every sense and orifice. Miguel was playing with his voice, practicing long open vowels and a "grr." Julia told me how he looked at an electric switch by her bed. He looked at it and then at her and then back to the switch. He then reached for the switch, and Julia told him "no" and he stopped. "Oh, you two are really talking. He knows that if he looks at you and then at some object, you will follow his gaze and you can both look at the same object. He already has a lot to show you. He is saying 'let's look and think about the light switch.' Imagine how much more he will have to tell you as he gets older. He enjoys these games with you," I observed to her.

Miguel rolled over onto his belly in response to Julia's squeals. I then showed her how to help him begin to creep by letting him push off his legs against her open hand. Miguel was so interested in the wobbling apple toy with a smiling face that he obliged my experiment by pushing off with his legs, lunging forward to the toy and getting up on his knees for a brief moment. "Oh my God!" shrieked Julia. "He is moving!" We were all excited. I was pleased to see how Miguel's new strength gave her so much happiness. This was the highlight of the day for all of us, I would guess.

Miguel began to fuss. I asked Julia what he was telling her. "He is hungry," she said and she produced a bottle of milk and held him in her arms to feed him. As she fed him I asked her how she was doing this week. "You had said that you were angry." "I'm okay," said Julia. "I am managing," she said. "I went and saw my stepfather. My stepfather is my mother's second husband. He told me that my mother said that she respects me. That despite everything I carry on." Julia raised her voice as if she was addressing an unseen crowd. "I told him that this is me. I am not going to let my life go down. Having a baby and being a 16-year-old mother is not the end. I was so sad when my baby's father and I split up. I was pregnant and I lost interest in everything. I couldn't even watch TV; it was boring. I just cried and cried. My foster mother at the time couldn't believe the change. Before, I was out all the time, going to the mall, going to parties, going to get my hair done. But I was changed. I didn't want to leave my room. It felt bad to know that the one person you cared for did not care at all about you. Then one day, something I saw on TV made me think. I would end up in a dead-end job paying very little if I didn't finish high school and go to college. I did not want that for me and now I don't want it for Miguel. I have to be strong and show him how to manage his life by my example. My mother and her family think I am wrong for having Miguel. My mother would hurt me by referring to him as a mistake. A mistake! 'His name is Miguel,' I would tell her. This is not the end of my life. I will show you. No one will be able to tell by my face what I have been through."

I noted that Julia's dramatic delivery was similar to the time she recounted her personal history. Her wish to keep her private pain within her has been a theme, sometimes imposed by the adults of her family, sometimes, I conjectured, as a way to distance herself from her history of loss and rejection by those who were close to her.

"Has this happened to you before?" I asked. "That you felt you had to hide how you felt?" Julia looked carefully at me. "Yes, I often have to hide how I feel. If people knew how angry I was feeling, they wouldn't like it. I have to go on and not let these things pull me down."

I look straight at her and told her, "I do appreciate your strength. From what you have shared with me, you have had a lot of painful losses."

"A lot of letdowns," Julia interjected.

"Yes, your anger and determination have helped you keep on going and survive. But hiding your real feelings has a cost. You are not true to how you are really feeling. I was pleased last week when you allowed yourself to be sad and cry when you learned your uncle had just been shot in Santiago. You said that you were not going to keep this inside yourself and that you were going to go to your room and cry. So I wonder if you know what it means to keep something inside yourself that is painful?"

Julia nodded. "Mandy [the court investigator, a social worker] says she wants me to be evaluated and have medication. Drugs is what she wants for me." Julia rolled her eyes.

"I see you don't agree with her," I observed to her. "No sir!" exclaimed Julia. Miguel had finished the bottle and wanted her attention. I sensed that it was late and time to leave; we had exchanged enough for one visit. I told her "this is important" and "we can talk about it more next time." We arranged that I would meet her next week at their pediatrician's appointment.

"So you think I should give him iron in his formula?" she asked me as a part-ing question at the door. I answered. "It sounds like you checked this out with your pediatrician. This was good thinking on your part. I would go with your pediatrician's advice. I look forward to meeting you next week at the clinic, and you can tell the pediatrician all that Miguel can do now."

"And he'll be crawling," laughed Julia.

## Attachment and Abandonment

Julia continued to enjoy playing with Miguel in our sessions. Miguel was very responsive, and a reciprocal dynamic was established. I showed Julia that her baby was able to enter into complex social and affective interactions. It was a pleasure to witness how Julia would respond to his action by repeating it or changing it slightly, such that he continued to expand his social, language, and cognitive repertoire. How would Julia respond to Miguel as he initiated his own baby plans, such as reaching for something she had not expected, like the light switch as mentioned earlier? Sander (1962) wrote of a 6- to 9-month-old infant's need for a more passive response from his mother than earlier in his development in order to allow for the infant to assert new ini-tiatives. So far, Julia did not intrude or impinge unnecessarily on Miguel's creative actions. Would Julia find his growth and emerging autonomy a threat or another experience of abandonment? Would Julia be able to pro-vide Miguel with a reliable and trustworthy environment when she has not experienced this in her relationship with her own parents? I found myself speaking for Miguel and his need for his mother, such as when he was returned in a van at the end of the day at child care. He often arrived asleep in his car seat, and Julia would ask me if I wanted to hold him. I would respond that I would like to hold him later but that I thought he would want to wake up in her arms. Would Julia's love–hate relationship with her parents be expressed in transference to the therapist? Did she expect her infant to take care of her needs, the way she took care of her mother's needs? How much conflict would there be between Miguel's emerging selfhood and his mother's adolescent development with its normal adolescent narcissism and self-preoccupation (Fraiberg, 1987)? For now, all this was in the future. Yet, all of these thoughts swirled around in my mind as I played on the floor with Julia and Miguel, watching and listening for what would happen next, waiting and thinking carefully as I connected with them both.

I wanted to support Julia's mindfulness of her son by using interactive play to increase her understanding of child development and of Miguel's experience through interactive play. The light switch game was an opportunity for the therapist to show Julia that the game is saying, "We are doing this together" (Tronick, 1989). The play to encourage and then to see the infant make his first move forward on his belly was an opportunity to show positive delight and appreciation of the importance of Julia's play with her infant (McDonough, 2000).

Three months after Julia and Miguel arrived at foster care, the foster mother told me that recently Julia had not been home in time to meet the van that dropped Miguel off home from day care. I raised this with Julia, explaining how Miguel needed her to be there for him when he returns from a day in child care. This was a new development in Julia's parenting. It occurred after a harrowing day in court when Julia heard the judge pronounce that her parents had officially abandoned her. Julia asked me to go with her to court, and so I had accompanied her. I did not want her to sit alone on the bench as strangers decided her fate. The judge declared that Julia's parents had put her out of the family. At the time I felt punched in the stomach as I listened to the judge. I asked Julia afterward how she felt listening to the judge; she said she felt nothing. How could Julia know how to be there for her infant if her own parents had rejected her? Both Julia and Miguel were now in the legal custody of the state. I explained to Julia over and over that it was not a reflection on her that Miguel was in state custody. It was because she was a minor, and in protective care herself, that her son became the responsibility of the state. Who would pay for the costs of his needs otherwise? I explained to her. Julia now needed the support of a range of adults (e.g., judge, lawyers, CPS, foster care placement) who had authority and responsibility for her and Miguel in order for her to keep Miguel with her. I noted both to Julia and myself that throughout the harrowing proceedings, Julia had tended to Miguel and kept him content during the long day in court. Her inner strengths under such stress and her ability to keep Miguel in mind—to follow his lead and respond appropriately to his infant needs—were impressive. The court scene became another chance for me to witness and then explore with Julia how she managed her pain, hiding it inside and putting on a brave smile.

## Mother's Internal World

After Julia's foster care placement, I discerned that, although Julia was unable to feel anything in herself, she could talk about it in displacement through Miguel. Yet, if she were to feel how intensely Miguel loved and needed her, she would have to face the painful loss of her parents and the fact that no one kept her and her feelings in mind when she was young.

During this foster care period, Julia worried that she might be missing something that was wrong with Miguel. She was afraid that she would find out when he was 2 years old that there would be something to worry about. When I asked her if she was concerned that there was a problem with Miguel now, she answered that "maybe there was something I could help him with now so he wouldn't have problems later."

I addressed this issue with her the next week, and told her I had been thinking of her fear that Miguel may have a problem that she does not understand. I repeated that she was a very thoughtful mother. Her wish to understand her baby and how he was feeling with all the changes they had experienced was very important.

"Look at how these changes have affected you. Miguel feels them too." Julia responded immediately by talking about herself: "It feels like no one understands me. No one knows what it is like for me. Everyone wants me to have counseling." Julia then told me how she had once talked with a counselor in confidence. The counselor wrote a report of the therapy, showed it to her father, and her father had not talked with her since. So talking could be dangerous for Julia: "I don't feel anything. I don't want to think about it. I don't let it in. I must move on and not let it get me down." Julia's wish to change Miguel's formula so that he did not spit up had metaphorical significance for Julia's working model of keeping things inside her, even if this perpetuated her emotional malnutrition.

In retrospect, the court hearing when both of Julia's parents did not respond or show up, or at least show an interest in what was happening to her and Miguel, marked a downturn in Julia's stability. Julia's inability to self-regulate emotionally, especially about relatedness, gives some indication of the nature of her own implicit memory of her early attachment relationships (Amini et al., 1996). She was no longer attending school and not reliably home to collect Miguel after child care. Soon after, Julia ran away by herself, and CPS called me. The worker said that they planned to move Julia and her son to a specialized shelter for adolescent mothers. From the CPS perspective, foster care was not working, as the foster mother was unable to take care of Julia and Julia was unable to take care of Miguel.

I tried calling Julia repeatedly after this conversation, but was unable to reach her. Two days later she returned to her foster home and returned my call. We had a long phone conversation in which she shared her fear of moving to the shelter. Julia told me that she had been thinking of hurting herself, and blurted out a long rambling discourse of suicidal ideation, dissociated images, and paranoid feelings. Her thoughts jumped from topic to topic, from one period of her life to another, without transition, with the incoherence that is the hallmark of disorganized states of mind regarding attachment (Hesse & Main, 1999).

"Everyone is out there to get me." She told me she had been riding trains and buses all night, going back and forth, crying, lost in her fears and painful memories. She was so sad that this was affecting Miguel and that she couldn't be home for him. Her mind could not take it. She said she knew she needed help. She saw Miguel laughing in his crib, reminding her of his father and the hatred she felt for him. "I want to control myself and my anger. I just can't." She talked of her rape at age 9 years. "I used to lock it in a box and put it away. I am taking it out now; I want to open it up and I want to fix it. I don't want to endanger Miguel. I wanted this baby so much. Babies always love their mothers, no matter what. Everything fell apart. My perfect life is breaking to pieces and nothing is there. I was so rapt in this man. I was blind until the last Sunday we were together. Someone cut my heart to pieces. 'If you truly love me our love will last,' he told me. The father of my son is leaving. Something happened to me. I am here with Miguel but not really here with him. I am not making it right. My mother got up and left. Something happened to me in Santiago. She told me it was my father or one of my uncles. I can't function the way I used to. I was an adorable child. No one wants to tell me what happened to me in Santiago."

I encouraged Julia to talk with her CPS worker to let her know how she wanted help and how troubled she was feeling. Julia asked me to help her talk with the worker. I agreed to be there the next morning when she was coming to take them to the shelter.

When I arrived at the foster mother's home, Julia and Miguel were waiting with their belongings stashed in plastic bags. The worker arrived and Julia was able to tell her with my support that she was feeling very troubled, and that she had experienced thoughts of hurting herself and that she wanted help. Julia was serious, sad, and articulate. We had a long talk about her history, and I filled in some information about trauma and dissociation, validating that Julia's state of mind was both seriously troubled and dangerous. I spoke to the CPS worker directly about her need for evaluation, possible medication, and intensive therapy. I raised the possibility with the worker that Julia needed to be hospitalized. The worker did not want to lose the bed in the shelter and wanted to take Julia there initially for an intake. I raised concerns about Julia entering a new environment in such a fragile state. To myself I wondered: Who will help Julia hold herself together at the shelter? Who is going to put the pieces together for her? The worker said she would inform the shelter director, a psychologist, of Julia's current mental status and that she wanted me to continue to see Julia and Miguel at the shelter. The shelter would be responsible for finding therapy and a psychiatrist for Julia. I told Julia I would visit her the next day.

## Pressures Upon the Therapist

Extra pressures on the parent–infant therapist marked this foster care period. In this new setting, I wanted to maintain a therapeutic relationship with Julia and Miguel in order to help stabilize and secure their own relationship, to continue to maintain a relationship with the CPS worker, and to engage and support Julia's foster mother and Julia's relationship with her. I also kept an eye open to the possibility of reengaging Julia's mother so that I could assess whether and how to support a reconnection with her daughter and grandson.

The foster mother worked full time and had two, sometimes four, other foster children in her care. The gaps of care or support for Julia as a young teen mother increased. I wondered about where to best use my role in the interest of Julia and Miguel, both together and individually. I became more actively involved as Julia and Miguel became more vulnerable. The court hearing in which the judge officially pronounced that Julia's parents had abandoned her was painful for me. While sitting in the court with Julia and Miguel, I was aware that Julia had not given up on her mother and was even then holding on to a fantasy, looking for her mother to walk into the court and claim her. Amini et al. (1996) wrote, "If the therapy is to be successful, this will result in the evocation in the therapist of genuine affective responses matching the pattern of the melody that the patient knows by heart" (p. 234). In the courtroom Julia could not feel the pain, but I had a visceral response and felt it for her.

The more Julia became dissociative and fragmented, the more I became aware that I was trying to send her a lifeline, which was in reality only a phone line. While speaking with her on the phone, I thought about our long conversation, trying to assess her potential suicidality. I spoke with her foster mother that evening; the next morning I went to see Julia and her CPS worker at the shelter. I tried to help the worker, as Julia's guardian, understand that Julia needed careful professional help—possibly hospitalization. The worker felt that Julia needed the safety of a specialized shelter and that the shelter would be responsible and obtain any psychiatric emergency intervention. Julia was afraid of the shelter, yet professionally I had to trust the systems. I felt ambivalent about trusting them and anxious about handing over Julia and Miguel to their worker who was in turn handing them over to the shelter, yet a new set of providers. In her extreme fragility, was another abrupt departure the best choice for Julia?

## INTERVENTION: THIRD PHASE IN THE SHELTER FOR ADOLESCENT MOTHERS

The next phase found Julia and Miguel in a complex separate world with the challenges of a resident population that shared Julia's history of trauma, constant crises, chronic depression, stress, anxiety, dissociation, and amnesia. The rotating staff was subjected to vicarious and secondary trauma as they struggled with insufficient resources to integrate the needs of infants and young children and high-risk adolescents. Julia told me she was afraid of the other girls. Safety considerations were an issue at all levels, especially for the infants and young children whose young mothers drained the staff of energy and attention.

It was difficult for me to surmount the many barriers at the shelter in order to support and sustain Julia and Miguel over the next 12 months. Communication at all levels was difficult. There was no way of directly calling her, and I had no way of knowing if a message I left for Julia was delivered. Her case manager would often not return my calls and would forget my regular weekly visits, scheduling other appointments for Julia at our appointed time. I would arrive at the shelter, sign in at the front door, and the security person would call staff to ask if Julia was there. Only then would I learn if I was to be let in.

### Observation of Toddler

In the new surroundings, Miguel sought out the security of his mother's side. They both beamed and hugged each other when they were reunited after Miguel returned from day care. It felt as if they both needed to cling to each other. Julia reported to me that Miguel initially did not eat or sleep well in his new home. His day care was changed despite Julia's protests. The shelter staff decided that the on-site day care at the shelter was preferable because the transportation to his previous day care was too difficult to coordinate. Miguel now had to relate to changing day care staff shifts as well as to the changing house staff shifts.

Miguel seemed to grow up quickly in the shelter, as he walked early and became an active toddler. He was often sick and was frequently absent from day care. The shelter staff questioned Julia's decisions to keep him in her room and not attend her own schooling. Julia reported that Miguel would not go to sleep at night and would be awake for hours playing and talking. They both became very dysregulated. Their interactions grew more intense. As Julia became more disabled by depression, Miguel's behavior became more insistent and demanding. As a result, Miguel adapted to a variety of adults and a variety of caretaker interactions. He gave up the idea that his mother alone could satisfy his needs. However, he still preferred his mother to other caretakers. Miguel grew into a smiling toddler, running the hallways, happy to go to anyone who took an interest in him. He was still spontaneously joyous and sought out activities of pleasure, mostly in movement. He liked to bounce to music, throw balls, run, and climb. He had a toddler's fearlessness and excitement—the world was there for him to explore. Miguel was easy to enjoy, yet I wondered how much of Miguel's happy persona was a toddler reflection of his mother's masked gaiety, the beginning of a false self (Winnicott, 1971). He would cry loudly and protest when it was time for me to leave. This was the only time I saw Miguel in persistent distress. Julia was unable to contain him or bear his feelings. Initially she wanted to divert him and not deal with the emotions of his loss, as was her own internal model. Julia's need to not know her son's helpless and raging state was embedded in Julia's and Miguel's relationship, as well as part of Julia's own history. For her, the only way to respond to Miguel's pain was to not know it (Lyons-Ruth, 2003). During each visit, I worked with Julia on how to help Miguel with this separation, how to name it and acknowledge his sadness, plan our next meeting, and help him transition to their next activity together. I hoped this routine experience of a planned separation would resonate with both Julia and Miguel.

## Observation of Mother

Julia was tense, sometimes sad, and sometimes forcefully gay when I saw her at the shelter. She was now further isolated from her family and familiar world. She stopped going to school and attended an alternative school at the shelter. Julia's own trauma therapy was never solidly established. When Julia was placed in the shelter, the shelter took over Julia's care. As an outsider I was unable to work within its system to influence options and procure something sustainable for her. She kept missing appointments with a hospital outpatient clinic therapist, but did have a doctor who prescribed antidepressants. She also suffered from migraines. Julia repeatedly told me she did not feel safe, and it was difficult for me to assess how much was real and how much was a manifestation of her paranoid projections. She accused other residents of threatening her, poisoning her food, and stealing her passport and money.

## Notes of a Visit to the Shelter, Mother, and Toddler Aged 16 Months

One cold winter afternoon, I arrived at the shelter to find the door to Julia's room closed. A staff person told me that Julia was in bed in her darkened room, with a migraine. Miguel was inside the room with her. I knocked hesitantly on Julia's door, indicating who I was. After a pause, she responded by asking me to come in. I found her lying on her bed under the covers. Miguel was in his crib, which was full of toys. He was standing up against the railing closest to his mother. He greeted me with smiles as I entered.

I asked Julia if I could play with Miguel in their room; she said "sure." I removed Miguel from the crib and played with him on the floor. Miguel was very animated and joyous, a contrast to the stillness and quiet of his mother. He demolished the blocks and stacking cup towers with relish (some aggression on his part that needed to be expressed) and yet was also able to carefully balance the blocks as he built a tower. He was laughing and Julia began to watch us from under the blanket. She began gradually to comment on Miguel's play. "Good papa," she said softly as he placed the third block. She told me she had been prescribed an antidepressant, but she wanted to make sure it was okay to take with her migraine medication. She had put calls in to her different doctors to find out. I praised her for being alert and a good advocate for her own health care. I noted also how she understood that it was helpful to have good communication between her doctors. I remembered that she had asked me to teach her and Miguel some American children's songs, so I began to sing "The Wheels on the Bus." Miguel responded with the actions he had learned in day care. I continued to sing, and Julia began to sing softly along with me. She finally got out of bed and we held hands with Miguel and danced the circle dance of "Ring Around the Rosie."

I was aware of how fragile she was and of how hard I had been working to hold her and Miguel together in this dark moment. When we fell to the ground together at "we all fall down," she and Miguel were laughing. I could feel the pressure in my chest lighten. Maybe our work together would lead to somewhere good for both of them. Julia then took me on a tour of her room crowded with piles of clothes and toys while she held Miguel in her arms. Julia wanted to show me the poems that she had hung on her walls, some of her own poems and others of her favorite writer, Maya Angelou. I could see how Julia connected to these poems of honest rage, love, and pain that had been written with Angelou's vitality and passion. Julia's own poems were also about love and pain.

### Parent–Infant Interactions and Intervention

When Miguel was crawling and an early walker, Julia was able to absorb my example and distract Miguel when she felt he needed to stop what he was doing or change his actions or feelings. Then Miguel became more agile and could easily leave Julia's side. Did she internalize this as meaning that Miguel could now abandon her? I noted that at the same time that Miguel was mobile and we discussed safety concerns, setting limits, and saying "no" effectively to a toddler, Julia was experiencing perhaps a parallel safety concern for herself as she spoke of being threatened by the residents. It seemed that, in Julia's experience, the world was no longer safe for the both of them. The staff noted to me that Julia left Miguel and would instead carry a younger infant of another resident, making Miguel jealous and uneasy with her unavailability. Was Julia abandoning Miguel before he was taken from her? During my visits I rarely saw Julia fail to respond to Miguel, but once we left the shelter playroom on my way out, I could see Miguel was on his own and she did not always respond to his distress.

How would Julia respond as Miguel got older and had a tantrum? Would she respond with her parents' pattern of rage and shaming? As Miguel became a separate individual, could she handle the feelings of abandonment this evoked with less hostility than her own mother had? If Miguel was too fearful to be separate, the relationship system would be repeated in this next gener-ation. I worked to affirm the strength of her bond with Miguel, noting how their reunions after day care were happy occasions for Miguel. I continued to value Julia's understanding of Miguel's behavior and his feelings. I linked her actions with Miguel to her past history and encouraged her to think about this with me and with her own therapist—when she had one. I told her it was impossible without good help not to repeat the abandonment she had expe-rienced. I continued to take photos of Julia and Miguel, as I had since they were in the foster home. I gave the photos to Julia with a photo album from the program so that she could keep a picture history of them together. For Miguel's first birthday party, which was held soon after they had arrived in the shelter, Julia decorated the party room walls with copies of these photos of Miguel and herself. She cooked a meal for the party, decorated the room with streamers and pictures, and invited all of the residents. Her resilience to pull herself up and celebrate her son's first birthday by herself without her family or close friends was magnificent.

## Mother's Internal World

Julia seemed so vulnerable in this setting. "I don't trust anyone," she told me again and again. Her anguish continued to emerge; it went back to the unresolved impact of her parents' failure to protect her, which allowed her to be raped. When her mother could not maintain connection, it was difficult for Julia to be connected with Miguel. The wound was kept raw. The bond between Julia and her mother was very complicated. She often complained about her mother, and then startled me with her generous understanding and clarity about her need to have her mother be the mother she needed and wanted. Julia was able to see both good and bad aspects of her mother. She acknowledged that her mother loved her but was not always able to be there for her. "My mother was there for me when my son was born. My mother tried. She tried. She took Miguel to day care; she was helping me out. She did not agree with the life I chose, but she was there helping me."

I tried to feed Julia's need for a caring presence. I encouraged Julia to look after herself, to go to therapy as well as to turn to others (e.g., the shelter staff) for help, and to write poetry, exercise, and think of future goals for herself. She wanted to be a nurse, doctor, or lawyer. I brought her copies of Maya Angelou's poetry, as well as positive hip-hop songs. She in turn invited me to Miguel's birthday party at the shelter, the shelter Thanksgiving Dinner, and the day care's holiday party.

## Pressures Upon the Therapist

The communication barriers with many different helping providers made this phase particularly difficult. While dealing with the day-to-day crises, there seemed nowhere to go with my concerns about the larger picture. My role was very marginalized by the shelter, and I was rarely informed of staff concerns.

Her CPS worker, the court, and the shelter all pressured Julia to be in therapy to address her trauma history. Although I agreed that Julia needed intensive therapy to help her with the depth and severity of her past, I felt she needed to be in a safe holding environment to do this deep, painful, uncovering work. The shelter did not seem safe to Julia, and she was still reeling from her parents' abandonment. It seemed unhelpful to mandate therapy and judge Julia's "cooperativeness" by her inability to engage in trauma therapy at this time.

Yet Julia needed so much more with her deteriorating mental health and daily threatening crises. It was hard to focus on the impact of all this on Julia and Miguel's relationship. Sometimes our play sessions seemed to create an oasis of protected calm and pleasure, and I hoped they both took nourishment from it. Other times, Julia was so tense and distracted that I felt very inadequate with what I had to offer them. Julia was unable to contain consistently Miguel's affect regulation. I found myself wanting to leap in and put out all the fires around them.

## TERMINATION

Eventually I too had to leave Julia and Miguel when I left my position to accept another job. When I told Julia I would be leaving, she responded that Miguel would miss me as he was attached to me and looked forward to my visits. She then said she was not happy about this, as she wanted me to stay with her until Miguel was grown up. We reviewed all we had done together, and Julia told me how much she had felt the support and care and how much she now understood about Miguel. She shared with me that when she first had Miguel as an infant, she was afraid she would not be able to be a parent. "Yet you believed I could be a parent and that helped me." She refused to be transferred to another parent–child home visitor. I fantasized privately for a while that despite the realities of a full-time job in another area, I would continue to see her myself. I soon realized the pitfalls of not having a program to legitimize my presence and work. It had been difficult enough to gain access to the shelter with my role in a program, and I did not want to promise Julia something I could not confidently ensure. It was a wrenching leave taking for me, and I felt I had betrayed her.

## REFLECTIONS

The hardest of the brick walls that I faced in this case was attempting to do infant–parent psychotherapy with an adolescent mother while she was being abandoned yet again by her own parent, then again by the foster mother, and then again by the rotating shifts of the shelter staff. The limitations of the work can be located in both Julia's internal and external worlds.

## Risks and How to Work With Them

It was a challenge to meet Julia's overwhelming needs along with Miguel's ever-present needs. It was clear that Julia was better able to parent her infant when she was initially living with her mother, as she didn't have to worry about being abandoned and could use all her capacities to care for her infant. The institutionalized caring systems that were then set in place to be responsible for the young mother and her infant were unable to provide the safety and stability she needed. Julia deteriorated, became dissociative and suicidal at worst, and at best was depressed and hostile. Miguel's experience during this period must have been overwhelming to him, as Julia was unable to be emotionally available to contain or mirror his own reality (Arons, 2005).

## Limiting Realities: Factors in the Family

Julia presented as an adolescent with a history of unresolved trauma and a pseudo-maturity, the mask of a false self that covered her painful sadness about loss and abandonment. The task of adolescence is to separate from one's parents while the parents remain there. It was extremely challenging to try to find a protected space for the continuing developmental needs of both Julia and Miguel while Julia's own parents were in the process of abandoning her yet again.

Julia's relationship with her mother was ambivalent, full of love and pain. Their relationship had the stressful complexity of forced separation as Julia's mother initially left Julia as a young child in order to go to work in the United States. During these forced separations both parent and child were left with fantasies of their relationship that may not be lived up to when the parent and child are reunited. The disappointment may lead to further disconnection and complicated attachment relationships (Bragin & Pierrepointe, 2004). For Julia, the stress of separation from her mother was compounded by being unprotected and sexually abused. In retrospect, I now see how Julia's hopes for her mother's love and protection when reunited with her mother before the birth of Miguel were bound to fail because of their history of unresolved separations. Julia's relationship with her mother was toxic, intense, and full of disappointment and longing. They longed to be together and then their hopes dissolved in pain as each could not live up to the other's fantasy. The fight with her mother that led to Julia and Miguel being placed into foster care was a pivotal moment and marked a spiral downward for them.

Maybe there were inherent limitations to the work of affecting the relationship of Julia with her baby while her own relationship with her mother was unresolved and abandonment continued to be reenacted. Julia had experienced her mother's rejection three times and told me her mother sent her away. I heard her mother threaten Julia with being sent back to foster care. Julia told me a few times that her mother told her that everything that happened to Julia in Atlanta was Julia's fault and that Julia had to "live with it." Yet Julia's mother did try to be there for Julia when she had her baby. I noted that when I visited Julia in the hospital after the birth of her son, her mother had already visited and left Julia her favorite home-cooked food. Julia did not give up on her mother and tried to call her mother at different times, including on her mother's birthday. No parent contacted her for her birthday or for Miguel's first birthday. During the 2-year period that I worked with Julia and her son, neither parent tried to contact her after she was removed and taken into state custody. Neither parent called CPS to inquire after her, and neither parent showed up in court to claim her or their grandson. Both her mother and father were reported by the CPS worker to easily become disruptive in anger when contact was made. The parents' anger with each other easily led to violence.

## PROFESSIONAL BOUNDARIES AND FACTORS IN COMMUNITY

In my work with Julia and Miguel, I developed relationships with a host of people: her mother, her foster mother, her CPS worker, her close girlfriend who was also Miguel's godmother, her family day care provider, her pediatrician, her guidance counselor at school, Julia's and Miguel's court assigned attorneys, the court investigator, the many different shelter staff, the other shelter residents, the day care staff, and her church mentor. Many of these people in Julia's life were angry with her, just as the adolescent mothers in Fraiberg's work (1987) had everyone angry with them.

Julia's relationships with her foster mother, CPS worker, and then shelter staff were fraught with conflict, which disrupted her stability again and again. I tried to prepare Julia for this and talked with her about the possibility that conflict could erupt and how difficult this was because it brought up times when her own mother did not understand her. The foster mother, CPS, or shelter staff may have their own reasons for being judgmental of Julia's behavior. At times Julia would sob as she retold some misdemeanor, perceiving it as another time when she tried so hard and still messed up.

There were so many appointments and providers, each with his or her own agendas to manage. All of the pieces in this house of cards were vulnerable to falling down. Communication between all was sporadic at best; often there was no sharing of information. There was no framework to hold it all together for the providers, let alone for Julia. How could she feel safe and supported? The inability of the various providers to integrate their work and support for Julia only added to Julia's fragmented sense of self. It underscored the uproar and disruption in her life with no one holding responsibility for it all. At 16 years of age, it was too much to expect Julia to be responsible for everything. For a while, Julia placed me in the role of holding it all together for her. She asked me to keep copies of various documents for her, such as court documents, her lawyer's letters, and a list of Miguel's completed vaccinations from his doctor.

A serious limitation of my own work to support an at-risk parent–infant relationship was the chronic difficulties and frustrations in coordination and communication with other providers and systems that played a role in Julia's life. To be effective, I felt I needed to address the foster care system, welfare system, family court, shelter, and public school system to help develop their understanding of how to support parent–infant relationships. Without such communication and coordination, the work I was doing with Julia and Miguel was too much for one person alone.

## COUNTERTRANSFERENCE AND THERAPEUTIC USE OF SELF

When I first met Julia, I had a sense that we liked each other. Our relationship seemed to flow, and it was mostly easy to engage with each other in a range of circumstances. This therapeutic relationship made me feel hopeful that we could work together and maybe make a positive difference in her life and her infant's.

My own countertransference responses to Julia and Miguel provided useful information and helped me in various aspects of parent–infant psychotherapy. First, my responses to Miguel's nonverbal communication allowed me to mentalize the infant's unique self and verbalize for him so that his mother could begin to access his separate mind. Countertransference informed my work in every session. It guided me as to the level at which I expressed the work and the way it was done (Acquarone, 2004). Paying attention to my own response helped me make meaning creatively in the moment as I interacted with Julia and her infant. It also informed me when it was clear that Julia should have her own psychotherapy to help contain her flooded and overwhelming feelings and flashbacks to her traumatic history.

Strong countertransference responses were especially evoked in the absence of any parent or parent substitutes for Julia. The absence was always present, and at times seemed shocking to me. I absorbed all of the pressures and responsibility of intervening in two vulnerable lives: an adolescent and her infant. I found myself wanting to cook her a meal and take care of Julia and her baby when the gaps felt difficult to bear. I procured a sling and later a stroller donation through my program so that Miguel could be safely transported and so Julia could better manage the logistics of going to day care on two buses and then school, twice a day. I tried to carefully time when to act and when to wait. I was constantly considering what Miguel needed at that moment, even if his young mother could not provide it. When can the infant or toddler wait and when is it critical that his needs take precedence? Miguel's dependency on such a young and at times so fragmented mother added to my sense of urgency and constant vigilance. I felt I had to keep them both in mind, and it made me anxious that no one else was doing so with a long-term commitment. During the last portion of their time at the shelter, Miguel's attachment to his mother was becoming more disorganized. I felt helpless watching an intergenerational pattern repeat itself. Even worse, the helping systems and fragmented providers who were responsible for Julia and her child unwittingly provided her with a reenactment of abandonment and danger over and over again. Knowing that funding for my position was unstable, I unsuccessfully worked to get Julia connected to a clinic, a safe place where she could continue longer term therapy for both herself and her parent–infant work. During this whole period that I had been seeing Julia and Miguel, my program was vulnerable to state budget cuts and imminent closure. My position was insecure, and I was very aware of my possible abandonment of Julia. At one point I was one of only two staff who were left to carry the program for several months. Julia was one client I was able to continue to see during this stressful period of too many needs and too few staff to meet them. As I continued to see Julia, I was aware that she was affected directly by this, but as her infant mental health therapist I was aware of my limitations as I felt very stretched, marginalized, and unsupported in the work on many levels. I was fortunate to have skilled infant mental health supervision to process the material and my feelings. However, during the last year, while Julia was in the shelter, I had no clinical supervision. In retrospect I can see how the lack of regular supervision through a shifting and harrowing period made me feel more vulnerable and helpless. There is an uncanny parallel between my own work situation and that of Julia in that we both were feeling abandoned, stressed, and unsupported by our "parent." There was a potential risk for me to be overzealous to heal Julia and Miguel as a reparative action in the face of my own insecurity.

Being present when the judge announced that Julia had been abandoned by her parents compelled me to take on the responsibility that I should not abandon her. Eventually and painfully, I became another of the many who had to leave Julia and Miguel, knowing that whenever Julia felt abandoned she found it difficult to be there for her son.

In retrospect I see that my box of attachment intervention tools was not sufficient in Julia's and Miguel's precarious world. My presence in a caring attentive relationship to allow Julia and Miguel to find and experience pleasure in their own connection with their own melody was not enough. Both their relationship and my work with Julia and Miguel required a safe home and the connected grounding of a caring team working thoughtfully together.

> I couldn't tell fact from fiction
> or if my dreams was true,
> The only sure prediction
> in this whole world was you.
> I'd touched your features inchly
> heard love and dared the cost.
> The scented spiel reeled me unreal
> and found my senses lost.
>
> —Maya Angelou
> *Oh Pray My Wings Are Gonna Fit Me Well*

## ACKNOWLEDGMENTS

I wish to thank my teachers, supervisors, and colleagues at the infant–parent Training Institute of Jewish Family and Children's Services of Greater Boston. Individuals to whom I am most grateful for their support, insight, and review of early versions of this chapter include Judith Aarons, Gaby Cavallacci, Ann Epstein, Francisca Guevara, Bianca Shagrin, Simon Shagrin, and especially, and always, Steve Joshua Heims.

## REFERENCES

Acquarone, S. (2004). *Infant-parent psychotherapy: A handbook.* London: Karnac.

Amini, F., Lewis, T., Lannon, R., Louie, A., Baumbacher, G., McGuiness, T., et al. (1996). Affect, attachment, memory: Contributions toward psychobiologic integration. *Psychiatry, 59,* 213–239.

Angelou, M. (1975). Senses of insecurity [poem]. In M. Angelou, *Oh pray my wings are gonna fit me well* (p. 17). New York: Random House.

Arons, J. (2005). "In a black hole": The (negative) space between longing and dread: Home-based psychotherapy with a traumatized mother and her infant son. In R. A. King, P. B. Neubauer, S. Abrams, & A. S. Dowling (Eds.), *The psychoanalytic study of the child* (Vol. 60, pp. 101–127). New Haven, CT: Yale University Press.

Bragin, M., & Pierrepointe, M. (2004). Complex attachments: Exploring the relation between mother and child when economic necessity requires migration to the north. *Journal of Infant, Child and Adolescent Psychotherapy, 3*(1), 28–46.

Fonagy, P. (2001). *Attachment theory and psychoanalysis.* New York: Other Press.

Fraiberg, S. (1987). The adolescent mother and her infant. In L. Fraiberg (Ed.), *Selected writings of Selma Fraiberg* (pp. 166–182). Columbus: Ohio State University Press.

Fraiberg, S., Adelson, E., & Shapiro, V. (1975). Ghosts in the nursery: A psychoanalytic approach to impaired infant–mother relationships. *Journal of the American Academy of Child Psychiatry, 14,* 387–422.

Hesse, E., & Main, M. (1999). Second generation effects of unresolved trauma in nonmaltreating parents: Dissociated, frightened and threatening parental behavior. *Psychoanalytic Inquiry, 19,* 481–540.

Lieberman, A. F., Padron, E., Van Horn, P., & Harris, W. (2005). Angels in the nursery: The intergenerational transmission of benevolent parental influences. *Infant Mental Health Journal, 26,* 504–520.

Lieberman, A. F., Silverman, R., & Pawl, J. H. (2000). Infant-parent psychotherapy: Core concepts and current approaches. In C. H. Zeanah (Ed.), *Handbook of infant mental health* (2nd ed., pp. 472–484). New York: Guilford Press.

Lieberman, A. F., & Van Horn, P. (2005). *Don't hit my mommy! A manual for child–parent psychotherapy with young witnesses of family violence.* Washington, DC: ZERO TO THREE.

Lieberman, A. F., & Zeanah, C. (1999). Contributions of attachment theory to infant-parent psychotherapy and other interventions with infants and young children. In J. Cassidy & P. R. Shaver (Eds.), *Handbook of attachment* (pp. 555–574). New York: Guilford Press.

Lyons-Ruth, K. (2003). Dissociation and the parent-infant dialogue: A longitudinal perspective from attachment research. *Journal of the American Psychoanalytic Association, 51*(3), 883–910.

McDonough, S. (2000). Interaction guidance: An approach for difficult-to-engage families. In C. H. Zeanah (Ed.), *Handbook of infant mental health* (2nd ed., pp. 485–493). New York: Guilford Press.

Sander, L. W. (1962). Issues in early mother-child interaction. *American Academy of Child Psychiatry, 1,* 141–166.

Slade, A., Sadler, L. S., & Mayes, L. C. (2005). Minding the baby: Enhancing parental reflective functioning in a nursing/mental health home visiting program. In L. J. Berlin (Eds.), *Enhancing early attachments* (pp. 152–177). New York: Guilford Press.

Stern, D. (1985). *The interpersonal world of the infant.* New York: Basic Books.

Stern, D. (1995). *The motherhood constellation: A unified view of parent–infant psychotherapy.* New York: Basic Books.

Tronick, E. (1989). Emotions and emotional communication in infants. *American Psychologist, 44*(2), 112–119.

Wakschlag, L. S., & Hans, S. L. (2000). Early parenthood in context: Implications for development and intervention. In C. H. Zeanah (Ed.), *Handbook of infant mental health* (2nd ed., pp. 472–484). New York: Guilford Press.

Winnicott, D. W. (1971). *Playing and reality.* London: Routledge.

# CHAPTER 3

# COMMENTS ON SUSAN SKLAN'S CASE

*Marian Birch*

As I read and reread the story of Susan Sklan's work with Julia and Miguel, I am struck by how little Miguel himself comes into clear focus as a "character." It is Julia who haunts me, and who calls out to my wishes to protect, rescue, or pray. Julia herself is a child, forced—literally—into motherhood far too soon. In offering her treatment *as a mother*, by not offering her treatment *as a child*, does the system become complicit in the abuse and neglect she experiences, as well as the foreshortened future she faces as she heroically attempts to mother without education, income, or life experience as an adult? The question at the heart of this heart-wrenching story is whether and how much Julia, as an adolescent mother, can be helped. Can Julia, whose traumatic losses and brutal deficits in protective care are *not* ghosts, but alive and well in the present, be helped to give her baby the safety, unconditional love, and developmental facilitation that she still needs and never receives? Are Miguel's needs compatible with his mother's needs? Who decides? Who is responsible?

These very serious questions may not be adequately addressed by our standard intake assessment procedures. Although the use of the *Diagnostic Classification of Mental Health and Developmental Disorders of Infancy and Early Childhood* (DC:0–3R; ZERO TO THREE, 2005) can give us a fairly rich picture of the infant's functioning, and of the state of the infant–parent relationship, it lacks any systematic process for evaluating the precise nature of the parent's impediments to parenting. It is a system that takes the infant as its subject and the parent as a component of the infant's functional competence. In this way we

67

inadvertently mirror the egocentric worldview of the infant who is quite unable to picture his parent as a complex and multifaceted human being with many things on her mind besides him.

When we take the parent as a subject, there is, of course, a wealth of clinical research and literature that can help us be more realistic and aware of the grave impediments many people face in becoming parents. Some kinds of psychiatric disorders that parents experience do not, at present, have known "cures," although they do have both pharmacological and psychotherapeutic interventions that are often successful in helping afflicted individuals manage their illness and lead happier, more productive lives. These include the major psychotic disorders such as schizophrenia, schizoaffective disorder, bipolar disorders, and major character disorders, particularly of a borderline or narcissistic type. Because infant–parent psychotherapy does not purport to be a therapy for parental psychopathology, it behooves us to understand the nature of that psychopathology. We should be mindful of the outer limits this may suggest for progress, and when parental mental illness is a factor, we may need to set goals that are more compensatory than curative in their outlook.

For example, with a parent who was blind we could work until the end of time to establish reciprocal visual cuing and get nowhere. However, we could help the parent learn compensatory, nonvisual ways to engage in reciprocal interaction with her infant. This skill would be enormously valuable and would contribute to a far healthier psychological outcome for the dyad. It would not, however, take away the reality that such a child would have a mother who had never seen his face.

Sklan conceptualizes the work thus:

> The essence of the work is to develop the mother's capacity for mindfulness and reflective functioning so that she can take in the baby's needs and intentions in order to "keep the baby in mind." This is a key to parental sensitivity and to the development of a strong, positive attachment relationship between parent and child . . . I hoped that this type of attachment-based intervention would be an instrument of therapeutic

change and support for Julia, helping her ensure the safety and protection of Miguel and not repeat her own parents' lack of protection for herself. (p. 31)

Might a "colder" or, at least, "cooler" look at Julia's psychological profile have helped Sklan titrate her goals, passion, and hopes so that she felt less crushed at the end? Might that have helped her to keep in mind Seligman's (2000) deeply important but oft-overlooked description of the real goal of infant–parent psychotherapy:

> Interventions should maximize whatever potentials for progressive development can be located within the caregiving system, *rather than reaching some extrinsic criterion* (italics added). (p. 212)

Julia is a young adolescent whose state of mind concerning relationship (Hesse & Main, 1999) is profoundly disorganized. The disorganized relationships with her parents are not "ghosts." They continue in the present to keep 16-year-old Julia in a constant state of "fright without solution" as she goes on craving love, affirmation, and protection from her parents, who in turn continue to brutally annihilate her value and to exhibit shocking indifference to the dangers she faces. She becomes pregnant, while in foster care because of her parents' inability to care for her, by a much older and violently abusive man who abandons her. She chooses to leave foster care and return to her mother's home to have her baby in the hope that this, finally, will enable her mother to mother her. It is not clear if anyone was able to explore with her other options for herself and her baby.

Her expressed hope that Miguel, as *her* baby, will always love her and never leave her is actually more ominous than hopeful. It is likely that it mirrors the hope her mother had for her, a hope that the baby, finally, will validate that the mother is a lovable and worthy human being. Louise Kaplan (1991) warned of the infant's inevitable and catastrophic inability to carry such a burden:

Every mother looks into her child's eyes for an image of her own goodness. But when she is expecting that her very soul will be saved by her
child, we can be sure that violence is in the offing. (p. 412)

Furthermore, Kaplan added:

It is in this unquenchable thirst to be recognized as a worthwhile person
that the recycling of child abuse from one generation to the next begins.
The mother who was abused in childhood will be looking in the eyes of
her baby for proof of her own worthiness. (p. 432)

If our therapeutic focus is too exclusively and uncritically on supporting this
longing for validation as "a good mother" in a girl who has never felt deeply
"good" in any other way, we may be colluding with her wish to shut out and
ignore all of the dark and terrible thoughts, feelings, and impulses that, given
her situation, she must have. This danger is foreshadowed in the conversation Sklan and Julia have when Miguel is 6 months old. Julia is giving Miguel
formula without iron so that he won't spit up, although her pediatrician has
told her that he needs the iron and the spitting up is not worrisome. Sklan
supports her in her thoughtful seeking of advice, but does not address her
ignoring the advice. As Sklan notes, Julia's difficulty tolerating her baby's
spitting out what she feeds him is certainly tantalizing as a metaphor for the
issues in their relationship and in Julia's inner world.

At the end of this exquisitely rich and tender case report, Sklan states:

In retrospect I see that my box of attachment intervention tools was not
sufficient in Julia and Miguel's precarious world. My presence as a caring
attentive relationship to allow Julia and Miguel to find and experience
pleasure in their own connection with their own melody was not enough.
(p. 62)

The use of the word *enough* inevitably evokes Winnicott's (1952, p. 38)
concept of the "good-enough mother"—the mother who presents her infant

with her only-human mixture of love and hate, attentiveness and neglect, sensitivity and denseness, and finds that it is "good enough" or, perhaps, as the movie title goes, "as good as it gets."

In what sense did Sklan fail, as she laments, "to allow Julia and Miguel to find and experience pleasure in their own connection with their own melody" (p. 62)?

This treatment cannot be seen as a failure if we frame its narrative as a thera-peutic experience of relationship in which, for both members of the dyad, "reality" and "truth" are mutually cocreated, by means of empathic listening, sensitive responding, gentle challenge, negotiation, and reciprocity (Lyons-Ruth, 2006). Such a mutual creation of a shared world of affects and meanings stands in stark contrast to the tangled web of projections and impingements that constituted Julia's early and continuing experience in her family.

Furthermore, in the clinical material Sklan offers, there are several "moments of meeting" (Stern, 2004). These are moments when Julia and Miguel do find and experience pleasure in their connection, and they are created by the dynamically containing presence of the therapist.

One such moment occurs when the therapist shows Julia, in a wonderfully concrete way, how to be a "secure base" (Bowlby, 1988) for Miguel's explo-ration of the world, by giving him the firm support of her hands to push against as he learns to crawl. The delight mother and baby show here, in an activity that embodies the possibility of integrating connection and separateness, is nearly miraculous for such an abandoned and unsupported dyad to experience.

A second moment of meeting occurs when the therapist finds Julia and Miguel in the dark in their room at the shelter, desperately disconnected. Miguel is standing, wide-eyed and silent in the dark. He is frightened (I imagine) that any overt bid for his mother's attention will only drive her deeper into the darkness of her cave of blankets and her depression.

Here the therapist shows Miguel and Julia several important things. First, by asking for and receiving Julia's permission to play with him, she affirms, for them both, this young mother's desire for her son's happiness, despite, and without denying or minimizing, the anguish that renders her unable to tolerate and respond to his needs. The therapist then offers herself only as a gift from mother to son. She becomes the love Julia longs to and cannot give to her son.

Second, by gently and playfully engaging Miguel, without pressuring or lecturing Julia, the therapist creates an island of warmth and light in her dark room that draws Julia out of her lair and into the "magic circle" (Fraiberg, Adelson, & Shapiro, 1975) of relatedness. In doing this, she also shows Miguel something important about how to find his mother when Julia withdraws into her depression. Even though wooing and cajoling and being cheerfully but undemandingly available have real limits as an attachment strategy for a toddler—requiring the inhibition of affective intensity, of anger, fear, and distress that, optimally, could be expressed—they are, arguably, a step up from frozen, watchful waiting.

Third, in a flash of intuitive genius, the game the therapist chooses for this three-way reunion in the dark is Ring Around the Rosie. This is a game about falling down and getting up again and again. It is believed that it was invented by children in the years of the Black Death in the fourteenth century (Opie & Opie, 1969). It is a game about the way that, if you fall in a circle of loving relatedness, holding hands, it leads to shared laughter instead of lonesome tears.

In a sense, the whole treatment can be seen as a combination of Ring Around the Rosie and Hide and Seek, games that evolved to master the developmental challenges of standing on one's own two feet, coping with separation and frustration, and finding the help and connection one needs. Sklan, in a very active and dynamic way, creates a small space for this motherless child–mother and her child, a space for play, reflection, and the shared creation of meaning. In such space, called "transitional space" by Winnicott (1952), falling, losing, struggling for balance, reaching for another's hand, finding, losing, and refinding can all be thought about and metabolized.

Christopher Bollas (1987) wrote that the most tragic loss for victims of childhood sexual assault, such as Julia, is the loss of the capacity for fantasy and imagination. In the magical thinking of the child victim, to imagine or dream of something is to make it happen in reality. Therefore, thinking imaginatively and playfully is frozen. There is no distinction between thinking and doing, between feeling and enacting. Sklan's work with Julia and Miguel helps both of them keep the capacity for play and creative imagining alive. Julia is writing and reading poetry. She is not, at least by the time we lose sight of her, involved in another brutalizing sexual relationship. She is not pregnant again. Despite the devastating disappointments in her own mother, and the minimal emotional support she feels in foster care and in the shelter, Miguel has as much of her as it is possible for her to give. He is not sharing her with a violent boyfriend or a needy baby sibling or an addiction. These are not small achievements.

So, is this "good enough"? I doubt we would ask this question if we were discussing the psychotherapy of an adult. With adult patients, we have become relatively comfortable with the idea that therapy can provide certain experiences of emotional learning and growth, and that it is the patient's responsibility to make use of them to the best of his ability, as he navigates, like Hamlet, "the slings and arrows of outrageous fortune," and meets whatever opportunities life offers him. With adults, therapists do not, as a rule, feel responsible for intercepting the blows and finding the opportunities on their patients' behalf. When therapists do feel this way in work with adults, their training strictly enjoins them to refrain from acting on these impulses. Instead, they are encouraged to contain them and to reflect on them. We try to sort out unresolved longings, needs, conflicts within ourselves that are being activated in the present relationship with the therapist, as well as subtle (or not so subtle) interactional cues from the patient that pressure us to assume a particular role in the patient's internal object relations. These cues may include words, gestures, posture, prosody, and expressions of emotion.

Current thinking about the therapeutic process (e.g., Bromberg, 1998; Clarkin, Kernberg, & Yeomans, 2006) has emphasized how such containment and reflection inform us about the internal relational dynamics of the patient and how these dynamics uniquely dovetail with those of the therapist. This understanding guides our moment-to-moment responses to the patient.

Yet comfort with this attitude and this approach seems to decrease with the age and vulnerability of the patient and the stability of his life circumstances. Sklan describes an overwhelming sense of responsibility, and feelings of helplessness, that are common in therapists working with infants in dire psychological peril. It is very difficult to bear, let alone "contain" the sense of a baby falling out of the net of the world. Sklan had to contend with internal object relations that were nothing short of formidable. Both Julia and Miguel utterly lacked any secure sense of protection and nurturance. Julia, in addition, had repeated experiences not only of abandonment but also of brutal and savage sexual exploitation by adults. In addition to the good side of her feelings about her therapist whom she, realistically, experienced as kind, reliable, enlivening, and safe, there had to be a darker side, less conscious and less acceptable, that hypervigilantly monitored Sklan's every move, anticipating that she, like the mother, the aunt, the grandparents, and the foster mother, would allow (which in a child's magical thinking is the same as to cause) her to be traumatized again.

Miguel, whose emotional needs were not being adequately met, made strong bids to the therapist, who was probably the most predictable and consistent caregiver figure in his life. Although Sklan showed exquisite tact in respecting Julia as Miguel's parent, she, like all of us, is built to fall in love with a baby who makes such appeals. States of mind like Miguel's, of highly activated attachment need, are extremely contagious—for good evolutionary reasons!

Furthermore, the members of the dysfunctional social network—comprising the foster care worker, the shelter staff, the biological and foster families, the court, the mental health therapist, and the agency staff where Sklan worked—may also have been feeling anxieties stimulated by dealing with two children, one of whom was a parent, who were expressing overwhelming attachment insecurity, either directly or indirectly. These anxieties were also experienced directly by Sklan, as she took on the case management and advocacy roles so common in work with infants, rather than only secondhand as would be the case if the therapist merely heard about them from the patient.

One common result of all these pressures is a very intense *maternal counter-transference*, in which the therapist feels, as mothers often do, an overwhelming responsibility for circumstances that, in reality, are unimaginably beyond her control. These feelings, in my own experience as both a clinician and a supervisor, can be extremely intense, so much so that it is almost, or actually, impossible to think about them as feelings rather than being driven by them into increasingly frantic and heroic rescue efforts.

In this case, it is not the therapy, but those heroic rescue efforts that were not and could not be enough. Sklan is not Julia's mother, nor Miguel's. No one, not even a real mother, can actually match the absolute nature of the maternal omnipotence and omnipresence that the anxious child seeks, just as no baby can actually match the expectation that Julia had of newborn Miguel—that he would always love her and never leave her.

What the therapist was able to give Julia and Miguel was something less magical but more useful and terribly important. She gave them a co-created relational world in which they could both see and feel that she saw them and had feelings for them. They sensed that she felt responsible and wanted very much to help this appealing pair of children who had no one else in their lives willing to feel the feelings of responsibility and regret that she had for them. It is a humble gift, but a priceless one.

## REFERENCES

Bollas, C. (1987). *The shadow of the object: Psychoanalysis of the unthought known.* New York: Columbia University Press.

Bowlby, J. (1988). *A secure base: Clinical applications of attachment theory.* London: Routledge.

Bromberg, P. (1998). *Standing in the spaces: Essays on clinical process, trauma and dissociation.* Hillsdale, NJ: Analytic Press.

Clarkin, J., Kernberg, O., & Yeomans, F. (2006). *Psychotherapy for borderline pathology: Focusing on object relations*. Washington, DC: American Psychiatric Press.

Fraiberg, S., Adelson, E., & Shapiro, V. (1975). Ghosts in the nursery: A psychoanalytic approach to impaired infant–mother relationships. *Journal of the American Academy of Child Psychiatry, 14*, 387–422.

Hesse, E., & Main, M. (1999). Second generation effects of unresolved trauma in nonmaltreating parents: Dissociated, frightened and threatening parental behavior. *Psychoanalytic Inquiry, 19*, 481–540.

Kaplan, L. (1991). *Female perversions*. New York: Doubleday.

Lyons-Ruth, K. (2006). Play, precariousness, and shared meaning: A developmental research perspective on child psychotherapy. *Journal of Infant, Child and Adolescent Psychotherapy, 5*, 142–159.

Opie, I., & Opie, P. (1969). *Children's games in street and playground*. London: Oxford University Press.

Seligman, S. (2000). Clinical interviews with families of infants. In C. Zeanah (Ed.), *Handbook of infant mental health* (2nd ed., pp. 211–221). New York: Guilford Press.

Stern, D. (2004). *The present moment in psychotherapy and everyday life*. New York: Norton Books.

Winnicott, D. W. (1952/1987). Letter to Roger Money-Kyrle. In F. R. Rodman (Ed.), *The spontaneous gesture: Selected letters of D. W. Winnicott* (pp. 38–43). Cambridge, MA: Harvard University Press.

ZERO TO THREE. (2005). *Diagnostic classification of mental health and developmental disorders of infancy and early childhood: Revised edition (DC:0–3R)*. Washington, DC: ZERO TO THREE.

# CHAPTER 4

# BEN: THE BOY WHO WAS SWALLOWED BY FEAR

*Marian Birch*

This is the story of my work with a boy I'll call Ben, who was 2 years old when I met him at the home of his foster–adoptive parents, and who was 6 when our work came to a sad and disappointing end.

Ben was seen in infant–parent psychotherapy with his adoptive parents for 4 years. After an enormously hopeful beginning, which saw Ben, in 2 years, transform from a rigid, unresponsive, wordless automaton to an animated and intensely expressive little boy passionately connected to his parents, the adoption of Ben's biological infant sister precipitated a profound regression that neither the parents nor the therapist were successful in addressing.

In this chapter, I examine the unfolding of this failed treatment and reflect on some retrospective thoughts about its meaning.

I did my best, in working with Ben, to adhere to the model in which I had been trained at the Infant–Parent Program at San Francisco General Hospital. I was a proud second-generation heir of Selma Fraiberg's inspired legacy. This model, described in Fraiberg, Adelson, and Shapiro's (1975) seminal paper "Ghosts in the Nursery," as well as by Lieberman, Silverman, and Pawl in the *Handbook of Infant Mental Health* (2000), combines practical and emotional support, developmental guidance, and psychoanalytically informed interpretation with the aim of freeing infant–parent relationships from what Fraiberg et al. so evocatively called the "ghosts" of the parents' own painful early experiences. Fraiberg et al. worked primarily with infants and their biological parents. Her model does not specifically address the special circumstances when an adopted infant brings his own ghosts to his new family. Her work predated today's more open exploration of the therapist's ghosts and their impact on treatment.

Ben was referred to me by his social worker in Child Protective Services (CPS). The circumstances of Ben's conception, gestation, and the first 19 months of his life are all but invisible, but lend themselves to terrifying imagining. Ben was born drug exposed and 3 weeks premature, following an incident of domestic violence between his birth parents. At birth, he tested positive for heroin and cocaine, and experienced "mild withdrawal symptoms." He was discharged to his parents' "home"—a room in a transient hotel—when he was 5 days old. His first 19 months of life were spent with his birth parents, who were both actively addicted to drugs. Domestic violence at life-threatening levels and heroin addiction appear to have been his parents' primary preoccupations during Ben's gestation and infancy. His mother was hospitalized three times during his first 18 months following severe beatings by his father. There is no record of where Ben was during these hospitalizations. The very scanty medical records I was able to obtain noted that Ben received a diagnosis of "failure to thrive" during a routine checkup (the only one we had records for) when he was 5 months old. But he was not brought back for follow-up. We might speculate that his parents failed to feed him adequately or that his chronic levels of fearful arousal made it difficult for him to eat and metabolize what he was fed.

When we began our work, Ben was 26 months old and had been in out-of-home placement since he was 19 months old. After his mother passed out from an overdose in a shopping mall, with Ben in her arms, he spent 5 months in a shelter care home before being placed with the Doyles, a middle-class couple in their 30s. They had no other children and wished to adopt. It was the door of their pleasant and modest suburban home that I eagerly knocked on that sunny spring afternoon.

When Ben was placed in foster care, he had no language and was so unresponsive to his caregivers that he was assessed by a developmental clinic for a pervasive developmental delay. His evaluators were baffled by him, declared him untestable, and suggested that he be brought back in 3 months. Instead, a referral was made to me for infant–parent psychotherapy. When Ben's language and social behavior rapidly emerged, the possibility of pervasive developmental delay was tabled. Ben continued to receive speech therapy, but did not return for a comprehensive developmental assessment.

When he was placed at 2 years old with the Doyles, Ben was still a foster child. His parents' parental rights were not terminated for another 14 months. Weekly supervised visits were scheduled with each of his parents at the Department of Social and Health Services (DSHS) offices. His parents attended approximately half of these scheduled visits, but never gave notice in advance that they did not plan to attend. So Ben made weekly trips to the DSHS offices with Peggy Doyle. I was repeatedly assured by the social worker that parental rights were about to be relinquished or terminated. In turn, I opted not to engage with Ben's birth parents. In retrospect, this decision undoubtedly "protected" me from fully sharing Ben's experience.

His new foster–adoptive parents, the Doyles, had been married for 10 years. They were mature, sensitive people who appreciated Ben's intensive need for caregiving, and were prepared to rearrange their lives to provide it. Peggy quit her job to be a stay-at-home mother. In addition, Ben's child welfare worker was very engaged and committed to Ben. She thought that his flat affect and unresponsiveness to his caregivers might be the result of early trauma, and thought that infant–parent psychotherapy might help Ben and his new family to connect emotionally. She made the referral to me, and advocated vigorously for ongoing support for twice-weekly treatment for the next 4 years. She also worked very hard to counsel his birth parents toward relinquishment and tried to speed the court process of termination of parental rights, although with modest results.

We were all—myself, the Doyles, the social worker—quite optimistic about how much good, sensitive, responsive care with emotionally available and reliable surrogate parents could remediate the kind of profound early exposure to unrelieved fearful arousal that characterized Ben's first 18 months.

However, the fact that the story of Ben's infancy simply did not exist in anyone's mind as a coherent narrative had alarming implications for how Ben might experience himself and his world now.

I saw my primary goal in working with Ben as fostering a healthy attachment relationship between him and his adoptive parents. Profoundly influenced by Winnicott's (1952/1975, p. 99) dictum "there is no such thing as a baby" without the provision of maternal care, I simply had no other framework for working with a child who lacked an organized internal working model of relationship. I believed that repeated reliable experiences of sensitive, loving caregiving and mirroring from adults who were able to "keep the baby in mind" would inevitably stimulate Ben's movement toward health and toward love. I saw my role initially as one of helping the Doyles understand Ben and his needs while helping him feel seen and understood by them.

My first memory of Ben is of a tiny, solemn little boy with platinum curls, pale, almost translucent skin, and empty blue eyes. He looked like an adult with a big head and small body. I was reminded of Gollum, the cave-dwelling creature from *The Hobbit*. I had come to the Doyle's pleasant bungalow for our first home visit. When Peggy Doyle opened the door, Ben, his face expressionless, pushed in front of her. Without looking at my face, he took my hand, and silently moved to go down the stairs with me toward the street without a backward glance.

As I watched and played with Ben, and talked with the Doyles about what they were seeing in those first months, I learned that Ben had very few words. "Bye bye" was one of the most frequently heard. He seemed to lack any concept or any behavioral schema based on a belief that adults were available to help him, to protect him, or even to interact with him. He seemed only to know that they were there to take him away.

Ben never cried and never sought comfort when he fell or bumped himself. This happened quite frequently, as he was often shockingly reckless with his body, literally running into walls. He strenuously avoided eye contact. He alternated periods of stunned, silent immobility, staring vacantly into the middle distance, with episodes of violent careening around rooms, crashing into walls, knocking over furniture, and laughing all the while in a joyless, high-pitched voice. Ben's features were attractive and well formed, but his face and body had little of the softly vulnerable rounded tenderness typical of toddlers. His lean little body seemed to be in a chronic flinch, and his facial expression had a hooded, precociously hardened quality.

My hypothesis was that Ben's abnormal behaviors were defensive strategies to cope with severe emotional and physical deprivation, specifically experiences of chronic fearful arousal without relief from a reliable caregiver. I thought that if we could show him that loving care was reliably available, he would learn to relinquish those defensive strategies in order to respond and connect emotionally. The Doyles seemed amply suited to play their part. Warm, humorous, and tolerant, they were already deeply fond of Ben, even though he gave so very little back. I explained to Peggy and Paul that I wanted one or both of them to be present for all of his sessions, and that, rather than interacting with Ben directly myself, my focus would be on coaching and supporting their interaction with him. Ultimately, this work was done primarily with Peggy, as Paul's work schedule prohibited his regular participation, but he joined us when he could. Peggy was an excellent, sensitive observer. She told me of taking Ben to the neighborhood co-op nursery and watching him stand frozen in the middle of the room while other children clamored for her attention. She also told me of watching him "go totally blank" when he was led away by a social worker for his weekly visits with his birth parents.

Peggy was clearly stirred up by the numb suffering of this little boy, and she was eager and willing to participate in any way she could. She instinctively understood that his apparent lack of interest in her was a symptom of intolerable neediness rather than a personal rejection. Peggy was a creative and imaginative participant in our efforts to engage Ben with gesture, vocalization, and make believe, but she volunteered little about her own feelings or early history. Unfortunately, I was not yet aware, at this stage of my career, of the intensely painful ghosts that a child such as Ben could stir up in even the healthiest parents. Thus, I did not probe about her own childhood and never, in this early phase, explored what Ben's travails evoked in her own psyche. Ben's therapy was a powerful teacher in this respect. For a long while, Ben's numbness and avoidance did not seem to stir her up in any problematic way. She felt tremendous empathy and warmth and did not take his disinterest and unresponsiveness personally. It was later, when his anger, violence, and aggression emerged, that she began to have difficulty keeping her empathic connection with him—as did I.

We began meeting in Ben's bedroom. Peggy and I shadowed Ben, following him around while describing, imitating, and admiring him and his activities in the exaggeratedly inflected voices of motherese. When Ben fell, for instance, Peggy would exclaim animatedly, "Bam! Wow, you crashed! Does it hurt? Oooh, I bet it hurts." Peggy monitored Ben for "owies," and when she found one, or when, in our judgment, a normal child would have felt pain, she fussed, comforted, and applied kisses and bandages liberally. This would have been affective attunement as described by Daniel Stern (1985), except for the unusual circumstance that Ben expressed no affect whatsoever. Stern observed that normal mothers observe and comment on their babies' activities, vocalizations, and affective expressions in a kind of emotional counterpoint. They do not imitate the babies' expressions or emotions exactly, but they match them, as it were, harmonically. What Peggy did was mirror for Ben a reflection of himself as a feeling, confidently cared-for child—a misattribution, to be sure—but, we hoped a healing one.

In revisiting this case, second thoughts about this approach haunt me. Could we, or should we, have found a way to mirror instead Ben's *actual* feeling of frozen dissociated terror in a way that would have made him feel that he was not alone in that dark place, but that he had a hand to hold? Why didn't we try this? Was it because we ourselves could not imagine how that state of mind could be contained or regulated? In wooing him so vigorously, we may have hoped to reassure him and ourselves that the scar tissue of terror could simply be shed like a snakeskin. Christopher Mawson (n.d.) wrote of this dilemma in work with children.

When a little child is in the middle of a storm of painful emotion, and makes us share that pain and confusion, it can be very hard to stay with the child, to stay receptive and desist from "knowing" what is wrong, to reassure prematurely, or to intervene inappropriately in some other way. We may be made to feel quite often that we are cruel and heartless if we do not, and so this work may not be easy or comfortable for the part of us that needs consistently to be liked and thanked.

Mawson continues:

For some deprived children eventual communication on the part of the analyst of understanding of the content of their anxieties may for a while be of secondary importance to the basic need to find someone to contain and experience their unbearable and unwanted feelings for them. This may primarily be to actualize a sense of having expelled and disposed of an unwanted experience, or it may have the additional component of seeking to make the other person know it for themselves in the only way open to the child at that moment, namely through action. The foremost skill of the child analyst is the capacity, under strain, to transform the former towards the latter, to hold on and to process evacuations and enactments of emotional pain into meaningful communications using simple words.

It is extremely difficult to stay with a child's pain and distress without taking immediate steps to reassure and calm, but with traumatized children such reassurance may only convey that we cannot bear to see what they are trying to show us.

These challenges are intensified when we are working with a child such as Ben who utterly lacks a secure base. In such situations, we may feel, and the child may feel, in the words of an adult patient (recalling the hours she spent in a wrecked car with the dead bodies of her parents at age 2), "that the feelings were too big, bigger than I was, I could not hold them."

The most powerful tool, and, at the same time, the greatest countertransferential pitfall in work with young children and their caregivers, is the "right-brain-to-right-brain" (Schore, 2001; Siegel, 1999) connection between the disturbed attachment system of the child and that of the child's parents and the (invariably imperfectly resolved) attachment system of the therapist. Although most of our circumstances are far less dramatic than Ben's, we can all resonate with the unthinkable anxiety, the fear of the psychological chaos that ensues when the baby's capacities to muster an organized and coherent state, a "going-on-being," are overwhelmed. An infant has few tools available to ward off such psychic implosion. Inhibition and dissociation are among them, and they are blunt, destructive techniques that have enormous unintended consequences. The work of Karlen Lyons-Ruth (Lyons-Ruth, Bronfman, & Atwood, 1999; Lyons-Ruth & Jacovitz, 1999) meticulously traced the links between chronic states of fearful arousal in infancy, disorganized attachment, and dissociation and controlling/caregiving attachment strategies in later childhood and adulthood. *Working model of relationship* is a key concept in attachment research that describes the child's subjective set of expectations about relationships that reflect his or her experiences with caregivers. The infant whose relationships with caregivers are inconsistent and/or frightening in ways that make it difficult to consolidate an organized working model of relationship is at high risk for developing a set of expectations for relationships that calls for compulsively controlling the "other," either through aggression or through compulsive caregiving. Compulsive controlling caregiving might be the dark side of a therapeutic stance and a strengths-based approach, and may be an unflattering but accurate description of my attempt to help Ben by training him how to act as if he felt safe.

As Peggy tended to Ben, I, in a parallel universe, as it were, ministered in like fashion to Hokey Pokey, a small stuffed being of unknown species that lived in Ben's crib, utterly ignored by Ben. Hokey Pokey cried, protested, and responded to my soothing efforts dramatically, loudly, and expressively, unlike Ben, who stared blankly or pulled away for many weeks. One day, after about 8 weeks of twice-weekly home visits (during which Ben's play was entirely solitary and consisted of aimless throwing, banging, and handling toys), Ben picked up a toy shark with which he "bit" Hokey Pokey on the head while

Ben growled and made biting movements with his jaws. Now, for the first time, he watched intently as Hokey Pokey howled, called for help, and received and was comforted by elaborate first aid measures and sympathy from me. This sequence, with minor variations, was repeated many, many times in this and subsequent sessions. I took this to be Ben's way to signify his perception that relationships were interchanges between voraciously hungry predators and small defenseless prey. I assumed naively that he primarily experienced himself as prey, and that his flat inexpressive demeanor was his attempt, like the deer in the headlights, to escape notice. With hindsight it seems to me now that we all colluded in addressing *only* his feelings of helplessness and victimization, and gave insufficient attention to his equally intense though inchoate predatory rage fueled by actual early experiences of witnessing intense violence while in a state of unrelieved hunger, fear, and deprivation.

One of the core functions of the attachment behavioral system is to protect attachment figures from becoming targets of predatory behavioral systems (Bowlby, 1969; Mayr, 1976; Meloy, 1992). In predatory animals, like humans, the attachment system facilitates selective inhibition of predatory behavior systems so that attachment figures, and, in the course of development, members of the family, tribal, and cultural group, are not targets of predatory aggression. How fragile this process is, and how easily derailed, can be readily seen in the work of Meloy (1988, 1992) on attachment in violent offenders, as well as by a look at any daily newspaper. Main and Hesse's (1990) observations of predatory behaviors toward infants—like growling, baring teeth, and stalking—in mothers with disorganized states of mind regarding attachment are another window into this dark chamber. Ben's early experience, repeatedly watching as one of his caregivers brutally battered the other, was certainly a breeding ground for dysfunction.

However, happily innocent (or in denial) about these sinister implications, we rejoiced that Ben was now expressing this predator/prey representation in a symbolic form, as a communication to which we could respond. Paul and Peggy, with my coaching, found many ways to assure him that they would not hurt him or let him be hurt (perhaps indistinguishable categories for a 2-year-old), and that they would offer him protection, comfort, and even pleasure. We learned together how to pace our approaches to Ben to accommodate his hypervigilance and terror. Paul and Peggy made significant changes in their routines so that Ben was rarely separated from them. As weeks and months passed, Ben emerged from his protective shell of numbness. He began to talk, going from near muteness to constant fluent chatter in a few months. He became extremely preoccupied with even the slightest possibility of injury to his body, and made constant, urgent demands for bandages, antiseptic cream, and hugs/kisses for both real and imagined owies. He became very clingy and resistant to separations from his parents, interrogating them exhaustively when separations were inevitable. The Doyles responded unstintingly to this new Ben. Their supportive parental presence had suddenly become vitally important to him. They minimized as much as possible situations in which he would have to cope without them. Ben's transformation, from the expressionless little automaton he had been into an almost operatically expressive little boy, was remarkable. His parents and I were very happy and hopeful. Peggy and Paul loved being so needed and important to him and gave their love and attention wholeheartedly.

One type of separation was beyond our power to avoid, however. I was repeatedly reassured by the social worker that the birth parents were on the verge of relinquishing their parental rights, and that, if they failed to do so, termination of parental rights would swiftly follow. However, weekly visits with them continued to be scheduled throughout the first year of Ben's treatment. Ben was clearly disturbed by the visits, and, as they continued, I made a strategic choice to ask a colleague to perform an evaluation of Ben's relationship with the biological parents and make recommendations about visits and services. I "outsourced" this task to another clinician for two reasons. First, I felt that I had already become so aligned with the Doyles that it would be difficult to find or defend the impartiality that such an evaluation required. Second, I no longer possessed the open-mindedness needed to work with the birth parents to improve their relationship with their son. I had accepted the case and worked for a year on assurances that they would not be an ongoing part of his life. Again, in retrospect, all of these choices seem questionable and possibly driven by the same unwillingness to know the real darkness of Ben's world.

A colleague met with the birth parents, Jason and Louise, and observed them with Ben. Her evaluation concluded that the visits were intensely distressing to Ben, and that his birth parents seemed frequently oblivious to his physical and emotional needs. The evaluator recommended that visits be discontinued. Furthermore, Ben's social worker was still recommending that parental rights be terminated, because of their chronic noncompliance with court-ordered requirements for counseling and drug treatment. She met frequently with the birth parents to counsel them toward the voluntary relinquishment of their parental rights that would free Ben for adoption immediately. However, the birth parents clung tenaciously to their claim on their little boy, and were therefore legally entitled to regular visits while the very slow process of moving toward termination of parental rights went on its cumbersome way for over a year after we began treatment. With benefit of hindsight, I know I should have included the birth parents somehow in my initial treatment plan.

The visits continued weekly. Each Tuesday Peggy Doyle drove Ben downtown to the vast, labyrinthine offices of CPS. There, if either birth parent had managed to come for the visit, the social worker would take Ben's hand and lead him away from Peggy and through the maze of tall desks (higher than Ben's head) to the elevator. They would take the elevator downstairs to the small, cluttered, windowless playroom where the visits took place. Jason and Louise would often bring Ben a small present, usually a toy car or truck. (Ben saved these gifts, and years later, they formed the core of his obsession with collecting things.) They were glad to see him, and embraced and kissed him demonstratively, but neither was able to be consistently attentive to him. Both mother and father alternated frantic, often intrusive attempts to engage Ben with prolonged periods of withdrawal or distraction. They often appeared stoned, and at times nodded off. At times, Louise was very sensitive and loving with him, while at other times she used the visit to pour out her troubles to the supervising social worker.

Ben never openly protested being taken away from Peggy for these visits. Instead he appeared to glaze over into a dissociated state. His face became expressionless, and his eyes looked empty and unfocused. He interacted with his birth parents in a way that was indistinguishable from the way he had interacted with me at our first meeting, with no verbal, gestural, or facial expression of how he felt or what he wanted. His affectless compliance and occasional behavioral disintegration during these visits became increasingly discrepant over time from his current behavior in his adoptive home. After the court-mandated hour had passed, the social worker, who had observed the whole visit (and from whose notes I gained my impressions of them), returned him, by the same route, to Peggy, who had been waiting for him upstairs. Peggy reported that for a day or two after the visits, Ben would be unusually irritable and clingy. He would become intensely angry and have tantrums over things that seemed insignificant at other times. I asked them to consider that, at Ben's age, to the extent that he had allowed himself to depend upon and become attached to his foster parents, he inevitably believed that they had godlike powers. Given the cognitive limitations of a 2- or 3-year-old, he was caught between the deeply dismaying options that (a) his attachment figures wanted him to have these disturbing visits that rekindled his earlier traumatic attachment to his birth parents or that (b) no one was in control at all.

The attachment system is so powerfully prewired in children that they will almost invariably opt for the first option, no matter how traumatizing the experiences they attribute to the attachment figure, rather than expose themselves to the unthinkable anxiety of being without any attachment figure at all to function as a secure base. It is a challenge to try to imagine the subjective experience of 2- and 3-year-old Ben during these visits. On the basis of the recurrent themes of devouring and being devoured that characterized his play for all the time I knew him, I conjecture that Ben experienced these visit episodes as a kind of "being swallowed up by something dangerous." The preverbal child forms schemata about what is going on between himself and the outside world using symbols or templates from what he truly knows, most importantly, his own bodily experience. Swallowing and, later, biting and chewing, are prominent, familiar parts of what young children experience, as are hunger and gastrointestinal distress. Ben, we know, was diagnosed as "failure to thrive" at 5 months, and spent his first 18 months with caregivers too stoned or otherwise preoccupied to protect him from intense experiences of hunger and fear. Is it too fanciful to imagine that such a little boy being led away from the only safety he knows, past rows of tall desks and down an elevator, might experience these as the teeth and throat of a monster? Human beings are "apex predators" like wolves that depend on social bonds and social organizations to inhibit predation within the family group. No such inhibition was present in Ben's first home, and it is no more than luck that he survived physically. Mentally, he had been and still was devoured over and over by terror too intense for him to metabolize or mentalize.

Ben's "play," as it developed during this period from the initial attack on Hokey Pokey, consisted exclusively of crude devourings of himself and others by anything at hand. There was little variation and no relief or resolution in his scripts, although he watched soberly when I attempted to provide this by grafting themes of rescue and comfort onto his dramas. I wish, in retrospect, that I had done less of this and shown a sturdier capacity to share his more disturbing play.

As he approached 3 years, the bouts of affectless, chaotic motor discharge that were characteristic of Ben when I met him were replaced by intensely affect-laden tantrums. These occurred principally when Peggy or Paul imposed a limit or initiated a separation. Tantrums were much more frequent and more intense after visits with his biological parents. Although these tantrums were less bizarre and more in line with normal toddler/preschooler behavior than the earlier affectless behavior, their intensity was truly remarkable.

One summer evening, shortly after Ben's third birthday, when Paul told Ben he had to stop playing with the garden hose and come in and get ready for bed, the little boy went into a particularly intense, raging tantrum. He picked up a tricycle larger than himself and hurled it with astonishing strength at his foster father. It hit Paul's shinbone. Hurt and badly shaken, Paul picked Ben up, none too gently, and put him in his crib, telling him in a loud angry voice that he must never do that again. As far as I am aware, this was the first time that Ben's behavior succeeded in evoking a feeling of rage in either of his adoptive parents. It was the first dreadful step toward what they later called "being turned into monsters" by their son.

Beginning that night and every night for 5 weeks thereafter, Ben had horrific night terrors. Without appearing to awake or be aware of his surroundings, he would scream in apparent terror for up to an hour. He would become drenched in sweat and shake violently. Paul and Peggy felt helpless to soothe him or even to make contact with him during these episodes. However, if one of them sat and stayed with him, gently touching him, he would eventually calm down and fall asleep. The Doyles were very frightened by how "difficult" their formerly tractable child had now become. They were troubled by the feelings that his rage and defiance stirred up in them. Paul and Peggy were able to hold on to my formulation that this was likely a phase in Ben's return to life and normal development as he became more "real" and less frozen.

Again, with hindsight, I know I was too eager to see this violence as a phase to be gotten through, for both Ben and his parents. I was still seeing Ben primarily as a helpless victim of his early traumas and potentially "curable" by love and sensitive care. I stressed comfort and reassurance. Now I wish I had had the courage and wisdom to plunge into that lion's den with them. A less reassuring approach might have given Ben the opportunity to enact this demonic anger in a contained setting before it had done its dreadful work of poisoning his relationship with his new parents. Looking back at my notes, I see that over and over again I chose to give a voice to the victims rather than to let Ben know that I understood that hungry monsters *have* to kill and eat to survive, and, more than this, that the killing is thrilling and enlivening.

During the period of these severe nightly terrors, I encouraged Ben, in our twice-weekly meetings at his home, to use his expanding vocabulary to order me to draw things on his chalkboard. At first he asked me to draw a moon over and over again. Each time he would erase or scribble over it. Each time he did so, I would say, "Bye bye moon! See you soon!" Next, Ben instructed me to draw "cow jumped over the moon," which he pronounced as one word. It took me some time to decipher this directive, and carrying it out certainly challenged my limited artistic abilities, but Ben seemed satisfied with the results. Producing his first sentences, Ben went on to ask me to draw "cow bite moon," and "cow hit moon," and "cow kick moon." This then expanded into "booboo moon" and "ouch moon." These utterances would be followed by Ben's erasing or scribbling over the pictures, and then an urgent demand to draw it again. In this game I understood that Ben was beginning to explore, cautiously, the relationships between his actions and feelings and the absence or presence of the objects of those actions and feelings. After what seemed like an infinity of repetitions of this drawing and erasing game, which apparently reassured him to some degree that it would be safe to act, Ben began to play in earnest. At this point, his mother and I decided to meet at my office. In choosing to shift to office-based play therapy, I was (consciously) thinking about providing Ben with a more contained space and carefully selected play materials to help him elaborate his affective themes in symbolic play. His mother participated in almost all of his office sessions for the next year.

For many months following, Ben's play during therapy sessions consisted of increasingly elaborate and emotionally charged dramas in which a hollow rubber shark swallowed all the small toy people and animals that its insides could hold, most importantly, a little rubber baby he named "Baby Ben." As Peggy and I both commented sympathetically about how hungry the shark was, and how scared Baby Ben was, we wondered aloud how things could be managed so that the shark could have a full tummy and Baby Ben could be safe too. It is important to note that we tried to be as concerned about the hungry shark as about the frightened baby. Just as Freud suggested that the therapist of adults must be careful not to take sides between id, ego, and superego, I knew that the child's therapist must be sure not to take sides between good guys or bad guys in the child's play—both of which are part of the child's inner representation of him- or herself. A too urgent therapeutic need to rescue the good guys will be understood by the child as an unwilling-ness to address or know about the darker, more troubling aspects of the child's identity. Despite my good intentions, however, I nonetheless made the mis-take of focusing more on the shark's very sympathetic hunger than on its less sympathetic bloodlust.

After several weeks of using the shark to terrorize his small alter ego, Ben introduced a new character, a soft white unicorn puppet. Unicorn's job was to hold Baby Ben very tight and to prevent the shark from getting him. Ben was clear that only Peggy was allowed to have the unicorn puppet. He snatched it angrily away if I tried to use it. I moved into the role of commen-tator and spectator of the blossoming collaboration of Ben and his mother. Together they created an ongoing drama in which the dangers and fears faced by Baby Ben and his growing circle of small friends were resolved by the resolute action of trustworthy and loving protectors. At this point we all felt encouraged. Indeed, it seemed that a significant transformation had occurred in Ben's internal representation of himself and others, which increasingly now included the possibilities of communication, help, protection, and dependency.

While Peggy was the primary focus of this transformation, Ben seemed to be using her as a kind of armature, or supporting structure, for processing and integrating all of his life experiences, including those that predated their relationship. In this setting, where the current caregiver was not the actual caregiver of infancy, it was particularly clear that a child's construction of both his inner representational world (Sandler & Greenblatt, 1987) and his working model of relationships (Bowlby, 1969) is an active and cre-ative process rather than a more passive recording of objective reality. It was fascinating to watch as Ben grafted pieces of his therapist and pieces of his adoptive mother onto his "memory" of his birth mother. *She* (his birth mother) had given him the stuffed lion I gave him for his birthday, and she, he asserted, had liked peach pie, just like his adoptive mother. More disturbingly, this grafting process could go the other way. Ben insisted that he "remembered" being frighteningly neglected by his current caregivers, for instance, when "you wouldn't give me my bottle." Having formed an attachment to Peggy, it was simply beyond comprehension for him that there had been a time when she had not been there and had not known him. At times he would refer to "when you lost me" or "when you hit me." Thus the dark side of Ben's burgeoning attachment to his adoptive parents was his tendency to assimilate his representations of them with his representations of his early traumatic experiences of unthinkable fear, deprivation, and neglect.

At 4 years, Ben's expressive language was only 1 year delayed, and he was now passionately attached to and possessive of his adoptive parents. His play was operatic in its richness, complexity, and affective range. It was still dominated by themes of terrible monsters threatening small children and animals, but sprinkled liberally and imaginatively with themes of rescue, comfort, and humor. Ben's affect now was anything but flat and constricted; in contrast to his former numbness, he was intense and volatile. In many respects, at 4, he seemed socially and emotionally like a child in the rapprochement phase (Mahler, Pine, & Bergman, 1975), both intensely possessive and concerned with testing the limits of the tie to the parents. His birth parents had relinquished him (after failing to show up for months of visits), and he was also, finally, free for adoption, with the legal proceedings under way. His parents and I felt very optimistic about his progress. They enrolled him in a private preschool where he seemed to do well, although tuition strained their one-income family budget.

Shortly after Christmas, when Ben was 4½, the Doyles were suddenly offered the opportunity to adopt Ben's newborn biological sister, who had been taken into protective custody at birth. They were told they had to make a decision within a week, or the baby would be discharged from the hospital to another foster home. The Doyles knew it would be difficult for Ben to share them with a new baby, but they weighed this against what they imagined he would feel if he learned that they could have adopted his sister but had refused. When Ben appeared to respond enthusiastically to the idea of a sister, they agreed hurriedly to a second adoption.

A couple of things are far clearer to me in retrospect than they were at the time. First, I am struck that the Doyles simply did not talk to me about the possibility of this second adoption until it was a fait accompli. As I had by then been meeting with them twice weekly for 2 years, and because they had consulted with me in exhaustive detail about many decisions, such as choosing a preschool for Ben or leaving him with grandparents for a weekend, I wonder now if there was an unconscious agenda involved in this second adoption that could not be talked about, felt, or known. I can only conclude, by how long it took me to notice this and by how incurious I was about my growing and uncharacteristic exasperation with the Doyles as the consequences of their adopting baby Julie unfolded, that I too had a part in this unconscious agenda.

The kinds of infantile agonies a child such as Ben experiences, tiny, defenseless, and starving, as he witnesses violence of life-threatening proportions between his only possible sources of nurturance and protection (described by Main & Hesse, 1990, as "fear without solution") are literally unimaginable. They are unimaginable because the mental organization of such a child is characterized by what Winnicott (1989) called "unintegration." That is to say, to be a starving infant witnessing violence between the figures who represent your only possible hope of survival is to be reduced to a lump of intolerably dysphoric protoplasm. Such an infant's human capacities to observe, anticipate, regulate, signal, or remember are utterly overwhelmed.

I now believe that the Doyles and I were frightened from the beginning by the powerful rages and the dissociated states we saw in Ben. We all very much wanted to make it all better. Perhaps on some level we could not bear to know how bad it had been, how it had been seared into his nervous system, and could not bear to know that we could not kiss or comfort it away. Certainly none of us had the courage or the wisdom to go with Ben into that terror-filled world where he came from. The baby sister represented to the Doyles a chance to do it right in the first place. She would never feel what Ben had felt, and so we would not have to either.

After a brief honeymoon period, Ben responded with profound and primitive rage and jealousy to the spectacle of his anxiously beloved parents tenderly caring for infant Julie. It was clear that his jealousy, certainly an expectable reaction for any preschooler with a new sibling, was intensely exacerbated by his utter conviction that his adoptive parents (whose faces were worn by the parents in his internal world) were responsible for his own infantile experiences of abuse and neglect. Thus, Ben was twice traumatized, first by the terrible neglect and terror of his infancy, and second by the sudden, unheralded appearance of a rival—an infant who could express unconflicted, undefended needs for dependency and love, confidently expecting them to be met.

Ben had no cognitive options at this phase in his development other than to attribute his first trauma—his unthinkably deprived and traumatic infancy—to the Doyles. He simply did not have the cognitive capacity, and could not absorb the concept that Paul and Peggy had not known him, let alone cared for him, when he was an infant. He was caught between two dreadful alternatives: either they had starved and terrified him, or they had (retroactively) abandoned him. Of these two, the first was more tolerable; at least it was thinkable. Despite this belief, after 2 years of the tenderest, most careful wooing by the Doyles, Ben had dared to risk "forgiving the past" and allowing himself to love and need them.

The second trauma, the appearance of a sibling, who was given in full measure everything of which he had been deprived, could perhaps have been avoided only at a very real cost to both children. Unfortunately, Ben's response to the adoption of his sister mobilized the overwhelmingly bad internal self-representation and objects of his early life. His poorly modulated anger and jealousy were projected onto his parents, who now became betrayers and enemies in his eyes. When Peggy tried to pick him up and kiss him, he screamed, "Don't hit me!" and curled up into a ball. He frequently hit, bit, and kicked them. He deliberately broke Peggy's most treasured keepsakes, accidentally fell on the baby or dropped things on her, and taunted his parents with precocious cruelty. He constantly accused them of abusing him, especially in public places. This violent, destructive, and sadistic behavior was deeply confusing and disturbing to the Doyles. They began to doubt their

competence to parent Ben, and wondered if they had made a terrible mistake. They were hurt when their loving overtures were repeatedly treated as
attacks. Worst, Ben's provocative behavior, often most intense in response to
his parents most strenuous attempts to be especially loving and supportive,
began to evoke reactions of intense rage and equally intense guilt in them.
At times, they said, they felt they were actually becoming the horrifyingly
rageful and punitive parents of Ben's inner world. Their struggle to maintain
a loving and empathic tie to Ben in the face of his sadistic rejection, and the
troubling feelings of hatred and guilt that he evoked in them, was extremely
difficult, and not entirely successful. To make matters worse, the real time
pressure caused by having a second child made the logistics of bringing
Ben to sessions and participating in them herself much more challenging
for Peggy. This, combined with our collective blindness, had the unfortunate
result that Peggy was now rarely able to participate in Ben's therapy sessions
and the frequency of treatment was reduced to once a week. Although I
objected to these changes at the time, I didn't see, with anything like the
forcefulness that I see now, just how devastating and crippling these alter-
ations were to my ability to help Ben.

To the extent that I failed Ben, I believe it was due to my own incapacity to
accept the true depth of his agony. Ben shut me out, too, soon after the adoption of Julie. Instead of rushing into the office, exclaiming "Me-me! Me-me!"
(his nickname for me), he came in sullenly, with his eyes on the ground. He
reverted to increasingly grim, joyless, and sadistic enactments of the devouring of small, helpless, soft, baby animals by large, powerful, cruel, and ruthless
animals. The victims were not portrayed as needy or lovable, but as pathetic
and contemptible. The big, strong, and cruel animals had large teeth and a
cold pleasure in blood and guts. There was no escape, and Ben ignored me
when I asked about this possibility. There were few variations in the apparent
narrative. I was only permitted to participate if I conformed to the script.
This play had the quality of a blood ritual performed to appease implacably
angry and murderous gods. I was not up to the task of joining him in that
terrible dark place where he had gone. Ineffectually, I kept trying to offer

reassurance about the availability of help, both by offering myself as a benign and helpful partner and by trying to convey the same message in my attempts to join his play. My rescuers were promptly and gruesomely dismembered by monsters, while Ben kept his eyes away from mine and often turned his back.

In health, play involves a constant "trying on" of transient self-representations or identifications, like costumes. The child may pretend to be a cowboy, or an astronaut, a witch, a water sprinkler, or a rabbit. In health, this is playful, that is, manageably exciting, fun, unconstricted, and flexible. Roles are chosen and can be relinquished or exchanged at will. What about the child who, for internal, external, or a combination of reasons, cannot play playfully? In choosing to be a children's psychotherapist, I imagined that I would be spending my days happily exploring a wondrous world of the creative imagination with my young patients. On a conscious level, I was choosing a life of play, creativity, and poetry. In retrospect, it is all too clear that, on an unconscious level, I was also choosing a life spent immersed, often quite helplessly, in the crippling and constricting grief and terror of small children. I often learned that the possibility of play must be held and protected in the therapist's heart despite the fact that the child cannot play until her or his world has become a safe place to do so. A child without an organized attachment (Main & Hesse, 1990), without enough sense of "existing in another's mind" (Pawl, 1995) and of being "contained" by loving caregivers (Bick, 1968/2003), cannot play. The child therapist who does not have the courage and perseverance to go on working to help troubled and overburdened families to provide this will not be much help.

Christopher Bollas (1989) described this state well when he wrote of the child who has been sexually abused:

> This internal space (where we dream, imagine, talk to ourselves and think) for the incest victim is not experienced as a good container which can transform the experience of life into nurturing psychic material. (p. 175)

It is important to remember that this condition, of not feeling sufficiently anchored and contained to play, is always the result of an interaction between the child's constitutional resources and the caregiving environment. From the child's side, this may include delays or difficulties of sensory and cognitive processing.

Ben's compulsive pseudo-play, his repetitive enactments, serve to ward off disintegration and fragmentation in a fashion similar to the behaviors referred to as "autistic stereotypies" that include head banging and rocking. They provide a focus so that the child's brain, eyes, and thoughts can stay cohesive and functional. A healthier child regulates herself in the context of relationships, both actual and internalized. Having experienced reliability, consistency, and responsiveness in her human environment, she has been able to build these qualities into her representation of her self and to use her social partners to bolster them when they feel shaky.

The therapeutic role can easily become a venue for a field of dissociative responses on the part of the therapist who allows the observer to overpower the participant in the participant–observer role. Perhaps this is part of what happened to me with Ben. My continuing performance as the therapist became rigid and artificial as I ignored my inner reactions to feeling powerless to reach Ben. I was frightened and revolted by the cold violence of his scripts. Simply put, I kept acting "nice" and "helpful" when I felt neither.

My time with Ben did not have the happy ending we had all hoped for. His parents grew increasingly frustrated and desperate with his continuing and escalating anger and violence. My belated attempts to address their distress were met with little response. They balked at examining their own inner darkness, evoked by Ben, as a route to helping Ben. A psychiatric consultation led to a recommendation of both medication and social skills therapy.

Ben's therapy had been funded by CPS for 4 years. There was not enough funding for both social skills therapy and continuing work with me; nor could the Doyles see a way to take Ben to two appointments a week. I did not feel I could argue that I was being helpful to them—and they left. Social skills therapy did not help either, and a series of medications had little effect. When I last heard from them, Ben at age 9 was in a residential treatment center. His parents visited him regularly and still hoped to bring him home someday. His sister Julie was doing well.

In my work with Ben, it was both painful and humbling to experience my inability to establish myself in his inner world as a benign and helpful and caring person. I came to question whose need was being met when I found myself so focused on establishing a good internal object.

Even though Ben had a better-than-average adoptive home with two devoted parents, the parents' efforts to connect and repair the broken (or never forged) link between their little boy and the human world seemed to have limited impact. Belatedly—too late for helping Ben—I have learned to shift my focus with such children. In play therapy, I try to accept, contain, and join in uncritically both the horrifying themes and their compulsive enactments. I try to prepare parents for the turmoil these dark places will evoke in them. I also try to prepare parents early on that they too, like all humans, have a danger-ous and destructive side, which if unaddressed will cause great peril. I am now proactive in preparing adoptive and foster parents for the ghosts within them-selves that these traumatized little ones will evoke, and for the possibility that some wounds cannot be fully healed. It remains a struggle to understand these dark motifs and to provide a reliable container for them despite my counter-transferential need and wish to change them, as well as to escape them by focusing on "strengths."

## ACKNOWLEDGMENTS

I have been very blessed with wonderful teachers; here I want to especially honor and thank Alicia Lieberman, whose gifts, as supervisor and friend, for being a "containing presence" and whose fearless but kind curiosity have taught me so much about myself and about how to be a therapist.

## REFERENCES

Bick, E. (2003). The experience of the skin in early object relations. In J. Rafael-Leff (Ed.), *Parent-infant psychodynamics: Wild things, mirrors and ghosts* (pp. 74–82). London: Whurr Publishers. (Original work published 1968)

Bollas, C. (1989). The trauma of incest. In C. Bollas, *Forces of destiny* (pp. 171–180). London: Hill & Wang.

Bowlby, J. (1969). *Attachment and loss: Vol. 1. Attachment.* New York: Basic Books.

Fraiberg, S., Adelson, E., & Shapiro, V. (1975). Ghosts in the nursery: A psychoanalytic approach to impaired infant–mother relationships. *Journal of the American Academy of Child Psychiatry, 14,* 387–422.

Lieberman, A., Silverman, R., & Pawl, J. (2000). Infant-parent psychotherapy: Core concepts and current approaches. In C. H. Zeanah (Ed.), *Handbook of infant mental health* (2nd ed., pp. 472–484). New York: Guilford.

Lyons-Ruth, K., Bronfman, E., & Atwood, G. (1999). A relational diathesis model of hostile-helpless states of mind: Expressions in mother–infant interaction. In J. Solomon (Ed.), *Attachment disorganization* (pp. 33–70). New York: Guilford.

Lyons-Ruth, K., & Jacovitz, D. (1999). Attachment disorganization: Unresolved loss, relational violence, and lapses in behavioral and attention strategies. In J. Cassidy & P. Shaver (Eds.), *Handbook of attachment theory and research* (pp. 520–554). New York: Guilford.

Mahler, M., Pine, F., & Bergman, A. (1975). *The psychological birth of the human infant: Symbiosis and individuation.* New York: Basic Books.

Main, M., & Hesse, E. (1990). Parents' unresolved traumatic experiences are related to infant disorganized attachment status: Is frightened and/or frightening parental behavior the linking mechanism? In M. Greenberg, D. Cicchetti, & E. M. Cummings (Eds.), *Attachment in the preschool years: Theory, research, and intervention* (pp. 161–182). Chicago: University of Chicago Press.

Mayr, E. (1976). *Evolution and the diversity of life: Selected essays*. Cambridge, MA: Harvard University Press.

Mawson, C. (n.d.). *An introduction to the psychoanalytic play technique and a psychoanalytic view of early development*. Retrieved December 18, 2005, from www.psychematters.com/papers/mawson.htm

Meloy, J. R. (1988). *The psychopathic mind*. Northvale, NJ: Jason Aronson, Inc.

Meloy, J. R. (1992). *Violent attachments*. Northvale, NJ: Jason Aronson, Inc.

Pawl, J. (1995). The therapeutic relationship as human connectedness: Being held in another's mind. *Zero to Three, 15*(4), 1, 3–5.

Sandler, J., & Greenblatt, B. (1987). The representational world. In J. Sandler, *From safety to superego: Selected papers* (pp. 58–72). New York: Guilford.

Schore, A. N. (2001). Effects of a secure attachment relationship on right brain development, affect regulation, and infant mental health. *Infant Mental Health Journal, 22*(1–2), 7–66.

Siegel, D. (1999). *The developing mind: Towards a neurobiology of interpersonal experience*. New York: Guilford Press.

Stern, D. (1985). *The interpersonal world of the infant: A view from psycho-analysis and developmental psychology*. New York: Basic Books.

Winnicott, D. W. (1975). Anxiety associated with insecurity. In D. W. Winnicott, *Through paediatrics to psychoanalysis: Collected papers* (pp. 97–101). New York: Basic Books. (Original work published 1952)

Winnicott, D. W. (1989). Fear of breakdown. In C. Winnicott, R. Shepherd, & M. Davis (Eds.), *Psychoanalytic explorations: D. W. Winnicott* (pp. 87–95). Cambridge, MA: Harvard University Press.

# CHAPTER 5

## DISCUSSION OF MARIAN BIRCH'S CASE

*Richard Ruth*

In Hebrew, the language of my prayers and my dreams, Ben means son. It fits. This little boy has haunted me as if he were my own, and the story of his treatment—although I work in a markedly different way from my colleague—is also very much my own. I have known young children who open unsteadily and then go backward, seemingly spinning beyond reach; I have tried everything I knew to retie the fragile bond, and watched as a child I have grown to love turns away. How do we make sense of children like Ben, and how do we help them? What do we do when we cannot make sense of such children, or see a clear path toward making their lives better?

After my first readings of the intertwined stories of Ben and of Marian Birch's (chapter 4) work with him and his adoptive family, my initial impulse was to protest that there were elements missing. To make clear why ultimately I do not believe this is so, I need to go with you down some of the initial paths that tempted me.

### THE PATH NOT TAKEN

I first wondered about Ben's brain. Ben's birth circumstances were horrific. His early months were compoundingly horrific. Such circumstances take a toll on the body, as well as on the mind and the soul.

We did not know much about brains when I started out in the business of therapy with young children and their families. None of my teachers and supervisors treated brains as other than dissociated organs—and it annoyed and infuriated me to the extent that I sought training as a neuropsychologist. I do not know that this was a fair tack; maybe more self-imposed burden than path toward clinical effectiveness. However, it was the path I took, and it certainly has influenced my thinking.

Our field has learned a lot about brains in the years since Fraiberg's (1959; Fraiberg, Adelson, & Shapiro, 1975) seminal work, and certainly since Klein's (1984a, 1984b). We can take pictures of brains now, and, oversimplifying a bit, see what is whole and what is broken, measure what works and what does not. We no longer speak about a unitary phenomenon known as "organicity," and treat it as something over the edge of the world knowable to psychoanalytically informed therapists. Neurologists have somewhat better tools for regulating the activity of brains that are dysregulated, and neuropsychologists have tests, and ways of thinking about test results, that—when we are on our game—can help children and those involved with them get a clear picture of how the workings/misworkings of a child's brain, even a very young child's brain, are part of how the child experiences himself and his world. We can develop clear understandings of what a child does well and what a child cannot do, or does only painfully and with limitations. Such findings can help trace ways of teaching children to perform necessary functions that come hard to them, and of supporting children as they undertake the sometimes torturous work toward mastery. Like therapy, it is painstaking work that does not always work out.

However, these are thoughts on the edge still of the known clinical world. I know of few clinical teams, working with very young children and their families, that contain a neuropsychologist, at least, one who can communicate meaningfully and work in an integrated, collaborative way with an infant–parent therapist.

What was more confusing to me about the stories of Ben and of Birch's work with him was how it came to be that the simpler questions of an earlier age seemed not to come to the center of the thinking about Ben (or at least its recounting here). Was Ben retarded? We know about his gross motor functions—he could throw a tricycle effectively—but what about his fine motor abilities, often seriously hurt when a child is born substance-addicted and does not receive good care and adequate stimulation in the earliest months? What about the areas of his brain responsible for language development, damaged, as his limited emergence of language with the months of therapy ("only 1 year delayed") might suggest, or whole but traumatized, as other data suggested and as was the hope? Cognitive, fine-motor, and language limitations can frustrate a child terribly and make negotiation of an emotionally charged developmental turning point all the more difficult.

I am not questioning here the story line but its undermodeling. Ben was traumatized and—before the adoption of his sister—could hold clearly in his mind, expressing in rich and evocative therapeutic play, how he experienced his trauma and its wounds. What about the neurological and neuropsychological functions underpinning this experience and its mental representation? How intact and how damaged were the mechanisms for experiencing and processing experience?

My implication is not that had Ben turned out to be neuropsychologically compromised and mentally retarded, his therapy would have been in vain. Anything but, as lines of research, to which I have contributed, show (Blotzer & Ruth, 1995; De Groef & Heinemann, 1999; Sinason, 1992), neuropsychologically compromised and developmentally disabled persons are fully capable of forming therapeutic alliances, and the analytic therapies are as effective with persons with developmental disabilities as they are with other patient populations. When therapist and child metabolize together in the therapeutic relationship the fantasies, beliefs, habits, and interactive patterns that organize around an organic deficit, and when the therapist, where appropriate, makes interpretations about what appears to be happening, children can be freed from what Sinason (1986) has called "secondary mental handicap," and much potential for psychic growth can open up. The only precondition for this, to my thinking, is that the therapist be willing to hold in mind that a child may have neuropsychologically organized limitations, know something about these and how they work (or obtain consultation from someone with this kind of grounding), and be willing to accept that, after a good therapy, a limited child may still be limited. This is not always easy for therapists, whose main work experience may be with people without central cognitive limitations or neuropsychological compromise; but it is an achievable starting place.

So, I wonder how neuropsychological thinking might have differently conceptualized what was at play in the work with Ben and his family, yet acknowledge that it may not have changed, fundamentally, the viability of the work. Another question, however, arises from the wondering: If it was not possible to know whether Ben was, or would turn out, retarded, what would have been the place in the treatment for such a question? What might have been different if such a question had been held in mind in a different kind of way? Might it have tempered the excessive optimism Birch rues had she pondered more systematically the questions included under the rubric of "organicity"?

## THE BOTTOM LINE

Traditional analytic therapies rely on the concept of neutrality, an often parodied and misunderstood concept. It does not refer to a cold, uncaring therapist, but to one who, in Anna Freud's formulation (Freud, 1967, 1971), takes a position neutral among the competing forces of id (impulses, desires), ego (rationality, self-control), and superego (morals, values), and, in Karen Horney's (1999) more socioculturally oriented formulation, a position neutral among conflicting desires to move toward, against, and away from people, feelings, and goals. In either case, the notion is about observational vantage point, the place from which the therapist thinks about the patient. Implied in this is one of the more radical notions in analytic thinking—that it is the patient, not the therapist, who makes the choices. The therapist's job is not to remove a symptom or steer the patient away from a dangerous life choice, but to help the patient, as much as the patient can and is willing, to think clearly about the choices they make and the consequences of those choices.

This way of thinking does not fit well when the patient is very young—just how much in search of meaning, and responsible for her choices, can an infant or a toddler be? How can the therapist be neutral when the issues are not of neurotic conflict but of life (or at least livable life) or death or something close to it, as is so often the case in infant–parent work with deeply troubled very young children and their families?

Complicating things further: In an earlier, more hierarchical, and less democratically minded age, therapists' expertise and authority were more likely to be assumed than to be questioned, and ethical requirements for informed consent near the outset of treatment were not part of our professions' values. Much as I welcome the move away from a more authoritarian stance in psychotherapy, it is difficult to live up to current expectations. It is easy to obtain informed consent for manualized cognitive–behavioral therapies that eschew looking at the shadow side of life, or therapies whose intent is to teach skills or reinforce strengths; it is much more difficult to obtain good-enough informed consent for therapies that, almost by their nature, cannot be easily described and whose course and consequences cannot be predicted at the outset, except for the certainty that, when successful, what is most dreaded will be revealed.

Perhaps a way of approaching this is to tell families, at the beginning of infant–parent therapy, that there are things that cannot be described or known, things that can only be felt toward, experienced, and discovered. The main reassurance is that therapist and family will negotiate such territory together, in relationship. Perhaps some families cannot tolerate such uncertainty; and perhaps they are among those we are least likely to be in a position to help. Implicit in this thought is that our help has a center of gravity that involves making sense of things and can lose its grounding when we feel its focus has to be on making behavior changes.

It is in this context that I was troubled by Birch's early decision that Ben needed to be induced, first, out of his isolation, then his terrors, and then his rage. From one vantage point, her intentions were unimpeachable—to help him accept the love that seemed amply available to him, from devoted

parents and committed therapist; to move from lonely and painful disconnection to the social connections that can foster development; to become
able to play; to calm the terrors that kept him up at night; and then to soothe
his destructive rage and deadly, unmanageable projections. How could anyone disagree?

However, the cost, as Birch herself came to wonder about in hindsight, was
that there was a part of Ben's affective and experiential world that seemed to
be excluded from the space of the therapy. Her work had been aimed at trying to model for Ben alternatives to his unbearable perceptions and to his
symptoms. This left a part of his experience, and even perhaps his identity,
cut off. It constrained the space available for work with Ben in the transference relationship, where perhaps some of his feelings could have come into
clearer focus, have been better contained, and then better understood. The
period of play among Baby Ben, the shark, and the unicorn (interestingly, to
me, the point in the therapy in which the therapist seemed most grounded in
the value of neutrality, and the point in which the transference relationship
seemed most alive), just before the arrival of the adoptive sister, seemed
almost achingly hopeful. Yet there too, there seemed to be a tendency for
therapist and mother to positively connote this line of hopeful play and fantasy, and negatively connote the projections that began to ensue. This
seemed to me a subtle shift away from neutrality; the danger, in good therapies, is always one of subtle shifts. It may have foreclosed the space for the
associated murderous accusations and negative affects to enter the therapy,
where perhaps ultimately they could have been interpreted—that is, put into
words, and thus softened.

Kleinians are accused of making interpretations beyond what children can
make sense of and that are thus either counterproductive or of limited transformative value. In analytic circles, the image of the nice Selma Fraiberg
being helpful in the kitchen is counterposed to the mean, remote Melanie
Klein, making odd interpretations of unconscious content to incredulous
children while their mothers wait outside the consulting room befuddled
about and excluded from what is going on inside.

I like to think I am a nice Kleinian, able and willing to talk to children in their idiom and keep parents in the loop. However, my main ways of working with young children are in meeting several times a week for individual therapy, or meeting less frequently for family therapy, and my main tool is interpretation. So I began to fantasize about what I might have said to Ben while he was making violent accusations toward his parents—false and defamatory based on lived history but accurate in terms of the organizing unconscious beliefs in his mind.

Here, however, my thinking reached another dead end. I have made plenty of interpretations that have not worked. I have also made interpretations that seemed right in the abstract, but that did not help a deeply hurt young child behave differently with steady enough momentum and a steep enough recovery curve for even very good parents to be able to tolerate. Birch's work with Ben was as creative and enduring as anyone could ever hope. A different way of thinking and a different approach to therapy could not have guaranteed any different results, which is the only relevant bottom line.

## THE COMPLEXITY OF SOCIAL CONTEXT

I am rereading my last sentence and thinking, consistent with my training as a family therapist, that life does not consist of lines but of complex interactive systems in context. So, what was the context of Birch's work with Ben? Her write-up does not tell us much about this, perhaps because, as therapists, we are used to thinking of our work as autonomous, taking place in closed, private space rather than in open, social systems.

Let me try to make my point by asking some questions: How much was my colleague paid for her work? Was her reimbursement sufficient to allow her to buy, in our often market-shaped professions, the advanced training, consultation, and time off for processing and reflection that she needed? As I write in my own case report (chapter 6), my reimbursement and practice setting/structure do not allow this, and I try to imagine that I can somehow make do, an assumption I now have to question. How was Birch's work life structured at this time? How did it make space, or not, for flexible, open time to respond to the family's changing needs? Did this affect what the family felt open to ask her for, or not ask her for, or what she felt able to offer? What was the impact on the treatment that it was paid for by social services? Also, we have limited insight about how the Doyles' or Ben's ethnic and cultural backgrounds or their socioeconomic status affected what happened.

There are questions of another order: What social supports were available for this adoptive family through extended family involvement, informal networks in the community, and formal service provision (e.g., pediatricians, special educators, connections with other adoptive families with young children with trauma backgrounds)? What child care options were available—a mothers' helper? Respite? A playgroup? Also, what was the local community's attitude toward children? Without opening the whole Pandora's box of our society's attitude toward children and how it affects parent–infant therapy, can we at least acknowledge that such a box exists and wonder about what opening it might reveal?

To be transparent, my feeling is simultaneously that posing such questions strains the boundaries of what is permissible discourse, beyond what is fair—all case histories have to leave out much in order to be manageable—and that these kinds of questions lie at the heart of what we have to think about together. Yet, even if pondering these questions should prove unhelpful in understanding the work with Ben, they nonetheless may help us think in a more inclusive way about our work with other families. I will advance a provocative hypothesis: Infant–parent psychotherapy grew out of developments within psychoanalysis that opened up new possibilities, but was embraced by systems with little interest in the possibilities of radical, psychoanalytic change because, as a modality, it is convenient for political purposes. If we offer therapy, but not housing, money, community, or social support, to families with little kids with big problems, we can make believe we are doing good. Yet we may be, instead, setting up both families and their therapists. I will leave this hypothesis hanging for sociologists and anthropologists to prove or disprove; but I want it to hang, and be present, and I want to listen to my thoughts, as well as the readers' thoughts, as a troubling but present fantasy consultant.

## THE THERAPEUTIC TASK

Every therapy has at least two centers of gravity: the patient's and the thera-pist's. Our psychoanalytic ancestors used to focus mostly on the patient, feeling that the insistence that therapists be well analyzed and avoid countertrans-ferences was sufficient to keep us on track. Current thinking, acknowledging relationality and intersubjectivity, sees this as a fundamental error, and yet does not go far enough, to my thinking, in opening space that helps us look at what goes on in the minds of therapists working at our craft.

When I reread Birch's chapter—and it is compelling work, that I find myself reading over and over and over in an attempt to grasp its richness and complexity—from a literary perspective, I am struck that she seems to be writ-ing, as in much good contemporary clinical writing, from a vantage point on the margin of where she, Ben, and the family meet. She steps at moments into Ben's experience and into her own, and writes evocative "postcards" at such moments. However, a fuller immersion into her own, internal experience of her work with Ben and his family seems to lie beyond the border of the pages. So, I will take that as an indirect invitation to explore.

I suspect—because I hear it in the story and because it resonates with my own experience of infant–family work—that my colleague felt pulled by the strong, competing tides of hating Ben's dark side and passionately wanting to help him and his family.

Cognitive science tells us that our apparatus for thinking is engineered to operate on the basis of preexisting assumptions. We assume that chairs are chairs, and do not fly, and we cannot organize and process our experience otherwise. When something comes along to challenge this kind of ground-ing, fundamental assumption, there is a unique kind of disorganization that is painful beyond painful to experience.

We cannot operate as caring professionals other than on the assumption that children have parents, protection, provision, love, and at least a grounding modicum of safety; therapy, in a sense, structures itself on the assumptions that something in the essential context of life has gone wrong and needs to and can be repaired. The clinical experience of work with severely trauma-tized and brutally neglected/abused children, however, involves a confronta-tion with realities that such children can be thrust into this world without any of this—that there is no context, for such children, against which to react and work at repair. When we do our work, we come to know this impos-sible reality not from the outside but from the inside. The child re-creates it in our presence, projects it into us, and depends on us to experience it. We have no good choices. In a way more like shamans than like surgeons, we have to either experience the horror and try to survive (first) and then make sense or reject what the child needs us to come to know. Either way, we find ourselves in a life or death struggle with hate, the deepest and most primi-tive kind of hate, the hate of life, or the possibility of life for death. To be very specific, I think my colleague had to face, and try to overcome, not just hatred for what Ben was doing, but hatred for who he was.

If this reading is accurate, then the problem with trying to be helpful comes into clearer focus. The usual way, and seemingly the only sane way, to con-front death and hate is by negation, replacing death and hate with life and love or at least care. However, this could not have worked with Ben. If he had no preexisting framework for knowing what life was—wholehearted, passionate, and secure life as opposed to a perilous existence in permissible and tolerable small doses—no framework for knowing what real love was—as opposed to moments of interest and attunement—then confronting a fully alive, loving therapist or parent would have been an encounter with the unknown. It would be responded to as something inherently challenging and terrifying. Worse still, he would be encountering it at a developmental point when he lacked still the capacities and mechanisms for making sense of the deeply unknown. So trying to save Ben from his dark horrors may have come to have an as-if quality, a kind of *ur* countertransference as negation. What I am trying to talk about—and it is a complicated thing, so despite my efforts I'm not surprised if the words feel abstruse—is that when Birch kept trying to save Ben from his dark thoughts, overwhelming feelings, unbearable fears, and identification with the most evil and destructive of his persecutory fantasies—when she tried to "show him the light" (i.e., that life can be better and have a light side), her efforts seem to have had unintended effects. These unintended effects include negating that he was feeling what he was feeling, as well as acting as if life was different from how it had been and was for him.

I am counterposing the alternative possibility of being *with him* as he experienced the very basic, primal, primitive conflicts he was feeling, and working toward interpreting his conflicts. This would be in lieu of presenting him a way out that may have felt to him as if it were not fully real/realistic. This way out may also have been felt to negate or judge him as he experienced this part of what he experienced.

I am positing that Birch may have been in a very intense and (in the Kleinian sense) primitive countertransference that pushed her to negate rather than feel in a neutral vantage point toward his experience. Reaching primitivity, in some Kleinian circles, is the highest compliment. Although then you have to find your way out of it, which is never easy.

The best solution to such a conundrum I can suggest is to return to what the child is experiencing. We must do this as often as we have to and with as much clarity and support as we can muster, being in this kind of moment with severely traumatized and severely neglected children, immersed in the experiences of the child and the family, and our own experience, until we can formulate empathically in our minds—and I am speaking here about empathy with the darkest of horrors. We must do this until the child feels that we get it, and until he is willing to try to craft with us a fantasy of the first steps of emergence. Then we help to re-create it in play and then in words, in tolerable, small doses.

What I am suggesting here goes against classic psychoanalytic wisdom, which advocates interpretation of what is rather than creation of what is not yet in the children with whom we work. Perhaps Fraiberg and Klein had a sense of this when they undertook their groundbreaking work, or at least had a glimpse before turning in other directions, more classically supportive and educational, in Fraiberg's case, and more classically interpretive, in Klein's.

However, we live in different places and in different times. When we work with infants, even more than with older children or adults, we must take care not to make the mistake Winnicott (1958) described of "assuming that the patient exists as a person."

I do not know of any theoretical writing that lays out how to do the kind of work I am describing or at least imagining. However, I know that there are brave, committed, and wise clinicians, like Birch and the others writing here, who are trying to find their way. I ask that we make space for ourselves and for each other, which implies a willingness to fail over and over and over again, and to tolerate failing, and thus learn.

## REFERENCES

Blotzer, M. A., & Ruth, R. (1995). *Sometimes you just want to feel like a human being: Case studies in empowering psychotherapy with people with disabilities*. Baltimore: Brookes.

De Groef, J., & Heinemann, E. (Eds.). (1999). *Psychoanalysis and mental handicap*. New York: Free Association Books.

Fraiberg, S. (1959). *The magic years: Understanding and handling the problems of early childhood*. New York: Charles Scribner's Sons.

Fraiberg, S., Adelson, E., & Shapiro, V. (1975). Ghosts in the nursery: A psychoanalytic approach to the problems of impaired infant-mother relationships. *Journal of the American Academy of Child Psychiatry, 14*, 387–421.

Freud, A. (1967). *The ego and the mechanisms of defense*. New York: International Universities Press.

Freud, A. (1971). *The writings of Anna Freud* (Vol. 7). New York: International Universities Press.

Horney, K. (1999). On *the therapeutic process: Essays and lectures*. B. J. Paris (Ed.). New Haven: Yale University Press.

Klein, M. (1984a). *Envy and gratitude and other works, 1946–1963.*
New York: Free Press.

Klein, M. (1984b). *The writings of Melanie Klein.* New York: Free Press.

Sinason, V. (1986). Secondary mental handicap and its relationship to trauma. *Psychoanalytical Psychotherapy, 2,* 131–154.

Sinason, V. (1992). *Mental handicap and the human condition.* London: Free Association Books.

Winnicott, D. W. (1958). *Collected papers: Through paediatrics to psycho-analysis.* New York: Basic.

CHAPTER 6

# IN THE HEART OF DARKNESS:
# LEARNING AND RUNNING OUT OF TIME

*Richard Ruth*

A colleague—a European psychoanalyst whose thinking and work are watched by different ghosts from those who observe our work on U.S. soil—once likened mental retardation to Africa. He meant that both mental retardation and Africa too easily go unknown, and are too easily disparaged by professionals who should know better. I like his metaphor precisely because it is so uncomfortable in a U.S. context. It gets me thinking about the divides I live among. I stepped into one such divide when I became the therapist of the Jones/Muhammad family (not their real names, but names with resonances that ring true), and, in another way, when I undertook the task of thinking through why my work with them failed.

Sometimes I begin figuring out what I am thinking by finding out what music I am listening to. In trying to think about my experience with the Jones/Muhammad family, I have been listening to the blues—a genre rising from the African American experience of trying to find meaning by somehow making pattern or sense out of the complexities, impossibilities, absurdities, and horrors of life in a world in which the odds are impossibly stacked against them.

Many blues songs talk about what happens at the crossroads—places, metaphorical and real, in which major lines of development reach choice points, and subsequent events can play out one way or a very different way. My work with the Jones/Muhammad family took place at several simultaneous crossroads. I am White; the Jones/Muhammad family is Black. I work in private practice; the referral to see this family came from the child welfare system. I do psychoanalytically informed work with families; at least four members of the Jones/Muhammad family have mental retardation, a condition some believe cannot be helped by the approach to treatment I believe in and practice.

Singing and hearing the blues can be at least a partial antidote to having the blues. So here is my song and my story, and here is the only reasonable starting point. Every single encounter in the United States between a White man and Black people is alive with potential to be intensely complicated, and charged, in ways that are difficult to capture and impossible to evade—clinical encounters especially so. Whether the White participant is thoughtless or thoughtful, unaware or conscious, a lifelong battler against racism or someone proud of their prejudices, the ghosts of the victims and the perpetrators of the Middle Passage, slavery, and segregation are right there with us. If we are therapists, then these ghosts supervise our work—silently, like wise old supervisors who hold us to the task of thinking through.

Do White/Black differences between therapist and patient matter? If so, how do they play out? If, as some have written (Williams, 1991), sometimes such differences color the content and process of therapy, and in other cases seem to matter little, how can such a paradox be understood?

What happens when a young child, or a parent, or both have a developmental disability and present for therapy? Do we reject the case as untreatable, treat the disability as if it does not matter somehow (and consider the parallel "color blind" assertion—that White people and Black people are completely the same), or do we change what we do somehow? If nothing else, I have learned something about the salience of these questions—and something about what I do not know about them—from my work with the Jones/Muhammad family. At first, the case felt tantalizing, both theoretically and clinically; culture and disability seemed to show something of themselves more clearly in juxtaposition. Then, time ran out, and things fell apart.

Except, with the invitation to write about the case, the desires to think and to learn were salvaged.

## THE FAMILY

The Jones/Muhammad family was referred to me by a family court. Ms. Jones, in her early 50s—my age—was raising her adult daughter, Ms. Muhammad—something she would have done naturally and willingly but now was doing by court order. Ms. Muhammad had five children, ages 2 through 8 at the time of referral. Ms. Jones came to Washington, DC, from farther south. The children have, between them, three different fathers: all are absent, some are unknown.

At the time of referral, Ms. Muhammad's children were living in three different foster homes. The four older children had been placed in foster care, because of allegations of maternal neglect, almost 2 years earlier while Ms. Muhammad was pregnant with the youngest. The youngest was placed in foster care at birth on the grounds that Ms. Muhammad's living situation and economic resources at the time were inadequate for her to be able to raise children.

Ms. Jones has borderline average cognitive ability. Ms. Muhammad has moderate to mild mental retardation. Of the five children, the youngest two are moderately retarded, the oldest is mildly retarded, and the other two have tested with borderline retardation, but the testing reports on these two are so internally contradictory and so poorly written that it is difficult to know much about their cognitive abilities. In the 2-plus years I worked with this family, requests for retesting never received a response.

Because history matters, White/Black therapeutic couplings cannot meet, in the United States, as Bion (1965, 1970) wisely advised, without memory or desire. However, I tried by asking to see them before reading the court papers. Here are some first and enduring, impressions:

Ms. Jones is an overweight, middle-aged lady. Her way of dressing—cardigan and dress, neat but shabby, hair carelessly done—seemed to ask that I think of her, with sympathy, as poor and Black. Her manner of speaking reflects a

Deep South accent of an earlier generation; her usage, tone, and style of communicating struck me as simultaneously friendly, verging on subservient, and intended, in some part, to shield from me what she was really thinking. Conflicting notes seemed to establish themselves in our first encounter—we liked each other, and silently acknowledged to each other that there was much that was going unspoken—and sustained themselves throughout our contacts.

Ms. Muhammad marked herself as a woman of a different generation from her mother. She wore jeans and T-shirts. Her accent was more local and more modern. In the limitations of her vocabulary, her passivity, and her naïvete, she seemed observably retarded. Her eyes did not move in tandem. She was more overweight than her mother. In contrast to Ms. Jones, whose reading of a clinical situation seemed sharp, Ms. Muhammad seemed lost in my presence. She reacted to my soft voice and seemed to perceive me as nonthreatening, but had little sense of why we were meeting.

The oldest child, whom I will call Jacques here, was the only one of the children with a first name of European linguistic origin. He was slim and communicated passivity and oddness. He said little, but what little he said almost always had a remote quality, as if he were being reluctantly summoned back from the world of his own in which he lived. He was mannerly, difficult to engage, but not disruptive.

The other children had names of Arabic linguistic origin. (I wondered if the fathers were Muslim, or if Ms. Jones or Ms. Muhammad was Muslim. I hoped, by the open-hearted asking, that I was communicating this would not be a problem, but I never got a clear answer.) Next came 7-year-old twins, whom I will call Akil and Khadijah. They are attractive and have a vigorousness about them that the other members of the family lack. Their expensive, fashionable clothing communicated (accurately) that they had foster parents who spent money on them and who were more affluent than Ms. Jones and Ms. Muhammad. This seemed not just an objective, socioeconomic reality, but one that the foster parents were aware of and wished to underscore. They seemed to know they were dressing the children in a way different from the style of dress of the other members of the Jones/Muhammad family, who could not afford such upscale clothing and likely would not have chosen such clothing even if the money had not been an issue. Another way to say this would be that, both objectively and by subjective choice of their foster parents, Akil and Khadijah were living in one world and the rest of the family was living in another world—one that was socioeconomically less advantaged and culturally different. This was reflected in the children's manner of dress, among other ways.

Akil seemed to tune me out, but in a friendly manner, without animus. He seemed intent on giving an impression that he was happy and "normal." Khadijah seemed to want to be admired and to be the center of attention. Had she pushed her intent more, she would have come across as intrusive and flirtatious, but she held back and stayed safely within the bounds of politeness.

Mahmoud, almost 5, seemed even younger than his age. Like Jacques, he was slightly built. His skin did not look healthy. His movements were tentative, and his words were very few. He seemed not to know what to do in an office full of play materials. He seemed a bit frightened but reassured by his grandmother's nonverbal communication that the situation was safe.

Abdul was 2. I like 2-year-olds, but I found it painful to be with him. He seemed to have difficulty with the most basic aspects of motor functions and relatedness. I wondered whether he had fetal alcohol syndrome. (I still do.) He seemed ambivalent about the comfort of a standing posture. He said nothing, although I was assured he could speak. He did little, rarely straying from physical connection to his grandmother or, less often, his mother.

From the referral phone call, I knew that the Jones/Muhammad family had come into the child welfare system when Jacques was found running around outside Ms. Muhammad's home. Neighbors called social services; the investigating social worker found that Ms. Muhammad had run out of food. The theme of "running out" (in both senses: exhausted resources and escape) was a psychic as well as a practical theme that ran through the case.

Ms. Jones and Ms. Muhammad had regular visitation with the children. Some visits took place at the agency and some at the home they shared, mostly unsupervised at the time of referral. The social worker involved felt uneasy about what was going on, and thus made the referral. I was chosen because I am a known quantity to workers in the child welfare system and because I have a reputation for connecting well with African Americans. I am Latino.

I wrote the first draft of this chapter over the course of a summer. A good summer, actually. In the fall, I began a new job, as a professor of psychology, and I got married. However, in writing and rewriting, reading and re-reading the previous paragraphs—a process that took most of the fall and into the winter—I had a consistently queasy feeling. The paragraphs, and the Jones/Muhammad family, took up too much space and too little. I spent the summer living with the notion that life could be good. My initial encounter with the Jones/Muhammad family, several years ago now, seemed eerily to predict this happy summer feeling. They met me with a sense—communicated by Ms. Jones, primarily, but reflected in the others—that life could be good, and they wanted life to be good for them. They also communicated a sense that life was not good, and might never be good for them. There was no escaping that. No running out.

## THE INITIAL PHASE OF THERAPY

Stories about therapy are not therapy; sometimes the dissociations necessary to the written rendering do not matter. However, important truths in the story of my work with the Jones/Muhammad family would be derailed by such "innocent" dissociations of seemingly minor moments. This risk is even greater in the context of this book, in which *what* got derailed and *how* is the organizing theme. So, if the pace and tone of what follows seem painful, it reflects that there was much that was painful in this work, which is what I am trying to capture and think about here.

The court papers initially provided me added little to what the social worker told me in our first few phone calls. The papers described accusations of inadequate food and inadequate maternal supervision, but the wording was odd. Either horrible stories were being sanitized or these were accounts of poor Black people from the city who somehow found themselves in a White, middle-class suburban neighborhood where they made others uncomfortable. I found myself trying to hold both possibilities in mind, and to think clearly about how they fit together or clashed.

The initial 10 sessions were painstakingly arranged by the child welfare system, which financed the travel of Ms. Jones and Ms. Muhammad to my office, and that ensured that Jacques, Akil, Khadijah, Mahmoud, and Abdul were brought to sessions, more or less on time, from their three foster homes. This kind of orchestration, seemingly so basic to any therapeutic endeavor, is almost never brought off in the child welfare system. It was difficult not to feel celebratory and hopeful about this "success" while difficult not to feel wary: Was the system mobilizing to help us succeed or to prove that, even with this extraordinary effort, we would fail? I felt guilty for thinking such thoughts, and naïve when, in moments, I tried not to think them. Besides, showing up is the precondition for therapeutic work, not the work itself. On the other hand, showing up is the opposite of running out. So maybe something was going on here. What though?

The initial hours were full and active. I found it easy, almost, to be with the family. While there were difficult dynamics, they felt knowable and manageable. Ms. Jones was polite and agreeable to a point of excess. However, there was a bit of uneasiness with the easy feeling, and, as a therapist, I felt primed to tune in to it. Not only did Ms. Jones's manner contrast with the remoteness and limited engagement of the other members of the family; it made me feel like the "good White man" who is no better than the bad. However, on the hopeful side, there were also points at which her defendedness would yield to moments of genuine connection.

As in most things, the others followed her lead. Ms. Muhammad seemed incrementally more and more comfortable in my presence, and trusting, although with something edging into possibilities of uncomfortable passivity and emptiness.

The children and I got on. Jacques, Mahmoud, and Abdul played too quietly, with too much limitation in their imagination and self-assertion; Akil and Khadijah would intrude on moments of adult conversation and demand attention, but in small, gentle ways, nothing that was difficult to handle. Like their grandmother, the children would "take vacations" from their distancing and show me important things about themselves. Akil showed me how he was learning to throw a football, and carefully refrained from throwing it in the office. Mahmoud drew me a picture, explaining it was of a boy reading. Abdul made more eye contact, and shared tentative smiles. These are the kinds of things that matter in therapy and, though it is less easily or widely recognized, in life outside therapy as well.

To make some implicit assumptions explicit, I made decisions early in my encounter with this family to see them as a family and primarily in the office. I live in an area where there is only a fiction of a public mental health system; there is no longer a system of established, adequately resourced clinics able to provide thoughtful, flexible mixes of family and individual therapies to people who are not affluent, and where experienced supervisors can support younger therapists as they learn the craft necessary for work with complex issues, including how to meet Black families fairly and effectively. There was, at the time, one well-regarded agency in the area that worked with families with infants and young children, but the referring social worker had had negative experiences with their sensitivity to Black families. So these were external constraints.

Another external constraint was that I was requested not to involve the foster parents in the therapy. The agency's policy did not promote this, and the referring social worker said the foster parents were unwilling.

In hindsight, I wonder why I accepted the social worker's word without investigating on my own, and why I accepted the agency policy, and the related parameter on the treatment, without protest or at least more vigorous questioning. I think my motives were mixed. I wanted to be this biological family's therapist, and implicit to this seemed to be a willingness to hold in mind, to believe—as Ms. Jones and Ms. Muhammad did and maybe the children too—and to act as if the Jones/Muhammad family could be and become more of a family. I also wanted to be a therapist the agency would accept with some degree of comfort, in part because I saw the family being held in the agency's good graces as essential to the goal of the family being able to be a family. The agency had the power and choice to allow the family's effort to be together to continue or to cease. If being seen as a "good" therapist meant accepting the parameter of not seeing the foster parents, I felt there was something valuable, potentially, to be gained.

There was also another dimension. Even publicly funded and court-ordered therapy does not, ultimately, stop being space (or at least potential space) for private, internal psychological work. Unless the treatment is arbitrarily limited to psychoeducation or behavior change—a limitation I would not have accepted—I go in with the assumption, to be proved or disproved in initial sessions, that a family can do and benefit from such internal work. My initial experiences with the Jones/Muhammad family seemed to confirm this assumption. So we chose to proceed, using a way of working I was trained in, know, and believe in. We worked in a circumstance at some tension from my comfort zone, but it was not stretched beyond a point I felt I could bear. I felt close enough to my training and my clinical instincts to feel some sureness to what I was doing. So I did not incorporate into the frame of the therapy an open question about whether the family in my office was *a* family, or *the* family, that should be seen.

Again in hindsight, this framing of the therapy forced me to simultaneously hold in mind two different kinds of beliefs about the viability of the Jones/Muhammad family and two different motivations for undertaking the therapeutic work. The family believed they already were a family, and the therapy could prove this to the agency; the agency seemed to believe the family was not yet a viable family, but also not yet a family to be definitively dissolved, and the therapy might help determine which way to proceed.

Was this clear to me at the time? No, not consciously or fully. However, it may help explain a feeling that was clear at the time: I was stretched professionally, and tired, limited in what I felt I could take on, and, because of this, limited in what I was willing and able to think about. Objectively, I was limited in what I was being helped to, encouraged to, and supported in thinking about; subjectively, I did not challenge this. What I was doing was a lot, more than many private practice therapists are willing even to consider. I was able to hold two different realities in mind and find a way to work. Parallel to this, the willingness of the family and the agency to have the family therapy proceed generated a space for working. I sensed this was a valuable opportunity, and I still think it was. Also, to be truthful, I resent even having to think this issue through; why can't family therapy just be allowed to be family therapy without having to think and work through at already overburdened moments what it is and how it can work? Yet, maybe this is part of the task, and space needs to be made for it. Hindsight is a blessing and a burden.

At a couple points further along I questioned the wisdom of not including the foster parents; although the agency then offered, without enthusiasm, that I could contact them, and I did, none of the three sets of foster parents seemed interested in contact with me, and I did not pursue the issue. Was this because they had not been included from the onset? Perhaps; but the fact was that they did not move into the potential space that was offered. So I came back to the organizing reality that the hours with the Jones/Muhammad family felt productive; maybe work with the foster parents was someone else's job, though I doubted that, if so, a clinician was meeting it. Is this a peripheral issue? Was something else going on that I still do not understand? I cannot turn back the clock, so I cannot know. Not knowing is my fate, and maybe it was also my work. To say this in a different way, and push the point a bit further: I am clear that, already in the initial phase of therapy, I created a therapeutic "home" for the Jones/Muhammad family and a generative space in which they did productive psychotherapeutic work, even without the participation of the children's foster parents. Could this have constrained where we ultimately got to?

External constraints, in my view, should be acknowledged but never should determine a therapeutic choice. In the Kleinian tradition in which I am trained (Box, Copley, Magagna, & Moustaki, 1981; Hinshelwood, 1994), individuals' behavioral choices are shaped by the relations among internal representations of key relationships—the mother-inside, the father-inside, and how one feels about and interacts with them, mentally and emotionally, in development and in the moment—and the job of the therapist is to observe, and engage the patient(s) in thinking about how these dynamics of the inner life affect behavioral choices and emotional experience. The framework of treatment is constructed to serve this belief. Thus the therapist does not, for example, intervene in pragmatic problems directly; to do so would move the focus away from this opportunity to take up inner experience and inner work. I question this assumption all the time; in the place and time in which I work, it is seen as impractical if not outrageous and counterproductive by many. Yet I am continually impressed by what can be gained by holding on to this more classical way of working.

As for decisions to see a family together as opposed to individuals alone, there is a line of thinking that says therapists often do well to respect families' choices (Box et al., 1981; Luepnitz, 1988), and some literature to suggest this has particular salience in working with Black families (Boyd-Franklin, 2003). It seemed to mean something important to the Jones/Muhammad family that, by my seeing them together even though they were living, not by their choice, apart, I was respecting their will to be a family and the possibility that they could be a family; they seemed to be using this as a way to engage in the beginning work of therapy and not to resist it.

Much current literature, including some pieces in this book, questions the value of office therapy for poor families and families with young children. Undeniably, there can be value in seeing, engaging, and intervening in "life on the ground." Other writers (Heineman & Ehrensaft, 2006) have written of the value of poor families being seen in private practice offices, where what the setting and the implicit frame of the therapy communicate is that, though the broader society may work in an opposing direction, the therapy and the therapist offer the provision of comforts, privacy, and space for reflection that society, or at least the media, hold out to all in the United States, even while they deny such provision to many.

In the current case, however, the point to be made is that I had no choice. The Jones/Muhammad family had no common space. Except in my office, and in their fantasies of what might be, they lived in four separate households. In this sense, my decision to see them together was simultaneously something not thought out and a radical holding back from questioning the family's self-definition.

I believe therapies have an organic shape that is the job of the therapist and the family to discover and eventually perhaps to examine (Mendelsohn, 2005). This shape was not difficult to discover with the Jones/Muhammad family, and it emerged in this earliest period of our work together. We worked on two levels. On one, perhaps more on the surface, we did useful psychoeducational work, talking about the children's needs and desires, what was going on in the services they were receiving (special education for all but Akil and Khadijah, developmental evaluations for Mahmoud and Abdul, and individual, behaviorally oriented agency psychotherapy for Akil and Khadijah), and issues in the open child welfare case. Both the adults and the children, especially Akil and Khadijah but sometimes the others also, even nonverbal Abdul, participated meaningfully in these discussions. On another level, we developed a sense of being comfortable together, in which each member of the family seemed to become more alive and more present, and we began to be able to think together about charged issues.

One moment stands out. In the fifth session, Akil knocked something over in my office, seemingly out of at least partial intent. Ms. Muhammad seemed ready to scold him harshly; Ms. Jones had an instinct to hold back. The two women, both looking at me but seeming to want me to watch more than intervene more verbally or actively, discussed their views of what he had done and how they might respond before doing anything. The conversation was good—heartfelt with mutual care and honest but controlled emotion. As so often happens, Akil backed down when he saw the parental figures collaborating, and tried to clean up the mess, not something objectively easy for him. These are far-along goals in most therapies that are not always reached.

How could I not feel hopeful? Yet it felt difficult to steer a course. Where were we going, in these pleasant-enough, good-in-the-moment sessions? What we were doing felt necessary, but perhaps not sufficient. I wondered about the question, which plagues psychoanalytically oriented therapists working in interface with contemporary public systems, of how "getting somewhere" would be seen and whether it mattered. Part of me wanted fiercely to protect space for what we were doing, to let the therapy evolve on its own terms, and see, in the medium-distant future, where it might go. Another part of me found myself wanting someone to give me clear behavioral objectives, something I usually reject—at least so I could fight against them, if that was what was needed. Both the possibility and the impossibility of what the family and I were doing together felt present in my mind, and I suspected something parallel was going on with the family. I felt both on course and impatient, with an underlying disquiet that never quite went away.

In my occasional contacts with the referring social worker, there was encouragement intermixed with a similar holding back. She was encouraged that the family was coming to see me, and that they seemed to like coming. She seemed to follow my descriptions of what we were accomplishing and to appreciate the importance of the work we had done in setting a foundation and establishing a good beginning. However, I would hang up from my phone calls with her feeling there was something, perhaps something important or perhaps not, that was not being said.

## THE MIDDLE PHASE OF THERAPY

The middle stage of therapy covered 67 sessions. Week after week, the Jones/Muhammad family would arrive at my office; weeks were missed more because of fluctuations in my schedule than variability in theirs.

It was virtually unheard of for the child welfare system in the jurisdiction where the family lived to support a therapy in this way. The Jones/Muhammad family did not seem to know this. I knew it, but did not feel that it was my place, or therapeutically strategic, to point this out to the family. I was conscious, and grateful, that an overburdened, underresourced system was extending itself and aware the family did not share my gratitude. They—including the children, insofar as their statements to me were credible—wanted to be reunited, with the system out of their lives. Their focus on this, rather than on the operations of the system in which they found themselves involved, seemed a therapeutic gain, an assertion of the family's subjectivity and self-definition. At the same time, it was a marker of what the family seemed unwilling and incapable of knowing, and thus, simultaneously, a limitation on their gains. I did not know what to do with this awareness, and thus followed my training: when you are not sure what to do or say, be quiet, listen, and spend more time thinking.

I had my own suspicions about what the child welfare system was doing. Always, I sensed a disconnect between what I would tell the protective services social worker (who remained involved in the case—another rarity) and what I suspected she heard. Did the subtle process and dynamics of inner realities that I was working hard to describe make sense to her? She spoke in a behavioral language; I spoke in a psychodynamic language. We were both, in this sense, bilingual—that is, professionals with respect for the other's observations and perspectives—but I never felt certain whether we communicated over a bridge or over a chasm, or whether it mattered. Looking back, I think I felt my hopes for a good outcome for the family needed a private space in which to generate. My sense of what I should communicate, as well as my sense of what I could properly and meaningfully communicate, was that it needed to be somewhat limited at this point.

I very much had the sense that I was working, as systems thinkers put it, in a system far from equilibrium (Hoffman, 1981). How often do deep conversations between White people and Black people sustain themselves in this country, much less clinical conversations? For all the family's dance between engagement and evasion, openness and guardedness, there was an unmistakable intimacy that endured between the Jones/Muhammad family and me.

An example: I once had to cancel a session with the family, on short notice, because of a serious illness in my own family. Some therapists keep their reasons for such actions opaque from their patients, which did not feel wise to me in this instance. So much in this therapy seemed to hinge on a will to work toward openness. In the following session, everyone told me they had been praying for my relative. The children each brought me cards they had made, each card reflecting something of that child's personality and unique style, as well as their sincere regard for me. Both Ms. Jones and Ms. Muhammad offered me deeply felt words of comfort. I have rarely felt so moved in a moment with a family. However, only later did the full impact register with me: This was a family in treatment because of accusations of uncaring neglect. Clearly, they knew how to care. Also their care for me reflected a sense, rightly perceived and explicitly recognized, that I cared for them. Again the question: necessary, but sufficient?

At the level of deeper currents, a contradiction in our work seemed to come into focus. A pattern became recognizable in which Ms. Jones and Ms. Muhammad would ask for and receive information (e.g., about a child's developmental needs or the purpose and status of a particular service or court process). We would discuss the information thoroughly and establish through clear feedback that we were understanding each other; then, in a following session, it would seem that both Ms. Jones and Ms. Muhammad had forgotten not just what we had said, but that the conversation had ever happened. It was as if either their ability to contain the informational contents of our conversation had become, in the moment or perhaps even over time, inadequate, or that the contents of the conversation were somehow experienced as so unbearable that they could not be held and metabolized.

One week, for example, the children played quietly in one part of my office: Akil and Khadijah were organizing the younger children on a project that involved building an elaborate house, with Jacques less involved but still participating; the symbolic meaning, building a place where the family could be together, seemed transparent and positive, while Ms. Jones and Ms. Muhammad and I spoke about a meeting that would be taking place before the next session at Mahmoud's school, to prepare his individualized educational plan (IEP) for the coming year. We talked about what an IEP was, how the process worked, the personalities of the key players at the school (Ms. Jones seemed to know them well), what Ms. Jones's and Ms. Muhammad's rights were, what they wanted to see in the plan, and what they might do if the school was not in agreement. It felt like a good discussion. Both women participated actively and had ideas, which they shared freely and which we batted back and forth in an open interchange.

The next week, I asked how the meeting had gone. Both women had forgotten the meeting was to have happened and also had forgotten our discussion about it. They were pleasant and agreeable as usual, but I felt them to be more distant and inaccessible. It was a supremely uncomfortable moment that left me feeling angry and frustrated, questioning the value of our work together. This was an example of such a moment. There were many others, confusingly intermixed with times when such forgetting did not happen, when the women met responsibilities and themes of discussion in the therapy were sustained.

I think these moments of forgetting had to do with Ms. Jones and Ms. Muhammad reaching the limits of their capacities for thinking—an objective more than a subjective limitation, but not necessarily a limitation that arose from deficits on their parts. In parallel to the way I did not easily show them my awarenesses of the dynamics of the child welfare system, I believe they did not show me their own private senses of deprivation and grief, except in brief flickers of nonverbally expressed emotion that were difficult to capture and to read. Neither woman talked about the men who had at some point been in their lives or all the other myriad ways they had done without.

My sense, at points when these dynamics entered my awareness, was to be empathically present and to witness and not to confront. Instead, I wanted to listen to what they were saying, and to hold nonreactively my awareness of what they were not saying, and perhaps as well their unstated sense that they were unready or unable to say it. My metaphor was that they could project into me for safekeeping and, over time, metabolizing these unspoken, unconscious bits. Something powerful could happen, but I could be nonreactive while remaining present and connected.

Concepts of containment and containing are considered crucial in Kleinian notions of development and of mental operations (Hinshelwood, 1994). In development, the parent's ability to receive, without vengeful response, the wishes and needs a young child experiences as too dangerous to hold inside is essential for the child to have initial experiences of feeling safe enough to move beyond the constraints of either/or magical thinking and begin to consider ambiguity and, thus, the possibilities of learning and mastering the dangerous and the complex. In adult life, it is necessary to move beyond moments in which what we have to take in feels overwhelming, and we hide from it or reject it out of grandiose suspicion, to moments in which we can think through difficult material in a more considered way.

Containment, to me, is a powerful tool. I have seen it produce transformative change and accomplish goals that skills building, behavior modification, and other tools of contemporary strengths-based approaches have not been able to achieve. Did I think it was an adequate tool in my work with the Jones/Muhammad family? I had my doubts, but I tried to contain them, with awareness, in my own mind, parallel to the work of containment I felt I was doing for the family.

In the service of helping these kinds of deep dynamics come to light, some therapists insist on conditions of therapy in which the sole focus is examination and interpretation of psychodynamics. They would see psychoeducational work of the kind I, like many parent–infant therapists, was trying to wrap in as antitherapeutic because of its potential to foreclose space and will for more focused self-examination. They would see the job of providing information as belonging somewhere else; if this kind of split, between educator and therapist, felt too fragmenting to a burdened family, then the family would be seen as unsuitable for psychotherapeutic treatment or, at minimum, the therapy would be seen as needing much more extensive supports than were available to me (Barrett & Trevitt, 1991; Boston & Szur, 1983).

Although I questioned how I was conducting this therapy, often and sometimes harshly, I had a different sense. I focused more on the way larger systems had brought me together with this family, something highly unlikely to have happened otherwise, and tended to see our struggle to take in together information coming from these larger systems more as our task than our obstacle. Part of me longed for a "purer" therapy, in which the family and I might not feel yanked away from a different, potentially more interesting task by perceived demands to make sense of confusing information flows of external origin. On the other hand, our reactions to outside information also seemed to make inner dynamics clear, and our struggles to contain and process information, even when they failed, seemed to facilitate useful lines of thinking and developmental momentum in the family.

For example: Ms. Jones long questioned whether any of the children were retarded. She reasoned that others saw her as more limited and less resourceful than she was. (On formal testing, she had a borderline average IQ score, but a 12th grade reading level, due to well-developed compensation skills.) She focused on what the children could do, rather than on what they could not, and questioned, not unreasonably, whether some of their difficulties had to do with being asked to live in different worlds simultaneously: her world and the more privileged worlds of their foster families.

One day, at a moment when the timing seemed right, we spoke about this. I said I thought her questions were reasonable, but that there were many reports of teachers and psychologists that several of the children had marked limitations, and that these reports also seemed credible. I suggested a reasonable goal would be to get good evaluations on each of the children. Ms. Jones was quiet for a while—Ms. Muhammad focused on watching the children play and did not seem to want to engage in this line of conversation—and then, in a less defended tone, Ms. Jones said she thought I was right. I wanted the concept of mental retardation to be explicit in this context, and said that children can have mental retardation and also be good children, creative, and able to do and learn many things. Ms. Jones looked me in the eyes, not angry or at all remote in the moment, and said she understood.

Very clearly, there was something beyond forgetting, and different from forgetting, that was also going on. I appreciated the depth and quality of Ms. Jones's thinking and her undefended willingness to share it with me. This felt emblematic of something else going on in the process of the therapy. In the sessions, I was finding Ms. Jones and Ms. Muhammad more lively, less formal, and less passive with me, with each other, and with the children. The children, too, interacted with each other more, the older ones taking considerable care to include the younger ones in collective play. I was feeling hopeful for the family again.

As much as, in my own reflections between sessions, I could trace this positive line of development in the family, in sessions I found myself feeling buffeted, conflicted, and uncertain. At times, I would feel that the positive moments would eventually carry us beyond the moments in which Ms. Jones and Ms. Muhammad would speak of their pained forgetting. I would also feel hope that Ms. Jones, in particular, could move beyond a dichotomous sense of her views of the children's potential and others' reasonable descriptions of the children's and Ms. Muhammad's limitations. Perhaps she could achieve a "both/and" way of thinking, and model it for the other members of the family.

On the other hand, I felt that, at least for the moment, after almost 2 years of dedicated work, I was the one who held, for the family, the sense of the multiple limitations that were present. I knew. They did not know. Perhaps this was part of my job, but the emotions it evoked were intense and difficult to handle. I would feel the most affected when Ms. Jones and Ms. Muhammad would forget something important that had been said or when one or another of the children "looked retarded" in a moment of their speech or play. I felt, very sharply, the tension between what was and what might or might not become. Inside me, there was the odd sense that when I felt good about the family and comfortable with them, this led to a sense of unease—what was I missing or denying?—and when I felt confused and pessimistic and in ambivalent connection with the family, I felt better, like I was "getting it." I tried to hold both sets of feelings in mind. It was profoundly not easy.

Beyond the tensions in the moments, I questioned whether the Jones/Muhammad family could ever have the good life I wanted for them, and that they said they wanted for themselves. Maybe the goal was beyond what this flawed society was capable of or willing to help them achieve, and maybe even holding out hope was a setup. In my darkest moment, I wondered whether the therapy was doing a disservice. We were making great strides, but in the slow time such strides often require, and, while we were far from where we had begun, we seemed equally far from an imagined end point where a court, rooted in the values of White, middle-class culture, would be likely to see the Jones/Muhammad family as well-functioning and competent. What if I had been successful in helping the family stop running out on each other and stop evading encounters with uncomfortable realities that had served them as successful defenses against awareness of limitations they had and that they found unbearable, which now they had little sense of how to *be*? Also, what if the women's patterns of forgetting information represented their way of letting me know this? Was crisis looming and, if so, would our bond equip us to withstand it?

I want to add a coda before concluding this part of the discussion. I am aware I have been speaking mostly about whole-family/systemic dynamics; I think these are central foci of work in therapy with some families, and they felt like the center of the therapeutic action here. However, to not remain opaque about changes in the individual children, I offer next observations of each of them.

Jacques was, at this point, much more settled in his foster placement and his special education program. He caused fewer disruptions, and was reported to be happier. In sessions, he said a bit more, and his play was more imaginative. He joined in more readily with his siblings, in both their social interaction and in their play.

Akil seemed to have grown tremendously over the time I had been seeing him. He, and his twin sister, had tolerated and adjusted well to a change in foster placements, from one where the foster mother's capacities for emotional attunement and provision had long seemed questionable to a home with loving, if somewhat rigid, upper-middle-class, African American parents. He was performing to expectations in classes for students thought to have average abilities, both behaviorally and academically. He no longer tuned me out in sessions; to the contrary, he probably related to me the most warmly among the children. Akil had expectable interests for a latency-age boy and a group of friends. His assertions that he was happy and well-adjusted seemed grounded rather than hollow.

Khadijah at this point seemed the most troubled of the children. Her demands for attention seemed more acute, and her capacities for attention and self-regulation seemed uneven. The school described her as too easily upset, anxious, and demanding in class, although more or less on track academically, and like her brother she was in regular classes for children considered to be of average ability. The foster parents, with their own spin, described her as "spoiled." Her agency individual therapist, an undertrained and overworked clinician, seemed unattuned to what was going on and unresponsive to me and to the protective services social worker. Despite this, suggestions that the therapist get some supervision, or that a change of therapist be considered, were not taken up.

Mahmoud and Abdul were in the same foster home, where they were described as easy children to care for, and in the same school—a special school for retarded children, perhaps not the most sophisticated but a loving, supportive place to be. Their developmental and pre-academic achievements were congruent with what is often expected for moderately retarded children. In sessions, they interacted well with their siblings, and engaged in simple, happy, age-appropriate play. There was no clinical impression that they were traumatized or otherwise emotionally disturbed.

In the sessions, the children seemed bonded to Ms. Jones and Ms. Muhammad. They did not fuss about being away from their foster parents or about being with their biological mother and grandmother. As I was working as a family therapist, it may be there were aspects of their inner lives that were opaque to me and would have been of concern if they had had a different sort of vehicle facilitating their expression. However, that was not what things looked like. The children seemed to be doing reasonably well in foster care and to be benefiting in appreciable ways from the family therapy.

In a way, these achievements are prosaic, though I fiercely valued them, as did Ms. Jones and Ms. Muhammad. These is nothing wrong, I think, with achieving prosaic goals—survival, more or less on-course development, and calm are good, considering the alternatives. They are certainly the kind of achievements our colleagues with different theoretical orientations look toward.

At the same time, I held inconvenient truths about both the family—their forgetting, their limitations—and about the system—its failed commitments, its shallowness in some of their oversimplified understandings. I felt grounded in my own sense of what therapy was, and grounded in a sense that I was holding important ambiguities, in more or less clear focus and at least much of the time. I kept asking myself whether these things were enough. I still ask myself, years later and after months of concentrated thinking. I kept thinking that, if we just had a little more time, things would work out. In parallel process, the same theme has gone through my mind as I have struggled to get what I think about this family and this therapy onto paper: It will all come clear if I just work on it a little more, but it never did.

## HOW THE THERAPY ENDED

Things inched along. In the eight sessions that seemed to constitute an abrupt ending of this therapy—interestingly, I originally typed "the ending of this family"—the family did nothing bad. None of the children—who remained in foster care—were deprived, abused, or mistreated by the foster parents, Ms. Jones, or Ms. Muhammad. No great revelations emerged in the hours, just the plodding work that constitutes much of therapy. No one solved the dilemmas in my head, but that is never the job of a family. They survived, and survival, especially in therapy with children, in therapy with poor people, and in clinical work with persons with developmental disabilities, is always a good thing.

There was one disruption. The social worker asked me to prepare an update letter for the court, something I had been doing periodically. I prepare such documents in consultation with families I work with in the child welfare system. To help me prepare for writing the letter, the social worker provided me some court documents she had not given me at the outset. These described Ms. Muhammad's neglect of the children as more severe and extensive than what either the social worker or the family had depicted to me earlier. It was reported, for example, that, when he came into foster care, at age 3, Mahmoud was caked in feces and would not walk upright. The source of this information was the foster parent who had been caring for him.

I took up these concerns with Ms. Jones and Ms. Muhammad. Ms. Muhammad's denial, and Ms. Jones's initial insistence that the foster parent was exaggerating, seemed unconvincing. After a few minutes, during which I was mostly silent, Ms. Muhammad soon acknowledged the truth of what had happened, and she and her mother had an honest confrontation. Ms. Jones told her daughter, in a stern voice that managed also to communicate that there would be no disruption of their relationship, that there was nothing defensible about not cleaning up a soiled young child, and that there was no reason Ms. Muhammad could not have told Ms. Jones, at the time, about what had been going on. Ms. Jones would have helped, she said. However, what, I found myself thinking, would "help" have meant at the time? Giving the boy a bath? Buying groceries? Cleaning the house? Watching the kids for a few hours so Ms. Muhammad could take a break? Surely these would all have been small, positive steps. Yet what about the larger steps: For instance, acknowledging that Ms. Muhammad's developmental disability left her deficient in basic parenting skills, or that Ms. Jones had been out of touch with what was going on in her daughter's household. These issues had gone unacknowledged at the time Mahmoud came into foster care, and, 2 years into therapy, they were still not finding their way into words. The therapeutic space felt safe and generative, but serious limitations in the family persisted.

I did not count this as a therapeutic setback. The microprocess of therapy is composed of backward and forward steps, and much of therapy seems to me to have to do with the accumulation of small, good moments and the positive momentum and trajectory they can come to define, and not with the rare moments of transformation that, although moving in the moment, may not lead to sustained change. The ability of mother and daughter to work past a fiction and engage each other seemed productive and suggestive of forward momentum and prognostic optimism.

This is the place to mention that the child welfare system at several points promised things to the Jones/Muhammad family and never followed through. Staff promised to help get Ms. Muhammad qualified for Social Security disability payments, so the chronic poverty in the family could at least be attenuated. (Ms. Jones worked as a paraprofessional, supplying the needs of the household, and some of the children's needs, from her modest income reasonably and as best as she could.) Staff also promised to provide in-home parenting assistance so that an objective observer could assess, outside the arm's-length reporting available in the family therapy sessions, how well Ms. Muhammad functioned in a parental role and how effective Ms. Jones was at backing her up, by providing training and support in these areas and seeing how well it was taken in. They also promised to get updated evaluations on each of the children so that there could be a sense of how limited they were (or were not), what they needed, and what could be expected of them.

All of this was promised explicitly enough, and none of it was ever done. Budgets were tight, social workers were busy, service providers could not be located; other systems mysteriously malfunctioned, and no one could figure out how or why.

In another rendition of this story, the promised services that were not provided might have been seen as more pivotal. It was certainly outrageous that the promised services did not come through, just as it was outrageous that my social worker colleague had painted a distorted picture of the family's history at the outset. However, in a story of this kind of layered complexity, the causal centrality of these factors at least needs to be questioned. I resisted tendencies to reduce therapeutic conversations to these questions, and, interestingly, at this point in the therapy, so did Ms. Jones and Ms. Muhammad.

The Jones/Muhammad family experienced the denial of promised services in the historical/political context of White systems lying to, and injuring Black people. This was clearly not the only relevant context, but also the system's failed promises did seem to be another example of a painful historical/political reality. This chapter is not the place to fully take up questions of the impact of the history of Black oppression, whether this remains a racist society, the psychology of class and poverty, or the psychology of Black rage. Suffice it to say that empirical evidence of these phenomena exist, and they are not unknown or irrational. Believing and acting in ways that are cognizant of these phenomena, while sometimes hard for therapists to grab hold of and therapies to stay in touch with, make sense. Perhaps more focally relevant to current context, although Ms. Jones and Ms. Muhammad may have been seen as not always attuned to subtleties and complexities, their grasp of the system's broken promises was nuanced, sharp, and clear. They saw the phenomena as both hateful and unexceptional, something to be borne. I was impressed and humbled.

At the same time, the thinking of both Ms. Jones and Ms. Muhammad remained firmly concrete. Their focus was on the Social Security assistance that never came through, for instance, and not a more reflective discourse about class and race. I found myself wondering what part of this kind of concrete thinking was "hard wired," a part of the neurological/neuropsychological substrate of learning and developmental disability that was unlikely ever to change, and what part was defensive—what has been called "secondary mental handicap" (Sinason, 1986)—and could, over time, potentially be understood, challenged, and worked through in therapy. I saw the process of the therapy as involved with my radical acceptance of the family as they were, seeing them as much through their own eyes as through mine. This was not a therapy the family had sought out on their own for their own purposes. They were coming to see me because the child welfare system had asked them to come. They found their contacts with me affirming and agreeable experiences, and this seemed to open up some space for Ms. Jones and Ms. Muhammad to think about things together with me and, seemingly, for the children's developmental trajectories to free up and move forward. However, they did not focus on these changes; they focused, to the extent they showed a subjectively determined focus, on showing the child welfare system they were complying with the request to come to therapy and their hope that this would induce the child welfare system to return the children to their care. I was reasonably comfortable, at the time, with seeing my role as a thoughtful witness and commentator, more anthropologist than commanding general.

In any event, the therapy did not end, at least in any direct way, because the system failed to provide needed, and promised, services. It ended because the child welfare system decided that the therapy should end.

There is an imperative in child welfare laws that children have a sense of permanence in their lives (Briere, 1992; Fine, 1993; Solnit, Nordhaus, & Lord, 1992). This is sensible and important, although the discourse of laws and the practice of systems is often at variance. Systems often throw up obstacles to permanency, and the complexities of people, and relationships among people, throw up obstacles as well. Systems often do not do what they say they will do, or are supposed to do, which is the same with both biological and foster parents. However, the consequences tend to fall inequitably. Professionals generally do not lose their jobs, or their families, when they fail to get a family assigned to their care back on track (nor should they). Yet parents "in the system" can lose their children. Sometimes they should, because a situation is untenable and beyond help, but sometimes the decision seems painfully unfair.

Laws establish deadlines for when parents whose children have been removed from their care are to prove they can safely resume custody of the children. In the locality where the Jones/Muhammad family lives, for a long time there was much flexibility in these timelines. If needed services, as was not uncommon, took a long time to arrange, or if a family was productively involved in therapy or other services, and the possibility of a good outcome seemed potentially reachable, then extra time was not difficult to get.

This changed in the course of the time I worked with the Jones/Muhammad family. Perhaps it should well have changed, but notice of an impending change seemed fair, and no one told us the change was imminent. So one day, seemingly out of the blue, the family and I were told the family had not established, to the satisfaction of child protective services and the court, that Ms. Jones and Ms. Muhammad had demonstrated they were capable of raising the children without risk of future neglect or abuse. There was thus no reason for the child welfare system to fund or support future therapy. Ms. Jones and Ms. Muhammad had no resources to pay for their travel to my office and for the therapy. Even if they were footing the bill, could they have orchestrated on their own for the children to be brought to sessions? I had no capacity to accept an additional no-fee case. After 83 sessions of therapy that seemed to be going somewhere, we had run out of time and space in which to work. In this sense we were recreating, in the therapy, a moment parallel to the moment when Jacques had run out of the household, and the child welfare system had determined the household itself could not go on being a household. I insisted on time to terminate with the family. We were afforded two more sessions.

In the two sessions that remained to us, the adults and I were angry, together but in our own separate ways, and the children watched us with compassion and some understanding. Ms. Jones and Ms. Muhammad smoldered with resentment, deflecting their feelings away from me. I appreciated this and admired their abilities to be articulate and show restraint. I saw these as important gains of the therapy. I put into words that I felt their clarity and self-control were important strengths, and that they would take these with them, but my words felt incomplete and lacking in emotional resonance. I choked getting them out.

Colleagues who reviewed drafts of this chapter have told me that in infant–child work and other kinds of family therapy with poor families with young children, it is highly unusual for families to show up for these kinds of termination sessions. The editor of this volume told me she thought this was a sign of the therapy's importance to the family.

I certainly agree that the family's capacity for relatedness with me, developed over the course of our work together—not running out—was a good and important achievement. I hope they can take this capacity into their inner experience, and into their lives in the world, and re-create it in other contexts and endeavors, whether or not their thinking remains concrete and constrained by the limitations of learning and developmental disabilities.

Yet I do not go quietly into this maybe-good-enough assessment and its accompanying trickle of hope. The Jones/Muhammad family, in the time I worked with them, remained a family intervened, a family trying to be a family—hurt, vulnerable, and underserved. The unavoidable fact is that something that was theirs, and mine, a therapy that at least at moments seemed to be helping them, was taken from them and from us. Our forced ending felt more like a murder than a success, abduction more than exodus.

Sometimes the role of the therapist is to advocate. I told the social worker I disagreed with her decision, speaking in a professional and articulate manner. At Ms. Jones's request, I spoke with the family's public defender, whom I knew to be good at her job. There was a court hearing, but what the family and I argued for did not prevail. Time ran out, and therapy ended. Possibilities of what could have developed for the family, and of me having time and space to sort out my tactical and strategic dilemmas, were foreclosed.

I think therapists should advocate when advocacy is necessary to save space for a therapy to continue—a more prosaic example may be when a child therapist confronts parents who want to pull their child out of a productive therapy that the child values—or when something extreme from outside threatens carefully nurtured space for work. Over the years, I have lobbied state agencies to prevent funding cuts for clinical services, and argued with insurance companies when they did not want to pay for care that seemed essential. Abstention, in such circumstances, strikes me as too-willing collusion with harmful forces, and has potential to convey to families, inadvertently, that backing down in difficult circumstances is preferable to struggling through. Advocacy, and talking to patients about advocacy efforts, can potentially throw therapy off track.

Therapist and patient can focus on externals that are easier to bring into focus than complex, often unconscious, inner dynamics. However, I think it is possible for attuned therapists to capture this when it is happening and to steer therapy back to its center of gravity and back on course. I did not feel Ms. Jones and Ms. Muhammad stopped thinking and exploring issues with me, or that the children stopped showing me what they were thinking and feeling in productive play, when I advocated on their/our behalf for the therapy to continue and for this family to have more time to show they could be a viable family unit. I think they appreciated what I was doing.

My own feelings were complicated. There was a note of relief, to be free of the burden of a difficult task, but it was not a predominant feeling. More fundamentally, and more strongly, I felt the child welfare system was mirroring, in its own behavior, what they were accusing the family of in a kind of morbid parallel process. Their actions were saying, in effect, that time had run out on their willingness to follow through on their promises, their explicit promises to provide services that failed to materialize and the promise, implicit in their 2-year history of supporting the therapy, that they would stay with this family and help them become what they could become. I struggled painfully with self-recriminations, wondering how the therapy I had had primary responsibility for constructing had or had not contained this parallel systemic process, and whether my own failure to contain, metabolize, and help transform what the system was doing somehow constrained the possibilities for Ms. Jones and Ms. Muhammad acquiring similar capacities.

Can psychotherapy do this kind of thing? I do not know. Here is what I do know: Ms. Jones stays in touch. Every few months, she calls me, identifying herself, in the old southern way, as "Miss Jones." A court appeal, at the writing, remains ongoing. She keeps me apprised, and asks my opinions about things to try. She tells me how the children are doing (well, in her view, but missing her and their mother). Her tone is warm and intimate. Something of our relationship endures. Might the therapy revive itself, and, if so, might we get somewhere further? Again, I do not know. I do know, as an objective personal fact, that while my elements of pessimistic feelings for this family's future have come into clearer focus over the years—that I have come to feel less idealistic and less naive—my coexisting hopes that they can be a family and have a decent life have never extinguished. They are still alive and come right to the surface, along with all the other feelings, every time I hear Ms. Jones's voice calling me.

## REFLECTIONS

Of all the questions I have been thinking about, in a summer's musings and an autumn's, and now a winter's, labor of writing, three stand out: Was it inevitable that this case fail? If so, is the story really worth telling? For that matter, did the case actually fail, given all that was done and that the case, was failed by others at least as much as it failed? What was my role? What could I have done differently? What might have happened if I did?

To the first of these questions: Despite the efforts of all the professionals involved, children in the child welfare system most often do not have good outcomes; speculations about why and how this happens go beyond the scope of this chapter (Heineman, 1998; Heineman & Ehrensaft, 2006). I do not believe that, in this area of clinical work, a single therapist can necessarily shield a case from all the forces that impinge.

Yet, as the Talmud says, while we are not required to finish great tasks, neither are we free from the injunction to do what we can. In writing this chapter, I have tried to delineate the many less-than-perfect conditions under which the family and I operated, all of which could have been challenged with more creativity, insistence, and passion, as well as the many therapeutic choices made in response; all of them are worth questioning and requestioning.

What precipitates out for me is the strong belief that things external to therapy can never be determinative of what happens inside a therapy, and the corollary, perhaps less intuitive, that as long as the process of what is going on in therapeutic relationships can be described and understood, it has potential to shift and to change. The Jones/Muhammad family and I did not exhaust these possibilities. Therefore, in my thinking, nothing was inevitable—and perhaps our ongoing thread of contact, fragile as it is, testifies to that.

So nothing, in the end, feels inevitable about what happened in my work with the Jones/Muhammad family. The story presses for telling, I think, for two particular reasons. One is because it is a common case, one of many cases of families who do not come out of the child welfare system whole, despite active desire, professional and thoughtful social work, and engaged therapy. We do not speak often enough about common and inconvenient realities. The other reason, which motivates this book as a whole, is that, as our subfield develops, we need to pool our experience and scrutinize the lessons we learn from it. Is my experience with the Jones/Muhammad family typical of good-enough work that family therapists who work with families with young children do? To the extent that it is, then the story needs a public telling, as we try to sort out together questions of best practices, pitfalls and how to avoid them, and the relevant common features of our work.

To the second question, of whether the case failed: There is a body of empirical work that psychodynamic therapies not only work but also have a relatively large effect size (Norcross, 2002; Westen, Novotny, & Thompson-Brenner, 2004). Although the question of why public mental health systems and managed "care" ignore or deny this goes beyond our present discussion (but a hint: resource allocations are at the heart of this particular piece of intellectual dishonesty), there is a finding from the years when clinics provided psychodynamic therapies widely that is of focal relevance. In public systems, therapies that proceeded to mutually agreed upon termination were rare; but objective, clinical gains in "incomplete" therapies were the rule, not the exception. To the extent there were definable achievements in this therapy, they seem quite similar to what happens in other kinds of therapies (strengths-based and cognitive–behavioral) often used with this population, but perhaps with a more humane framework that made for additive benefit.

This description seems to fit what happened in the work being described here. The children and the adults developed, and reliable markers seemed to establish that the growth went beyond what time alone would have been likely to yield. I do not feel ashamed of this therapy.

Yet, I cannot honestly describe this therapy as other than failed. The children are not living with their biological parents; Ms. Jones and Ms. Muhammad live with the grief of children whom they love living apart from them. That they take this in stride intensifies, not lessens, the pain. In the flicker of the moment when I question the case's failure, I feel complicit in a history and a politics I reject, and its too-ready acceptance in clinical life. I write in a time when political leaders of the right trumpet their commitment to families. What about this family? It is, in a way, the only question worth asking in current context. If we add up all the failed cases with similar elements in common, we would see we are addressing a large, and deeply troubling, social phenomenon. So examination of the salient component parts, those we can capture, is important in ways that are central to clinical life, and that also go far beyond it.

There is also another dimension to thinking through whether this case failed. It is interesting that framing the case as "failed" involves an expression in a passive voice, inviting the inquiry that always comes up (or should come up) when mention of a subject is not specified: Who is the subject of the failure? A colleague, helping me think through my thoughts on this case, looked at me sharply and said, "You were neglected." She is right; in not telling me vital information, in cutting off the therapy as it was, in not following through on commitments to the family, professionals involved in a system tasked with preventing neglect were neglectful. I was neglected, and so was the Jones/Muhammad family. So the failure is not that of a television medical drama, in which fantasy characters played by actors do or do not solve the mystery, but has qualities of pathological parallel process, in which the helping system became, at critical moments, a hurting system.

What do I think of my own role? Therapy based on notions of projection, containment, and metabolization has the feeling of something quaint and impractical at best. How does it work? Certainly, the mechanism is a subtle one, but no less powerful for that. Here is a story about an example: at one point, late in the middle phase of therapy, the social worker told me about a school meeting Ms. Jones and Ms. Muhammad had missed. It was an important meeting, and thus important that I speak with the women about what had happened. I felt this strongly, and raised it in the next session. Ms. Muhammad seemed not to track what we were talking about, but Ms. Jones seemed incensed. When I mentioned the missed meeting, she reiterated, with a fierceness not typical of her manner of speaking, that the children were doing well. She felt that the school and the social worker never acknowledged this, and she felt that it was high time that the children were returned to the family. The fragment of awareness that the children had needs for professional assistance, and that the missed meeting was a problem, was unbearable to her, so it was projected onto me, perhaps accounting, in part, for my feeling at the time that it was important to push for some resolution of the issue. However, after hearing the intensity of Ms. Jones's reaction, my sense was that it was not the right time to insist on a discussion. I acknowledged Ms. Jones's feelings, and thanked her for expressing them, and said that perhaps this was something that was complicated and that we would need to think more about together (containment). The fierceness eased, and there was a sense of a return back to calm, mutual appreciation, and close relatedness between us. I continued to think often about this powerful moment over the next few days. Ms. Jones called me between sessions, something not usual for her, and said with sincerity, the fierceness gone, that she knew the children had needs, beyond what she and Ms. Muhammad could meet on their own, and that—while she still felt it was important for professionals to acknowledge the children's achievements and strengths—she was also aware of the children's needs for "outside help." Ms. Jones said that she was open to this help as was Ms. Muhammad. That is an example, to my thinking, of the therapeutic gain from the therapist metabolizing what the patient cannot, in the moment, tolerate, much less think about. The shift had to do with this process, not just provision of information, argumentation, clarification, or reconsideration, in my view.

But how can one be this sharp at every moment? With the multiply painful luxury of hindsight—I have status and sustenance that the Jones/Muhammad family does not have, and I am asked to reflect on a personal failure—I am troubled that I did not insist on, and seek out despite whatever obstacles, more personal support as I worked with this family. In the thinking and the writing, I can tally my burdens of stress, confusion, and pain, as I did this work, and they are all too high and probably intruded in ways beyond what I hold in present awareness. I would be reluctant to take on a case like this in private practice again, at least without more regular consultation and more peer support than I had while I was working with this family. Beyond all my open questions, this stands out.

Finally, I want to come back around to a question I posed implicitly in the opening of this chapter: is it fair to ask clinicians to carry some of the weight of White/Black history in America into their clinical work? I think I might have asked myself this question more gently, more diplomatically, some of the times it came up in my mind during this work. I am pretty sure, however, that I will ask it wherever I go, in whatever work I do as a therapist, all the days of my life, and that my answer will always be, "Yes." We learn from our failures, or at least we can. Also our failures, like all our experiences as clinicians, sap our energies whenever we do not appreciate their larger connections and patterns, taking such possibilities out of the inevitably narrow places of our thought and our practice and into the nether life of our dreams.

## ACKNOWLEDGMENTS

My thinking about work with people in the child welfare system has been shaped by my conversations over the years with Toni Vaughn Heineman and Diane Ehrensaft; my colleagues on the Washington, DC, steering committee of the Area Chapter of A Home Within: Barbara Cristy, Mary Durham, Julie Gardner, Maurine Kelly, Beryce MacLennan, Jane Nielson, and Louise Volk; and the many dedicated professionals and families involved in the child welfare system of which I consider myself a part. I am also grateful to my colleague Dorothy Evans Holmes, and the other faculty members and students at George Washington University with whom I have the privilege to work and who have sharpened and deepened my thinking about race. Finally, I want to thank my married partner, James North, from whom I stole time when my work with this family kept me up nights, and then once more during the long hours laboring to write about the work.

## REFERENCES

Barrett, M., & Trevitt, J. (1991). *Attachment behavior and the schoolchild: An introduction to educational therapy.* New York: Tavistock/Routledge.

Bion, W. R. (1965). *Transformations.* London: Heinemann.

Bion, W. R. (1970). *Attention and interpretation.* London: Heinemann.

Boston, M., & Szur, R. (Eds.). (1983). *Psychotherapy with severely deprived children.* London: Routledge & Kegan Paul.

Box, S., Copley, B., Magagna, J., & Moustaki, E. (Eds.). (1981). *Psychotherapy with families: A psychoanalytic approach.* Boston: Routledge & Kegan Paul.

Boyd-Franklin, N. (2003). *Black families in therapy: Understanding the African American experience* (2nd ed.). New York: Guilford Press.

Briere, J. N. (1992). *Child abuse trauma: Theory and treatment of the lasting effects.* Thousands Oaks, CA: Sage.

Fine, P. (1993). *A developmental network approach to therapeutic foster care.* Washington, DC: Child Welfare League of America.

Heineman, T. V. (1998). *The abused child: Psychodynamic understanding and treatment.* New York: Guilford Press.

Heineman, T. V., & Ehrensaft, D. (Eds.). (2006). *Building a home within: Meeting the emotional needs of children and youth in foster care.* Baltimore, MD: Brookes.

Hinshelwood, R. D. (1994). *Clinical Klein.* New York: Basic Books.

Hoffman, L. (1981). *Foundations of family therapy: A conceptual framework for systems change*. New York: Basic Books.

Luepnitz, D. (1988). *The family interpreted: Psychoanalysis, feminism and family therapy*. New York: Basic Books.

Mendelsohn, E. (2005). Rules were made to be broken: Reflections on psychoanalytic education and process. *Psychoanalytic Psychology, 22*, 261–278.

Norcross, J. C. (Ed.). (2002). *Psychotherapy relationships that work: Therapist contributions and responsiveness to patients*. New York: Oxford University Press.

Sinason, V. (1986). Secondary mental handicap and its relationship to trauma. *Psychoanalytical Psychotherapy, 2*, 131–154.

Solnit, A. J., Nordhaus, B. F., & Lord, R. (1992). *When home is no haven: Child placement issues*. New Haven, CT: Yale University Press.

Westen, E., Novotny, C., & Thompson-Brenner, H. (2004). The empirical status of empirically supported therapies: Assumptions, methods, and findings. *Psychological Bulletin, 130*, 631–663.

Williams, G. (1991). Work with ethnic minorities. In R. Szur & S. Miller (Eds.), *Extending horizons: Psychoanalytic psychotherapy with children, adolescents and families* (pp. 183–208). New York: Karnac.

CHAPTER 7

# REFLECTIONS OF RICHARD RUTH'S
# JOURNEY IN THE HEART OF DARKNESS

*Julie Stone*

My reflections are penned on Australian soil, and in the last few years it has been my great privilege to regularly spend time in Africa. In Kwa Zulu Natal, South Africa, the ghosts from the years of apartheid ominously stalk the present decade, and the legacy of racial hatred and how it can divide a population is still starkly evident. Australia has its own shameful history, and her ghosts tell a different story, which is also the same. A story of people divided, one group dominating another by assuming the mantle of "knowing" what is right. For the dominated, there is little or no choice. The dominating and oppressive faction almost invariably believes "God is on their side." In chapter 1, Birch quotes Fraiberg (1980), claiming this blessing for the infant mental health clinician. Birch wisely cautions, "believing that God is on your side is a tricky enterprise."

So Richard Ruth's title and his courageous chapter, which bravely steps into the territory of racial difference and mental retardation, touch a chord deep within me. The chord, in a minor key, leaves me disturbed and humbled. The music of the chapter speaks of love and loss and of compassion and what is possible in any therapeutic endeavour. It asks questions, impossible to answer, that nevertheless must be asked.

In preparing to write his chapter Ruth found himself listening to blues, "a genre rising from the African American experience of trying to find meaning by somehow making pattern or sense out of the complexities, impossibilities, absurdities, and horrors of life in a world where the odds are impossibly stacked against them" (p. 117). In preparing to respond, I found myself reading Valerie Sinason's (1993) writing about her years of pioneering work, bringing the richness of psychoanalytic thinking and practice to those who inhabit a world that is often precarious and certainly stacked against them. She too seeks ways to find hope by making sense of the complexities, impossibilities, absurdities, and horrors of life.

Sinason's (1993) experience lights the way for us and helps us think about what psychodynamic and psychoanalytic theory and practice have to offer individuals and groups whose experience of the world is not easily comprehended and who might more comfortably, for the practitioner, be placed outside the ken of psychodynamic practice. In 1993 Sinason wrote a book titled *Mental Handicap and the Human Condition*. The human condition embraces all. For clinicians working within the psychodynamic framework, the dictum is that all things can be thought about and talked about. As these case histories remind us, this is not as easy as it sounds.

In his work with the Jones/Muhammad family, Ruth confronts, head on, the challenges and difficulties of thinking and of thinking about thinking. He refuses to take the easy option to decide that psychotherapeutic work cannot be undertaken with children or parents with mental retardation. He does not say: This family is Black, I am not Black, therefore I cannot understand them, I cannot work with them. Neither does he say that neither mental retardation nor racial difference will affect him or the therapy. He is very aware of their potential influence. In his reflections on his work with this family Ruth says, humbly and honestly, "If nothing else, I have learned something about the salience of these questions—and something about what I do not know about them" (p. 118). With his humanness he embraces each member of the Jones/Muhammad family in their humanness. Together, they struggle to make sense of the worlds in which this family lives.

Curious and at times daunted, Ruth offers himself as psychotherapist to this family. He shares with us his endeavor to hold multiple possibilities in mind, to be open to whatever story unfolded in their work together. He remains open to what is shared with him by the family while also remaining open to communications from the other complex systems involved. He is alert to and curious about what is not shared. From the outset, he recognizes that "either horrible stories were being sanitized or [this family was] poor Black people from the city who somehow found themselves in a White, middle-class suburban neighborhood where they made others uncomfortable" (p. 123). Ruth writes, "I found myself trying to hold both possibilities in mind, and to think clearly about how they fit together or clashed" (p. 123). They are not mutually exclusive truths, and I suspect both were true.

Ruth worked with the Jones/Muhammad family, all seven of them. He reflects upon what this meant. His making space in his mind and his office to embrace these seven family members and his willingness to see them as "family" were vital component of the therapy. Although Ruth says he was wary about the motive and agenda of the courts and other agencies involved, the pragmatic truth is they too were committed, at least in part, to this therapy and to this family. Over many months and many sessions, arrangements were put in place to ensure that five children, their mother, and their grandmother, were transported from four different households to Ruth's office, so they could be together. Precipitous endings are all too common in work with families entangled in a child protective system—sustained, effective, complex logistics much less so. It is more amazing that Ruth managed to see this family for so long than that this therapy ended so abruptly.

In speaking of the core concepts of infant–parent psychotherapy Birch says,

> We try to understand . . . and in our way of doing so we try to offer a different experience of being listened to, understood, and cared about. . . . We are trying to provide an attuned, supportive relationship, a holding environment, a container within which [the family] can reflect on and resolve some of the obstacles to attunement, mutuality, and growth. (this volume, p. 15–17)

Ruth states that "containment, to me, is a powerful tool" (p. 133). He continues, "I have seen it produce transformative change and accomplish goals that skills building, behavior modification, and other tools of contemporary strengths-based approaches have not been able to achieve" (p. 133). My clinical work has led me to a similar belief about containment.

The relationship between therapist and family is a relationship in which all things can be talked about and thought about, and in which there is room for uncertainty and not knowing. The therapist is not uncertain about his or her theory; the theory and experience give a structure in which to hold the uncertainty about what may unfold. Ruth writes about this well. His relationship with the family becomes the container for their work together. Using the metaphor coined by Ed Tronick, Ruth's mind provides the scaffolding for the thinking that he does together with the family, and it offers a frame for the family members' further thinking.

Ruth established a courteous and respectful relationship with all seven family members; he liked them, and he was interested in them and what they brought to share. In all his dealings with them he offered them respect and courtesy. As Sinason (1993) attested, this is fundamental to our work. Sadly, history tells us that for many Black people, and for people with mental retardation, respect and courtesy are not common experiences. Ruth speaks of moments of "genuine connection" with this family. He says "I created a therapeutic 'home' for the Jones/Muhammad family and a generative space in which they did productive psychotherapeutic work" (p. 126). This is to be celebrated and valued.

In his gentle and reflective style, Ruth writes of his decision to share with the family his reason for cancelling a session on short notice. He then tells of the loving and thoughtful response each member of the Jones/Muhammad family offered to him in their meeting following the cancelled session: "cards they had made" from the children and "deeply felt words of comfort" (p. 131) from the children's mother and grandmother. Their gestures speak of a genuine connectedness and a reciprocal respectful relationship in which there is love. In an essay titled *What Does It Mean: 'Love Is Not Enough'?* Coltart (1992) wrote about love and hate in the therapeutic relationship. She asserts that love is an important component of the therapeutic relationship, and reminds us also of how difficult it is to judge psychotherapeutic work by looking to an end product. Ruth knows this, and yet he is left with a sense of dissatisfaction with the work. One of the themes of his chapter is his recurrent concern about whether what was happening in the work "was enough."

Ruth tells us it was difficult "to steer a course" with the Jones/Muhammad family. At times he wondered about the achievement of these "pleasant-enough, good-in-the-moment sessions" (p. 129). Were they good enough? He writes "what we were doing felt necessary, but perhaps not sufficient" (p. 129). I wonder what outcome he might have deemed appropriate or successful in work with this family? What would have been sufficient? He writes, "The children seemed to be doing reasonably well in foster care, and to be benefiting in appreciable ways from the family therapy" (p. 138). He adds, "In a way, these achievements are prosaic," and much of life is prosaic after all, and says that he "fiercely valued them, as did Ms. Jones and Ms. Muhammad" (p. 138). However, Ruth was left with a haunting feeling that "if we just had a little more time, things would work out" (p. 138).

I think this was what Ms. Jones hoped, and she did not give up on it. She wanted more time, and she wanted things to "work out." It seems that for her "working out" meant she and her daughter and her daughter's five children would all live together in one household. Ms. Jones is the family member with whom Ruth forms the strongest alliance, and together, in my mind, they form the parental couple in the therapy. Despite Ruth's effort to include all members of the family in his writing, I find it very difficult to grasp what Ms. Muhammad ever really felt or thought. I am struck by the passivity and at times seeming emptiness that he describes in her. I am intrigued by Ruth's wondering whether Abdul, Ms. Muhammad's youngest, might have fetal alcohol syndrome. He leaves the question hanging. There is no other mention of Ms. Muhammad's possible substance abuse.

Is this one of the horror stories that is being sanitized? I wonder what blocked Ruth's exploration of this important possibility in the family story? He writes that Ms. Jones "was raising her adult daughter . . . something she would have done naturally and willing but now was doing by court order" (p. 119). However, there is a whole chunk of history missing. What was Ms Jones's place in the family when each of Ms. Muhammad's five children was born? What communication did she maintain with her daughter? When Ruth discovers, only after being deeply involved with this family and nearly 2 years into the therapy, some of the details about the evidence of 3-year-old Mahmoud's extreme neglect at the time he was taken into foster care, Ruth writes, "It was outrageous that my social worker colleague had painted a distorted picture of the family's history at the outset" (p. 140). Was it? How could it be otherwise?

Ruth tells us, "I saw the process of the therapy as involved with my radical acceptance of the family as they were, seeing them as much through their own eyes as through mine" (p. 141). So, would it have mattered what information the social worker shared with him? Radical acceptance is important, as is trying to hold the differences between the family's way of construing reality and our own way of construing reality—what we see as their distortions. How do we build on the foundations of respect and courtesy to challenge the entrenched positions or beliefs of our patients, in ways that do not shut down thinking, is the challenge in our work. How do we hold the horror stories and keep the hope for transformation in thinking and feeling alive, in ourselves and in the work?

Ruth is a seasoned kayaker–therapist, to use Birch's paddling metaphor. He negotiated the "privileged yet perilous intimacy" (Birch, p. 8) with the Jones/Muhammad family, and the perilous forces unleashed upon their journey together, in a masterful way. Yet, as it is for all kayakers, he claims that often he felt he carried along by forces over which he had very little control. He confronts gently and respectfully, perhaps at times a little too timidly.

Ms. Jones was a strengths-based grandmother. Ruth tells us that Ms. Jones

> focused on what the children could do, rather than on what they could not, and questioned, not unreasonably, whether some of their difficulties had to do with being asked to live in different worlds simultaneously: her world and the more privileged worlds of their foster families. (p. 134)

Ruth gently challenges her. He states,

> I wanted the concept of mental retardation to be explicit in this context, and said that children can have mental retardation and also be good children, creative, and able to do and learn many things. (p. 134–135)

He says that Ms. Jones "said she understood."

I find this conversation poignant and very sad. For despite Ms. Jones's seeming to understand, it is as though she had never really been able to comprehend, embrace, and accept her daughter's limitations or those of her grandchildren. Perhaps it was just too painful for her to acknowledge Ms. Muhammad's limitations and what they meant to her as mother to a child with such limitations. In strengths-based work, the therapist is often so enthusiastic to emphasize what can be done that no time is taken to mourn what may have been lost. Without acknowledgment of the gap between the longed for and the actual, the limitations that may be inherent in the difference between these two positions cannot be fully understood or worked with. Our failure to really explore this gap in work with families means the creative potential of "what is possible" will always be muted, filtered through what we have not acknowledged together.

I am left wondering what might have been possible if Ruth had worked more intentionally with the longing and the loss, just as I am left wondering what may have been possible if I had been courageous enough to work more directly with Jay's mother's hate and disappointment in her boy in the treatment described in chapter 8.

How do we join the family or infant–parent system, and also keep a clear perspective on how being part of the system must color the lens through which we look and understand what goes on within the system? Birch reminds us that individual supervision, clinical case review with peers, and consultants can provide some help with maintaining a clear perspective.

Ruth's sharing encourages us to confront mental retardation and racial inequality with emotional honesty. Like Sinason (1993) he knows that we must embrace the unfairness of life, honestly and without sentimentality. When we do, there is a chance for transformation and for the alleviation of suffering. Ruth courageously and lovingly engages in therapy with the Jones/Muhammad family. Good things happen by their being together and thinking together. Despite this, Ruth is left with feeling he was not able to do enough, that time ran out. Whatever the limitations of the work or the outcome, I see the family as richer for their relationship with him, and I feel enriched by his sharing his reflections with us.

## REFERENCES

Coltart, N. (1992). What does it mean: "Love is not enough?" In N. Coltart, *Slouching towards Bethlehem* (pp. 111–127). London: Free Association Books.

Fraiberg, S. (1980). *Clinical studies in infant mental health*. New York: Basic Books.

Sinason, V. (1993). *Mental handicap and the human condition: New approaches from the Tavistock*. London: Free Association Books.

CHAPTER 8

# CHARLENE AND JAY

*Julie Stone*

Winnicott (1960/1980) famously reminded us "there is no such thing as a baby." The parent or caregiver is central in the infant's world and well-being. However, there are times when the interpersonal world of infant and caregiver becomes fraught with conflict and miscommunication, times when the needs of the mother are in conflict or in competition with what her child needs for healthy development.

I have chosen to write about Jay and his mother, Charlene, because our work with them painfully illustrates the dilemma and difficult-to-resolve therapeutic challenge of keeping the needs and experience of both infant and caregiver in mind without being drawn into the sometimes destructive drama being played out between them and without colluding with one against the other. In our work, as a team of two therapists working with Jay and his mother, this difficulty became intensified rather than being highlighted and better understood.

Jay and Charlene's story also illustrates the central importance of finding a place in infant–parent psychotherapy to face hate and all its emotional force, to think about it, and to work with it. The theory is clear, the practice often more complex.

It is not easy to think about the place of hate in parent–child relationships. Winnicott (1947/1975) wrote that all mothers hate their baby "from the word go," and cited, by way of example, 18 reasons why. The reasons he offered are ordinary and fairly benign. By mentioning hate, however, Winnicott reminded us that ambivalent feelings—love and hate—are part of intimacy. Hate is love's shadow. Morgan explained (in Thomson-Salo & Paul, 2004) her understanding of the relationship between love and hate: "To me, love is in the depressive position, you've gone through the schizoid stage where you have to have the split and an acute getting rid of hate" (p. 35). To love, the hate has to be owned, tolerated, and integrated. Morgan reminded us that we struggle with such feelings for our whole lives.

For the relationship between mother and infant to be "good enough" and to serve the infant's healthy development, the loving feelings must outweigh the hateful. The loving and mutually satisfying shared experiences between mother and infant must outnumber the hateful and painful experiences of misattunement, miscommunication, and misunderstanding.

Griffiths and colleagues (Bolton, Griffiths, Stone, & Thompson-Salo, 2007) wrote of the resilience a mother must bring to her role if she and her infant are to survive the sense of insufficiency she will inevitably encounter in striving to meet the needs of her infant.

What resilience and emotional stability it takes to face being unable to give our helpless, distraught, dependent infants all they need and want; to face their rage at not having their needs met, to face our own rage at them; and to go on loving and caring for them.

When the mother is feeling that her baby is telling her she is not good enough, how can she manage to stay present to the baby? What happens? The mother may protect herself from the unmanageable or threatening experience in some way, by cutting off from the raw feeling, distancing from it psychologically, or dealing with the threat to self by externalizing it and blaming someone else.

Sometimes, she blames the baby.

Charlene's pursuit of a diagnosis to explain Jay's behavior and developmental delays brings into sharp focus the inherent tension in all therapeutic work between assigning a diagnosis and seeking a dynamic understanding of the child's experience of the world and his parent's experience of the world.

The place of the infant and his experience is one of utmost importance in work with infants and their parents. Despite rhetoric to the contrary, it is sometimes overlooked, and it seems the child and his experience of the world and of therapy become sidelined to the experience of the caregiver.

My clinical practice, influenced by the work of Serge Lebovici in France and Ann Morgan, Campbell Paul, Frances Thomson-Salo, and others in Australia, has, at its heart, working directly with the infant and offering a meeting with him in his own right. That the infant has a mind and seeks to make sense of his world through interaction with the minds of others informs all of my clinical work. Charlene's need for attention and narcissistic bolstering made it seemingly impossible for her to put Jay's experience and his imperiled development at the center of the treatment. She saw and experienced Jay as a burdensome child, difficult and damaged.

Charlene had come to believe that Jay "had autism." To her this meant that Jay had "something wrong with his brain" that rendered him unable to love and be loved like "normal children." She held little or no hope for Jay's development, and saw him as destined to a life of impaired communication, robotlike interaction, and bizarre—at times "out of control behavior"—that made no sense. Charlene believed that Jay's behavior was determined by his biology, and that there was little she could do except be supported in learning how to "manage him." Reputedly, her belief was shared by Jay's grandmother and by one of the staff at the child care center Jay attended for many hours every week.

Charlene's conviction that Jay was autistic had prompted her to seek eight assessments for him prior to our involvement. He had been assessed by three different pediatricians, working in different parts of the health service, as well as by a developmental psychologist, two speech pathologists, an occupational therapist, and a physiotherapist. None found his presentation consistent with a diagnosis of autism. Jay's hearing had been assessed; concern about his excessive dribbling had been investigated. Many organic illnesses had been explored and excluded.

The third pediatrician who was asked to assess Jay became alarmed as she gathered together all of the information available in the hospital and outpatient charts. She was concerned that Jay's frequent presentation to health services was communicating something important that needed to be thought about. She referred this troubled mother and son to the Mental Health Services to see if they could help Jay and his mother make sense of what was happening in their family. Despite the findings of previous assessments, Charlene held onto her belief that Jay had autism. I suspect she hoped the Mental Health Services would see what others had not.

My first meeting with Jay was when he was 26 months old and his mother brought him to a hospital Mental Health Services department, where I spent time consulting. Charlene and Jay alone came to the appointment. A child psychiatrist in training was assigned to meet Jay. He had limited experience in assessing children under 3 years, and asked that I join him for the interview.

My colleague and I discussed how we would cofacilitate the assessment. It was agreed that he would primarily engage with Charlene, focusing on her story and observing her and her interactions, and I would engage primarily with Jay, focusing on his story and observing him and his interactions. One of our goals for this initial meeting was that both Jay and his mother would experience that they and their story were important to us.

In *The Baby as Subject*, Thomson-Salo and Paul (2004) outlined the essence of putting the infant's experience at the center of infant–parent work. In any assessment, all those who attend are welcome as having something to share; the contribution of each person present is actively sought through the intentional communication of the therapist. As well as hearing about the infant's history and listening to the parents' concerns and impressions of his behavior, the child in the room is also closely observed. The therapist remains open to and interested in the way the infant affects her, as with any countertransference. Without this openness and interest in the infant in the room, the therapist puts herself at risk of being caught up in seeing only the infant in the mother. In so doing, she loses the baby before her.

Direct communication with the infant conveys clearly the recognition that the infant has a mind and life experience to share. The therapist honors the child as a person to be known, separate from and different from his parents.

The work of Colwyn Trevarthen (2001) and Anne Alvarez (1992), among others, stressed the importance of the therapist being present and lively in working with young children and their families. This does not mean being excessively active or upbeat in the clinical encounter. As Thomson-Salo (2004) said, "[It] translates . . . to an attunement to the infant's affects, underpinned by a quiet enjoyment of what the infant brings" (p. 135). With this openness and "quiet enjoyment" in getting to know the baby, the therapist offers the infant an important experience. Trevarthen believed that the infant's sense of being enjoyed as a lively and engaging partner is an important contributor to the infant's sense of pride and budding sense of self.

Finally, of course, the therapist brings together in his or her mind all of the pieces—history, presenting concerns, observations, and reflection upon the meeting—in the hope of bringing some new understanding that will serve the family and help alleviate the distress and suffering that have prompted their presentation.

In meeting a family for the first time, I always introduce myself to each of them, including even the youngest infant. As part of the intention to communicate with the infant, I also ensure that a simple narrative description of what is happening in the consulting room is offered to the child so that he is included as an essential part of what goes on. This narrative communicates to the infant that he is seen, that the infant is considered worthy of being spoken to, that the infant and his mind is held in the mind of the therapist. The young child often responds and enters the dialogue in a way that suggests he follows a good deal of the meaning; that it is the infant's story being told.

Parents and caretakers are asked to alert me if there is any aspect of our discussion that they feel is inappropriate to discuss in front of the child. In turn, I promise that we will find another time when we can explore such material more fully. Charlene scoffed at this and at my conversation with Jay. "Oh don't worry, Jay does not understand anything of what is happening around him. He is 'not there,'" she said, pointing to her head. I felt wiped out by Charlene's comments, negated, dismissed. I wondered if this was an echo of how Jay might experience his mother.

After introducing himself to Jay and to Charlene, my colleague engaged Charlene. He was warm and sympathetic, listening thoughtfully and asking pertinent and important questions. Engaging Jay proved more difficult.

We heard that from the time Jay was 2 months old, his young mother, just 19 when he was born, had taken him to many professionals for consultation. She was "worried about him." She wanted to know "what was wrong with him." Since birth, his mother said, Jay slept poorly, he fed and gained weight poorly, he responded and interacted poorly. She thought he was "angry and irritable with her." She believed her young son "hated her."

In telling us that she believed Jay hated her, Charlene was alerting us to something very important about her experience as Jay's mother. I wondered if she needed her son to carry her hate, and whether her belief about Jay's feeling toward her was a replay of the hateful relationship she had had with Jay's father and the heartbreak she experienced when her own father left "without saying good-bye" when she was 2 years old. Might she not have felt that he hated her too? What I did not think about was that Charlene might have firmly closed the door on the possibility of a loving connection with Jay.

Jay sat on the floor where his mother placed him. He was stiff and seemingly lifeless. He had no curiosity for the array of toys that were available to him, and he made no reference to me. He did not return my gaze, and seemed not to register my greeting. Indeed it seemed that I was not there to him, and that his mother was right in that Jay was not present to the world around him.

I was undeterred. I continued to talk to him quietly, commenting and trans-lating into simple language for him aspects and themes of the dialogue that my colleague and his mommy were having. My interest in Jay was not dependent upon his interest in me. I could wait quietly, undemanding in my expectation that, given time, his curiosity and interest would be aroused by my interest in him and his experience.

Toward the end of the interview, Jay made a few furtive glances toward me. He looked from the corner of his eye. His face did not register any emotion. However, as they were leaving, he briefly looked directly at me and said, "bye-bye." His mother was delighted, saying proudly that she had just taught him to wave good-bye. My heart sank. Charlene's claim to the one meaningful communication that Jay offered in our first meeting was an ominous indication that perhaps she experienced his accomplishments only in terms of their narcissistic value to her as an accomplished mother and not in terms of any empathic understanding of Jay's experience or wish to communicate.

Perhaps the most striking thing from this first meeting was how utterly enchanted my colleague was with Charlene. He was full of sympathy for her and very concerned about how she could manage Jay's "difficult behavior." He found her articulate, thoughtful, and "clearly a very concerned mother." The Jay alive in his mind—demanding, destructive, and difficult—was very different from the Jay I had been with. His enchantment with Jay's mother was at odds with my impressions of a needy, preoccupied, and self-absorbed young woman whose own needs seemed to leave little room for the needs of her child. My colleague and I had met a very different mother and a very different baby.

Working with a cotherapist offers a wonderful opportunity to model two independent minds working collaboratively: seeing and experiencing different things, and respectfully thinking about and discussing these differences. With curiosity and an expectation of a greater richness of understanding from the bringing together of two minds, new understanding can and does unfold. This is, of course, the infant's experience when he is cared for by two parents who are committed to each other and to caring for him. I suspected that neither Charlene nor Jay had ever had the experience of being thoughtfully held in the minds of a cooperating couple. The experience of being part of a working threesome, sometimes being a part of the main action, some-times being left out, is one of the ways that children learn to embrace the hating and the loving, to integrate them rather than to keep them split off from one another. At this stage, I did not know what resistance we would encounter in trying to bring the pieces together.

Jay's father, Errol, was absent from his life. He had been a heavy drug user, mainly intravenous amphetamines. Charlene reported that Errol's behavior was erratic and at times extremely violent. She said Errol's violence escalated after Jay was born. She finally left him, taking her son home to her mother. Charlene said Jay suckled at her breast "for hours." Errol would become enraged by this. On the occasion that precipitated Charlene's departure, she said Errol had grabbed Jay from her breast and flung him onto the bed beside her. She was shaken and shocked, and left quietly the following morning.

By contrast, her new partner, Al, she said, could not do enough for her. When asked about his relationship with Jay, she replied, "He loves Jay." This was at odds with her reporting how she once took Jay to the local hospital demand-ing some respite from Jay's constant demands and neediness. At that time, Charlene had explained that Al was at the end of his tether. He was threaten-ing to leave her unless she could "shut the kid up." Charlene told us she hoped to have another baby, and believed that Al would be a "wonderful father."

I was left with many concerns. My colleagues who had previously assessed Jay had identified problems in his relationship with his mother; Charlene and her son were clearly not relating well. My colleagues had noted the violent and trau-matic early months, and suspected that Jay experienced posttraumatic symp-toms and was extremely anxious. They noted developmental delays, particularly in his communication. Jay's expressive language was rudimentary, but he was building his vocabulary slowly and using the words he did have appropriately, sometimes using two and three words together. He articulated poorly and was sometimes difficult to understand, although his jargon had a communicative prosody and was thought to be used contextually and appropriately. Jay often seemed to "phase out," and his attention was variable. At times, he was difficult to engage. His receptive language was assessed as being disrupted by his variable attention, but he was observed to respond appropriately to simple requests and to follow the conversation.

After my meeting with Jay, I thought his flat, lifeless presentation suggested he might be seriously depressed. Charlene certainly seemed motivated to "get some help," and was rightly worried about how she would manage when she had another baby.

Charlene and Jay were offered a place in an infant mental health program where I also spent time. Charlene and Jay were told that the program would focus on helping them relate more enjoyably with one another, and that we would collaborate with them and all the other people and agencies involved in supporting Jay's development. Charlene seemed keen to come.

However, just prior to the first appointment, she telephoned to tell us that the family was moving to a town 100 miles away because Al had a new job. Charlene also wanted to share her happy news that she was pregnant. She said she would continue with Jay's speech therapy, and had a further appointment with the pediatrician.

I did not meet Jay again for more than a year.

Then, out of the blue, Charlene telephoned and asked if she could still bring Jay to the program. I invited her to come to talk about what was happening with her and Jay, and to see if the program had anything to offer them. Several weeks later, she brought Jay to see me. Charlene had put on a lot of weight, and she looked pale and tired. Jay too looked pale and tired. I greeted Jay and reminded him we had met before, saying it was "a long time ago, when you were much younger; you have grown." He stared at me wide-eyed and quizzical, seeming to listen, but he did not respond in any discernable way.

Over the course of three assessment sessions, Charlene explained she had walked out on her relationship following her discovery that Al had begun a sexual relationship with a woman at his new place of work. She said Al had become increasingly cool, preferring to spend his evenings with this woman than to be with Charlene and Jay. She said he seemed to have lost interest in her, adding, "he was never very interested in Jay." Charlene had returned to the city. She and Jay were again living with her mother until she could find "something that would suit them."

Charlene was hurt and angry. She felt overlooked and discarded by Al. Where once she had spoken of him only in glowing terms, now it seemed he was without any positive attributes. With the force of her anger and disappointment focused on Al, Charlene seemed softer in her concern about Jay. This may have been because she could "blame" Al, which gave Jay some respite.

Charlene now reported that Al had "never liked Jay", a very different story to the one she offered at our last meeting. She said he was very cruel to Jay, particularly when he had been drinking. Charlene reported he had been physically and verbally abusive of Jay. She said that Al would taunt Jay, ridicule him, physically provoke him, and then laugh before becoming angry. Al would hit Jay if he lashed out or became angry in return.

When asked what she had done when this behavior was occurring, Charlene replied that sometimes she would join Al in taunting Jay. She added, "I should have stopped him, or reported him for child abuse." I wondered what stopped her and if Jay was offered up to Al's violence as a way of protecting herself. Despite the anger she was now feeling toward Al, Charlene described a perverse coalition of parental figures against the child in saying that she sometimes joined Al in taunting Jay. I wondered if there was ever a time when Al had joined with Charlene in an alliance in which together they could think about Jay and his needs. It seemed unlikely. I wondered too what Jay made of his experience in this family and how we might make sense of this young mother's complex need to be loved and what experiences she had that led her to choose men who treated her and her child so cruelly.

Now reflecting on this case, many years later, I wonder what stopped me from further exploring the protective concerns that I had about Jay's safety in the care of his mother or from thinking more clearly and courageously about the limits to this young mother's capacity to provide Jay with a good-enough emotional environment in which to grow and develop. Was I seduced by this mother's seeming eagerness for help, and so rendered unable to think the terrible thought that Charlene really might not be able find in herself a sustained and genuine longing for Jay to be happy? Maybe Jay's delayed and stunted development might be meeting a need in her, and maybe, in turn, Jay's distorted behaviour had become his most potent and effective means of engaging his mother and so, in its way, it came to serve him too?

In our striving to identify the strengths—those qualities upon which we can build and encourage to develop—in a caregiver, it may be that sometimes we eschew or underplay the perverse, hateful, and split-off parts of the parent. In so doing, we collude with them and inadvertently reinforce the split rather than creating a space in which all aspects of the parent's and the infant's experience can be thought about.

In child protection work, hateful acts are not uncommon, yet it remains extremely difficult to think, unflinchingly, about hate. As therapists working with young children and their parents, how do we find a place of compassion in ourselves that allows us to think simultaneously about the parent and the painful history that typically sets the stage for enactments of parental hate, *and* to see clearly the force of the hate in such acts and its impact upon the infant and young child? Blaming the parent is not a creative position. Yet, as Griffiths and colleagues (Bolton et al., 2004) described, knowing this may mean we get caught in the pursuit of "not blaming," rather than thinking about what appears to be blameful. Do we, and did I, flinch from thinking about hate because I was afraid of my own hate and destructive potential? Fearful perhaps that I too might be hateful were I unable to find and nourish the place of possibility for change within this troubled infant–parent relationship? Charlene and Jay were not part of the child protection system. She came seeking help, and we wanted to help her and her son.

While Charlene was talking about the events of the past year, from time to time I spoke to Jay, commenting on the conversation that I was having with his mother. For example, "Mommy is just telling me that sometimes Daddy

Al got very cross and angry, and sometimes you got hurt. It sounds very frightening." One of the messages I hoped that Charlene and Jay would hear was that all things can be thought about and talked about, and that naming the probable affect would be helpful to them both. Yet, in our subsequent work together, I did not find a place to think about the hate; it remained split off and unnamed.

Jay remained aloof, but he seemed to listen closely. On the one occasion he reached out toward a toy, his mother remarked, "Jay doesn't play; he is not interested in toys." He soon let the toy drop. Even in a softer space with Jay, Charlene was unrelenting in her negative attributions of Jay and his behavior. It was painful to witness and to be with. I felt a deadening within myself and again wondered if this gave some clue to Jay's experience.

Charlene told me about the family's difficult year. She had delighted in being pregnant but "lost the baby" after 10 weeks, soon after their relocation. She said she had suffered from "depression." She became impatient with my questions about this and dismissed them by stating, "I'm better now."

Charlene said she continued to struggle with Jay and his "maniac behavior." She complained that Jay screamed "all the time," and reported that he was "always angry," frequently smashing or breaking things. Charlene also complained that, try as she might to reason with him, he just "would not listen." Charlene said she had continued to take him to speech therapy "most weeks," but felt it really was a waste of time as he was "getting worse, not better." She said he was clumsy and awkward, and believed that sometimes he did things just to "get at her."

Over the course of the year, when Charlene was struggling with Jay, her failed pregnancy and depression, her partner's increasing alcohol use and his absence, Jay's behavior had become unmanageable for Charlene. He spent long hours in child care. She said he often spent "a week or so" at a time with his grandmother, who drove to collect Jay to give Charlene "a break." Charlene said her mother also found Jay's behavior difficult to manage. Charlene said her mom thought Jay was "a weird kid," and shared Charlene's belief that Jay had autism.

With Charlene's permission, we contacted the child care center Jay had recently left. I spoke with the supervisor who said that she was pleased that I telephoned, as she was very worried about Jay. She was concerned that his mother was often "quite mean" to him and went on to say, "It's funny, some of my staff loved Charlene and thought she was the best mom in the world; others hated her."

The child care staff had observed that Jay was often silent and his language was developing slowly. At times he made an effort to communicate and was pleased if he was successful in making himself understood; he became very frustrated when he was not understood. Jay demonstrated clear favorites among the staff, had learned their names, and used them appropriately. They were sorry not to have had a chance to say good-bye to him.

The supervisor commented that Jay found it difficult to play. He often seemed fixed and preoccupied in rolling cars back and forth, and was reported to do so for long periods of time. However, he could tolerate interruption and was able to embrace another's elaboration of his "game." He did not interact much with the other children, but would join with simple group activities. He was rarely, if ever, seen as a happy boy, and his caregivers thought he was sad and worried.

She reported he was, at times, very aggressive to other younger children, and certainly when frustrated he could "scream the place down." He had also been observed to pat another little boy who was crying, saying to him in a voice that sounded kind, "No cry, no cry." Charlene indicated Jay demanded that routines be strictly adhered to. The child care center found Jay most often could accommodate changes in the day-to-day routines. The staff had not observed any repetitive or stereotyped mannerisms.

At times Jay seemed to be walled off, remote from the world. The child care supervisor reported that sometimes Jay seemed "lost" and was difficult to reach. I wondered if Jay was dissociating or if his disconnection was evidence of a protective shell, as described by Tustin (1990), grown to ward off the traumatic attacks he had experienced in his short life. Tustin suggested when the mother, for whatever reason, is unable to protect the infant from frightening experiences that impinge upon him and threaten him, some infants "originate their own protective covering" (p. 82) by wrapping themselves in their own bodily sensations. They become preoccupied with their own sensations and so can "ignore their dependence on others." This pathological self-sufficiency is what Tustin saw as at the core of the autistic child's difficulties in engaging with the world; their protective shell is their defense against the terror of annihilation and also their barrier to the world of relationship with others.

At times Jay's behavior did look autistic. It seemed that he had developed some autistic-like defenses to help him manage the sometimes impossible world of feelings and relationships; but there were many inconsistencies in his presentation. I thought that most of his behavior could be explained and understood as a response to the violence he had experienced in his early relationships and by the difficulties he and his mom had in meeting one another.

On our second meeting, again Jay hardly interacted with the toys at all. He did explore the playroom with a little more interest, and repetitively rolled some cars back and forth in a desultory and lifeless kind of way. He had been essentially silent throughout. After speaking with the child care supervisor, I decided I would like to observe Jay separately from his mother, to see what, if any, changes there may be in how he related to me or in how he engaged with the toys in the room.

Another colleague, Vicki, an experienced senior clinician, was invited to meet with Charlene to ask her more about her losses and to explore her hopes for the future. Whilst Vicki was talking with Charlene, Jay and I shared some time in the room where we had met previously with his mother.

During this third meeting, Jay seemed to gain some energy and was able to engage in some meaningful play for the first time. He offered me a glass, into which he poured imaginary coffee from the pot. He prepared a pizza from the Play-Doh and shared this between the two of us. I was touched by this interchange, and felt very appreciative of Jay's gesture, perhaps because it lit a glimmer of hope for his capacity and for the possibility of his engaging in therapy in a way that may help him more fully engage in the world. I felt a longing for things to be different for this boy, and I was aware of an intense sense of loss and sadness. Although I had no doubt of Jay's capacity for aggression, sadness/depression had been the dominant affect in our meetings. There was also the lifeless deadening I have spoken of. I felt this boy was in need of live company (Alvarez, 1992). *Live company* is a phrase used by Colwyn Trevarthan that Alvarez took as the title for her wonderful book detailing her long analysis with a young, troubled boy. In saying "I felt Jay was in need of live company," I mean that it seemed important for Jay to have the experience of being in the presence of someone who could avail their heart and mind to him, be open to him and his communication, and who could enjoy being with him and responding to him.

After a brief reflective discussion with Vicki, we offered to work with Charlene and Jay, both individually and together. In our infant–parent program we often worked in this way. Our experience was that the joint work, the child–parent therapy, was often enhanced when both parent and child had a space in which to have a therapist's undivided attention before coming together for the joint relationship work. Many of the mothers we saw were overburdened and needy; almost all of them would have benefited from individual psychotherapy. Most of these women, however, were not ready to consider such a referral, and services for them were limited. What we offered was a space in which the therapist supported the mother to think about her child(ren). The therapist helped the mother make links between past and present, with the hope that this thinking would lead her to a greater understanding of her contribution to the relationship dance with her children.

Some of the children also needed a therapeutic space in which they could explore their feelings free from their caregiver's habitual responses to them. Although individual work with children and their parents was often part of the work we did with families, it was always an adjunct to the dyadic or family work. The sessions always ended with bringing child(ren) and parent(s) together. Our usual experience was that the parent(s) was more able to respond warmly and empathically to her child(ren) when she felt that she had had some space for herself.

Charlene seemed to relish the opportunity to spend time with Vicki, who found her lively and likeable. Our hope was that Vicki would be able to create a space in which she and Charlene could think about Jay and their experiences together and in which they could together explore ways for Charlene "to have a life" and be a mother. I elected to work with Jay. Our hope was for Jay to become more alive to himself and to relationship through our psychotherapy, and that this, in turn, would enliven his relationship with his mother, who we assumed would be relieved and delighted by her son's increased liveliness. Looking back, they seem ambitious and somewhat grandiose plans. However, as Thomson-Salo and Paul (2004) noted, "Most parents, if they present with a distressed infant, want help for their infant and welcome the therapist's direct intervention" (p. 14). This was certainly our most frequent experience. Thomson-Salo and Paul stated that "working with the parents was seen [by those who do not work directly with the infant] to affirm them as parents and not to exacerbate guilt or envy" (p. 33). Not working with Jay directly may have avoided Charlene's envy, and yet I think that Jay would have missed out on an important experience. In families in which the mother's guilty or rivalrous feelings are stirred up in the therapy, perhaps it would be more helpful for both mother and infant if we could find ways to think about such feelings and work with them rather than avoiding them. Sadly, we did not manage to do this in our work with Jay and Charlene.

Although the therapeutic plans were discussed with Charlene and she appeared to accept them, we failed to appreciate how fervently she continued to hold on to the idea that Jay had autism or to understand why this was so important to her. Her goal of ultimately receiving this diagnosis for him was at odds with the one we had identified for him and thought we were working toward together.

From the outset, the individual time went well enough. Vicki and Charlene developed a strong relationship, and Vicki reported Charlene was appreciative of the support and of the opportunity to talk about what was happening in her life and with Jay. Charlene expressed her longing to find another partner and to have another baby, a baby girl.

After meeting weekly for several months, Jay began relate to me in a more robust way. He verbalized more, and his speech was becoming increasingly easier to understand. Jay showed his pleasure in greeting me, and ran ahead of me into the therapy room.

His need to test the limits of the therapy room was a constant challenge. A number of games developed out of this. One grew from my need to rescue Jay from climbing onto some shelves where the toys were kept. The shelves were not fixed to the wall and would have been precarious with the extra weight of a little boy. The first time he began to climb up, I firmly took hold of him and placed him on the floor saying, "No Jay, it is not safe." He looked surprised, and again made toward the shelves to climb them—again and again. Each time I would say, "No, no Jay, it is not safe," placing him on a small colored carpet square. Sometimes I would call him a "little monkey." Sometimes he crawled toward the shelves, sometimes he would walk. Jay loved this game, and would visit it for one or more rounds each time we met. It was as though he liked to hear me say over and over again that I would intervene to keep him safe.

His affect remained limited. Although there were shared moments of delight, overall he seemed worried and sad. During one session, he curled up beneath my chair and sobbed. I sat on the floor near him and spoke gently to him about his sad and lonely feelings. Sometimes Jay brought his rageful and destructive feelings into the therapy room. When this happened, Jay experienced that he could survive them, I could survive them, and that our relationship could survive them too. The rules of safety were, of course, paramount.

One afternoon Jay seemed more cutoff than usual. He began to throw the blocks, first in a desultory, directionless way and then at me. I reiterated that this was a space where he could throw the blocks, but no one must get hurt. He was not to get hurt, and I was not to get hurt either. I told him it was also a place where we would talk about and think about his mad and throwing feelings. He continued to throw toys, and then swiped all the toys from the shelf and went to stamp on them. I restrained him and said I would not let him break the toys. I held him while he writhed and raged against me physically. I spoke with him quietly, telling him I would hold him until his bubbling over hurting, throwing feelings had quietened down. I told him I would hold him until he could be safe and I could be safe and no one would get hurt. Eventually he quietened, and when we came together he went to his mother for a cuddle. Charlene seemed surprised and responded to her son's overture. I explained that Jay had worked hard in therapy today, and he had been exploring some very big feelings. It seemed the therapy was developing slowly and well.

Bringing Charlene and Jay together did not often go well. It was fractious and fraught. Charlene usually seemed disinterested in engaging Jay. Creating opportunities for "interactional guidance" was tough, and opportunities to build on mutual enjoyment and reciprocity in their relationship were scarce. Charlene wanted attention too from Vicki and from me. She became increasingly petulant with me, and complained to Vicki that I treated her "like a child."

Hopkins (2003) warned, in her article on therapeutic work with infants, discussing countertransference, "Unfortunately, countertransference can also be a source of difficulty in this work, especially when therapist's feelings become split between parent and infant" (p. 129). In working with Jay and Charlene, there were the feelings of two therapists that at times were split between parent and child. Bringing the pieces together proved difficult. Hopkins went on to explain that the mother "rightly" became angry with her when she "briefly took sides." Hopkins became exasperated with the mother, and "identified with the child's cries, and treated her [the mother] as the patient." I suspect Charlene's criticism that I treated her like a child meant that she felt I had lost sight of her as Jay's mother.

We did not spend enough time together thinking about these splits or the implications of them. Nor did Vicki and I engage fully with thinking about the difficulty we had in thinking together about this family. It was much more difficult than usual to come together to share our thoughts and reflect upon the therapy and how it was progressing. In our effort to heal the splits in the family relationships, we fell into them and seemed unable to breach them or to think about them. Reflective supervision with the team did not bring enlightenment either. Perhaps they too had become divided in a way that stopped us thinking creatively.

We did not give enough thought to Charlene's complaint that I treated her like a child, nor, perhaps, did I consider the gravity and importance of Charlene's complaints that I was too permissive with Jay, that I allowed him "to trash the room." She was angry that I did not insist he "clean up." She said she was afraid that Jay would expect her to clean up after him, complaining that I was undermining her authority. I explained that I never expect a child to clear up the therapy room; I see this as part of my role and my work. As I quietly restore the room to order for the next young visitor, I think over the play and what was communicated during the session. I believe that the child knows I will think about whatever he has left with me.

For Charlene it seemed that my containment of her son and his messy rageful feelings enraged her. She felt invalidated and undermined, and was suspicious that I was stealing Jay's love, which should be for her, his mother.

One week, Charlene arrived excited to share with us her pride in Jay. They had been invited to join in celebration for an uncle's birthday. Previously such occasions had been "a nightmare" for Charlene—Jay usually screamed and generally created havoc. On this occasion, all had gone well. Many people had congratulated Charlene on the "marvelous job" she was doing; Jay had been "great." Charlene had enjoyed him, and it seemed they had enjoyed the outing together. Vicki and I were delighted, and hoped that this was the promise of more harmonious family music to follow.

However, it did not last. Except for brief glimpses of the possibility of something being different, for the most part, Charlene took no pleasure from Jay or in his increasing vitality. She believed that he liked seeing me only because I "let him do what he wanted." It was not the case that I let him do whatever he wanted, though I tried to let him know it was all right to want whatever he wanted. The limits of the therapy room were very clear, and Jay knew them and accepted them. I do not think I was overindulgent of Jay, but his mother certainly did.

Writing about children with autism or who use autistic-like defenses, Tustin (1990) managed to explain the mystery of therapy to the mother of a boy she was seeing in therapy. She wrote a letter to the mother explaining the following:

> The child is in a situation where he can express his feelings, but he is not allowed to become overwhelmed by them. The therapist tries to hold these feelings in her mind and to talk with him about them and to express them to some extent, but he is helped to do this through such activities as talking, playing, etc. He is shown that it is all right to have feelings, but it is no good letting him just rampage around destroying everything, upsetting the therapist's capacity to think, and then deluding oneself that this will do the child good. It will do him a lot of harm. Psychotherapy uses the subtle way of helping the child to show his feelings and then helping him to pattern them. They do not go through the therapist like a dose of salts. They go into her mind, and she metabolizes them there by thinking. It is a very difficult situation to know how far to let a child go so that we know what he is thinking and feeling, and to know when to stop him and talk with him about his feelings. If children are left in the grip of their destructive feelings and nobody is helping them to pattern them, then it is a very frightening situation for them. They feel left on their own to deal with these feelings in their own naïve way, which may be extremely restrictive and repressive. Autistic strategies are an attempt to have a strong barrier against those explosive feelings. (p. 73)

This is a lucid description of what happens in psychotherapy with a young child. Jay was a boy left in the grip of his destructive feelings, and, for complex reasons of her own, his mother was unable to help him with them. In fact, she may have needed him to "carry" her own destructiveness. It seemed that Jay's destructive feelings had become intertwined with hers; their traumatic and violent history was shared. My work was to help Jay pattern these feelings, to name them, understand them, and so be freer to manage them rather to continue in their destructive grip. As well as working individually with Jay, in our work with the dyad we also made every effort we could to help Charlene and Jay better understand what was happening between them.

However, we were unable to facilitate Charlene becoming more able to see the world from Jay's point of view or to see the individual therapy as being in the service of his development and their relationship. Perhaps we could have been more helpful had we done things differently. Perhaps it was not possible for her to make the necessary shifts to embrace Jay or not in the time available for Jay.

Tustin (1990) described the recipient of her letter as "a very co-operative mother." In many ways Charlene also seemed very cooperative. She was responsible and always came on time, often early, for their appointments. If, for some reason, she was unable to come she would telephone in good time to let us know. She was very dedicated to "seeking help" for Jay; she brought him to see us, she took him to his continuing work in speech therapy, she drove him to two different schools. Yet there was also a steely resistance in her to seeing the developmental gains that Jay was making.

After 8 months of working together regularly, Charlene telephoned Vicki to announce that she and Jay would not be coming back. Finally Jay would receive some "proper help," as he had been diagnosed with autism.

I was flabbergasted, as was the rest of the team. Vicki admitted later she had an inkling "Charlene was up to something." She knew that Charlene had been seeing a psychologist who "was very helpful" to her because, she said, he knew she was "the mother and must be in charge." Charlene's sense of not being taken seriously by me was perhaps echoed in her rubbishing the work Jay and I were doing together by bringing it to an abrupt and premature end. She said they would not be coming back. It was as though she could not value any of the work we had shared.

Over the ensuing weeks, Vicki and I attempted to engage Charlene. We invited her and Jay to at least say good-bye. We were concerned about what sense Jay would make of never seeing us again; another abrupt and traumatic ending. In a telephone conversation with Vicki, Charlene said as it was some weeks since Jay had seen us, he had probably already forgotten who we were. What we had offered had been pushed aside, discarded, and reviled. This felt like the repetition of a destructive pattern we had not thought about clearly or fully enough in our work with Charlene and Jay.

Finally, brokenhearted, we had to concede we had been sacked and there would be no opportunity for reparation. We wrote letters: one to Charlene and one for her to read to Jay, in which we attempted to honor them and the work we had shared and in which we expressed our hopes for their futures.

Although Jay's behavior was, at times, very disturbed and challenging, and his language development significantly delayed, I was certain that Jay did not have autism. I was shocked that no one from the assessment panel had sought our professional observations or opinion about this boy. The psychologist Charlene had found whom she felt understood her had arranged for the panel assessment. He had provided the only report, and Charlene had refused permission for the assessment team to contact any of the services that had previously been involved with her and her son. Within the stark facts that were reviewed, Jay's reported and observed behavior and his delayed development led to a provisional diagnosis of autism.

I telephoned the pediatrician involved. He said the team had assigned a provisional diagnosis because the team members had been uncertain about a number of key issues. He admitted that he and several other panel members had found Charlene "very difficult." They had been surprised by Charlene's refusal to allow them to talk with other professionals who had been involved with Jay and his family. My colleague said that Charlene's refusal was very unusual. He said he was left feeling uneasy about her refusal and what it might mean.

Following our discussion, the assessment team made full cooperation from the parent(s)—including permission to allow the team to seek whatever collateral information they could to supplement their observations—a necessary condition to complete an autism assessment. A clearly articulated position about talking with others, he hoped, would avoid unhelpful collusion in the future.

Charlene had demonstrated a remarkable capacity to engage service providers and to split them into good or bad, helpful or unhelpful, supporting her or undermining her. Yet we failed to really see and think about the split that had widened in our team. The pediatrician who first made the referral to mental health services stated her concern that Jay's frequent presentation to health services was communicating something important that needed to be thought about. She was right. Despite our best intentions, we missed some very important opportunities to do this thinking, and so failed Jay and his mother.

A pediatric or psychiatric evaluation can and should bring fragmented experiences together, helping child and family better understand the complex interplay of biology, history, and experience across generations and in specific relationships. However, all too often a brief or simplistic evaluation leading to a diagnosis does not serve the child or his or her family well. *DC:0–3R* (ZERO TO THREE, 2005) is a very important and illuminating diagnostic classification system for young children and infants. However, as a psychiatrist often looked to make or endorse a diagnosis in young children, I am wary about the hasty assignment of diagnosis. It often seems that a diagnostic label does little or nothing to enhance thinking or understanding about a child's perplexing or challenging behaviors, doing little to help others see the world from the child's point of view or to offer understanding that may alleviate or diminish the child's distress.

It is possible for a diagnosis to impinge upon a child's sense of self and to leave him thinking or feeling that he is damaged in some way, that there is something wrong with him and his brain. Children can also be left with a sense that somehow all the distress and concern about their behavior is caused by them and so is "their fault." When funding for services is linked to diagnosis, some argue that diagnosis is a fair means to this end. I disagree, although I see the matter is a vexed and complex one.

A thoughtfully determined and well-supported diagnosis can bring enormous relief and enhanced understanding for parents. However, there are also times when it seems that in some cases for some parents, the assigning of a psychiatric diagnosis leaves them feeling victorious and with a sense that they are vindicated. I suspect that in some way this is how Charlene felt. I can only hope that her relief in finally getting someone to affirm her belief that Jay was autistic also led to greater understanding to help her and Jay relate in a more mutually rewarding manner.

## Acknowledgments

Heartfelt thanks to Jay and Charlene and all the families who taught me so much in my professional journey. Thanks also to Shirley, Ralph, Grant, and Denise, my family of origin, for my first vital lessons in loving and being loved and in knowing I would survive hating and being hated. To Peter, whose loving support facilitates all of my creative endeavors. Finally, thanks to my many wonderful colleagues, to the courageous Family Early Intervention Program team, and most especially to Frances, Carol, and Judy, whose sharing has enriched my understanding and my life.

## References

Alvarez, A. (1992). *Live company: Psychoanalytic psychotherapy with autistic, borderline, deprived and abused children.* New York: Brunner Routledge.

Bolton, C., Griffiths, J., Stone, J., & Thomson-Salo, F. (2007). The experience of infant observation: A theme and variation for four voices. *Infant Observation, 10*(2), 129–141.

Hopkins, J. (2003). Therapeutic interventions in infancy: Two contrasting cases of persistent crying. In J. Raphael-Leff (Ed.), *Parent–infant psychodynamics: Wild things, mirrors and ghosts* (pp. 131–141). London: Whurr Publishers.

Thomson-Salo, F. (2004). Summarising infant–parent psychotherapy principles: RESPECT the baby as subject. In F. Thomson-Salo & C. Paul (Eds.),

*The baby as subject: New directions in infant–parent psychotherapy from the Royal Children's Hospital, Melbourne* (pp. 134–138). Melbourne, Australia: Stonnington Press.

Thomson-Salo, F., & Paul, C. (2004). Some principles of infant–parent psychotherapy: Ann Morgan's contribution. In F. Thomson-Salo & C. Paul (Eds.), *The baby as subject: New directions in infant–parent psychotherapy from the Royal Children's Hospital, Melbourne* (pp. 27–41). Melbourne, Australia: Stonnington Press.

Trevarthen, C. (2001). Intrinsic motives for companionship in understanding: Their origin, development, and significance for infant mental health. *Infant Mental Health Journal, 22*(1–2), 95–131.

Tustin, F. (1990). *The protective shell in children and adults.* London: Karnac.

Winnicott, D. W. (1975). Hate in the countertransference. In D. W. Winnicott, *Through paediatrics to psychoanalysis: Collected works* (pp.194–203). New York: Basic Books. (Original work published 1947)

Winnicott, D. W. (1980). The theory of the parent-infant relationship. In D. W. Winnicott, *The maturational process and the facilitating environment* (pp. 37–55). London: Karnac. (Original work published 1960)

ZERO TO THREE. (2005). *Diagnostic classification of mental health and developmental disorders of infancy and early childhood: Revised edition (DC:0–3R).* Washington, DC: ZERO TO THREE.

# CHAPTER 9

# DISCUSSION OF JULIE STONE'S CASE

*Martin Maldonado-Durán*

Investigators in the area of evolutionary medicine tell us that there is always a conflict between the interests of the baby in utero and those of his mother. Mother and infant to some extent "struggle" during pregnancy for nutrients and blood supply. Once the baby is born, the human infant is considered highly "altricial," which means that the mother (and other caregivers) have to make an enormous investment of energy, time, and care to promote the survival of the infant. Compared with other animals, the human infant seems highly dependent, needy, and vulnerable for quite a long period of time. It is extremely "costly" for parents to support the development of such a large brain, from the evolutionary point of view.

It has been suggested that in species (like primates) that have very dependent and vulnerable babies with such large brains, an evolutionary strategy develops that has been called "cooperative breeding" (Hrdy, 2005). This strategy is thought to have evolved in humans (and other primates) many thousands of years ago. In cooperative breeding, other females usually assist the new mother in taking care of the baby and of the mother herself. Usually, it is the females with a closer biological relatedness to the new mother that are the most interested in the new baby and are the individuals who assist the mother, providing her with food, rest, care, and so forth. In many traditional human societies this is indeed what happens. Cooperative breeding in such societies often takes the form of highly ritualized sets of behaviors and "obligations" that relatives have to fulfill when a woman is pregnant and when she has delivered a new baby. Even nonmature individuals, such as cousins and nieces, are fascinated with the new baby, who exerts a powerful influence on those around her to elicit care and protection.

In situations when this help and support are not possible, the mother may lose interest in the baby and develop behaviors that are "not maternal" toward the child, in the form of rough handling, relative neglect, or frank hostility. In other words, the usual "altruistic behaviors" of the mother are deviated, do not develop, or are "perverted" somehow. This evolutionary/biological/cultural point of view throws light on the situation described in this case.

Furthermore, in traditional societies, these childhood experiences in girls (and boys) of observing "baby care" (handling, holding, feeding, playing, etc.) seem to be important learning experiences for the children once they become parents themselves. They would have been exposed to "models" of providing care for a small infant, and this would assist them when in turn they have a child. In societies with very "nuclearized" families; that is, where multiple generations do not coexist and the close observation of child care by concerned persons other than the parents is not possible, many new parents are "born as parents" (Lebovici, Barriguete, & Salinas, 2002, p. 167) lacking many important tools to face the multiple and exhausting demands of a small baby.

There is also a fair amount of evidence indicating that a new mother who herself has not been mothered in an empathic or sensitive way will experience more challenges in providing "maternal care" to her own child. This can be seen from the transgenerational and individual point of view, in terms of the life history of the new mother.

These two lines of thought may throw some light on understanding the situation presented by this young mother, Charlene, and her little boy Jay.

Unfortunately, the situation presented here is not at all rare but is, rather, a good example of what often happens in specialized services dealing with parents and infants. The clinician is faced with a mother who is very inexperienced in terms of providing care and who has hardly any support to be a mother. In the case of

Jay's mother, the caregiving system includes exclusively the young mother and her infant, without even marginal support from the child's father.

Although the evolutionary, biological, or even cultural considerations may not be immediately applicable in terms of understanding a dyad such as Jay and his mother, those perspectives are very important in understanding the context in which this child comes into the world.

In the description provided in this case, there are several quite difficult expectations and needs. The clinicians hope to fill "gaps" that are enormous, and this is to be accomplished through psychological means in a model that involves psychotherapeutic interventions. However, is this what this family needed? Can such gaps be filled in this way?

Emmy Werner, in her studies of follow-up of resilient individuals from infancy through the fourth decade of life, found that these resilient individuals had mostly stabilized their life, but even when many had been in counseling and psychotherapy, looking back on those experiences, only 5% of them thought that it was useful at all (Werner & Smith, 2001). That is, very few thought that seeing a therapist or counselor helped them in any way. The sad lesson from that study is that despite the best efforts from many mental health professionals, one's assistance may not be quite what the person needed at the time, or the type of assistance offered is not helpful, at least at that particular point.

What do families define as "help" or even more to the point "psychological help?" The case history appears to illustrate a mismatch between the needs and expectations of a very young mother and therapists with the best of intentions but with too few tools (and perhaps not the right ones) to assist the new mother and her infant in very limited and limiting circumstances.

These considerations are important in Jay's case, precisely because their situation is not at all unusual or unheard of. On the contrary, infant mental health clinicians everywhere struggle with the frustration of trying to help mothers to assume a more "maternal role," to feel tenderness toward the baby, and to trigger those altruistic maternal behaviors. Our tools for doing so are quite limited, however.

The case in question illustrates very well the struggles that these highly skilled, sensitive, and empathic therapists face in trying to help a young mother and her son. The lens with which the case is approached may be "too narrow" for the situation at hand. It would appear that we need different models to help this mother. The more "psychological" approach, in which the mother comes to appointments to talk about her situation, may not be the most helpful in promoting her maternal feelings and behavior. There is a world view of the therapists: They are interested in promoting mentalization, empathy, and compassion of the mother toward her child, and are motivated by a hopeful feeling that she could enjoy him. These feelings and concerns seem very muted in the new mother, and some seem nonexistent. In a sense she is also "autistic" in that that she is in her own world, her own space, and not so much thinking about the mind of her child. Her world seems "closed" to the beneficial effect of therapists and counseling. She is inside herself, perhaps mistrustful, scared, and "refractory" to outside interventions. This must be so for very good reasons. A thick protective shell has to form in children who are exposed to frequent disappointments, betrayals, and maltreatment. This is not easily permeable by the mere presence of a "helper." Her inner world cannot be easily reopened, and the invitation to do so may be quite painful. Therefore, the need to escape.

However, given the considerations mentioned above, this may not be at all unusual or strange, but quite understandable.

The purpose of understanding the young mother in the light of the lenses proposed previously is that this gives us a perspective of her not only as angry at her baby, but also unable to have empathic feelings toward him and to think about his emotional needs. If one understands why this would be so, there would be less of a sense of anger toward her. If one truly sees her situation, her reactions would be more understandable and less appalling, outrageous, and incomprehensible. In other words, one would not feel so frustrated and disapproving of her.

These considerations also lead to the question "what would this mother need to be able to empathize with her baby"? or "what would she consider helpful?"

Lieberman (2002) and others have explored and speculated about this issue. For all we know, the young mother might find it more helpful if someone offered to take care of Jay (for some periods of time), to buy things for the baby and her, to provide food, and so forth. In other words, it is possible that from her point of view "real help" might be much more concrete than the offer of reflecting on her internal states and those of the baby, reflecting on her (possibly) painful past. It may be that we need better therapeutic models to deal with these problems when the offer to come to group meetings, individual sessions, and playgroups is not experienced as helpful. These, when a mother and infant can profit from them, may be wonderful new opportunities to find joy in the child and in the interaction with the baby and with other mothers or professionals. However, when this is not occurring, something else might be necessary.

Obviously, this is not only a psychological or therapeutic matter. It would be necessary to rethink the strategies we use to "provide help" to people in very squalid and deprived circumstances: how to reach them and establish an alliance and a gradual move toward further psychological work. The models provided by home visitation, psychotherapy "in the kitchen," and providing concrete help might be closer to what this woman and child may have needed. However, even in these circumstances, there are numerous limits to what society is presently willing to offer to impoverished and deprived, traumatized new mothers. The dominant culture in the United States is very afraid of "creating dependency" and tends to think that everybody "should" be able to be on their own, in their own apartment, and somehow find happiness in that isolation and lack of support from other people. It would require a much more ambitious social commitment to reach the many mothers who find themselves trapped being the only source of support and satisfaction to their baby in very difficult conditions and having themselves received so little.

In this particular case, there are some additional issues that are worth exploring further. One is the issue of the "diagnosis" of the infant. The mother herself has long ago made a diagnosis of autism. She seeks confirmation with various professionals. The clinicians who deal with her disagree with this diagnosis. It seems that the deeper issue is whether the child is "psychologically dead" or not. The clinicians view the diagnosis as a "damning label" of the baby and do not see a reason for it, given the vivaciousness and communicational and symbolic gestures from the infant. They seem to fear this—unjustified—diagnosis, which has such ominous connotations for them. The worst fear is that the mother would see her son practically as a small animal incapable of human emotions and attributes. However, she is convinced of the correctness of her diagnosis, and the clinicians sense once more signs of "hate" toward her child in making this sweeping and unshakeable attribution. They hope to help the child by transmitting to the mother the notion that there is much more to Jay than just "autism." However, this does not seem to reach her. One would think that a mother would be utterly reassured by experts advising her that her son does not have that terrible condition. Instead, she seems to believe deeply that they are wrong.

Obviously, the mother holds on to her belief in her son's lack of abilities, limited range of emotions, and multiple disabilities. In hindsight, it might have been more profitable not to try to convince her or even question her "diagnosis" of him. In reality, her view of the child is the most important here. From the beginning of the interaction between therapist and mother, one senses the tension between the mother seeing the child in the autistic extreme, while the therapist sees him very differently. The same tension seems to exist when the mother insists that the child "should pick up toys" in order to be "trained," and the therapist insists that it is her practice not to expect this, that it is her job. These are just two examples of a "clash of views" about the child that seems to be polarizing for the mother and the child's therapist. It might have been better to "metabolize" her view of the child as quite impaired and her expectations of compliance on the part of the baby (e.g., picking up toys, not allowing him to yell intensely). In other words, the clinician may have to withstand, together with the child, the barrage of negative attributions, negative views and criticisms, high expectations, and harsh treatment. This empathic operation is very difficult. Only through a gradual resolution of these negative emotions might these attributions subside, but they do not go away by the mere contrary statements from a therapist.

This "metabolism" might help the mother feel understood and that the therapist was not "working against her" or undoing what she is carefully trying to construct ("My son is impaired" and "My son should be trained to function and pick up after himself"). These mismatches may be at the root of her fleeing the therapy in an abrupt way.

It is also very striking that some clinicians in the various teams have such a positive view of the mother and see her as very motivated, engaged, and likeable. Stone, as the child's therapist, views her very differently and emphasizes the mother's hate toward the baby and its multiple manifestations. With this line of reasoning, logically the therapist tries to at least help the infant himself through therapeutic experiences: being heard, listened to, attended to, played with, and so forth. These are very noble attempts that unfortunately might not be able to compensate, with 1 hour a week, for Jay's inundation with very different experiences that are his "real life" the rest of the time. That is, Jay really lives with his mother and she really treats him in a very different way. An alternative approach would be to respect her "rules" and concept of the child, and continue working with the child and the child–mother relationship over a more extended period of time, enduring and metabolizing her negative attributions, constant criticisms, and dismissal of any positive views of the baby.

The therapist wonders if they should have tried to save Jay from the experiences he will have at the hands of his mother, particularly in the long run. Of course, the ultimate obligation of the therapist is to be an advocate for the child and attempt sparing him maltreatment when this is occurring (e.g., by involving child protective authorities). However, there are many situations like this one, in which the treatment of the child is quite harsh, but not to the degree that one would try to protect the child by removing him from the mother. While she is harsh, negative, and sees Jay as a very impaired and animalistic self, it is doubtful whether he could have been removed from her care due to the regime of emotional deprivation or harsh treatment she was giving him. At least in the United States (and perhaps in many other countries) even if such a removal were possible, the clinician would have to think hard about the realities of alternative care (e.g., the "foster care system") and its vicissitudes, which sometimes are as or more undesirable than remaining in a harsh emotional environment.

At the present time, the reality is that we do not have very good therapeutic strategies to help in families in Jay's situation. We need such strategies, and it would appear that the models involving simply individual/group sessions in a clinic to explore emotional and psychological matters are often not sufficient or not what the family really needs. Our field needs to explore alternative models of intervention that might address the real needs of the dyad or family, even if they are costly, involving long-term interventions, and much staff time and effort. The cost to the family, and to society, of an untreated or unsuccessfully treated family like Jay's, or like Jonah's in the next chapter, is far greater. Babies, mothers, and fathers deserve these investments.

## REFERENCES

Hrdy, S. B. (2005). Evolutionary context of human development: The cooperative breeding model. In C. S. Carter, L. Anhert, K. E. Grossmann, S. B. Hrdy, M. E. Lamb, S. W. Porges, & N. Sachser (Eds.), *Attachment and bonding: A new synthesis* (pp. 9–32). Cambridge, MA: MIT Press.

Lebovici, S., Barriguete, J. A., & Salinas, J. L. (2002). The therapeutic consultation. In J. M. Maldonado-Durán (Ed.), *Infant and toddler mental health: Models of clinical intervention* (pp. 161–186). Washington, DC: American Psychiatric Press.

Lieberman, A. (2002). Treatment of attachment disorders. In J. M. Maldonado-Durán (Ed.), *Infant and toddler mental health: Models of clinical intervention* (pp.105–124). Washington, DC: American Psychiatric Press.

Werner, E., & Smith, R. (2001). *Journeys from childhood to midlife: Risk, resilience and recovery.* New York: Cornell University Press.

CHAPTER 1 0

A GIFT FROM GOD

*Martin Maldonado-Durán*

Jonah was a 20-month-old African American boy who lived with his biological mother, maternal grandmother, and an uncle. He did not attend
any form of alternative child care, and spent all his time with his mother and
grandmother. A team of early childhood interventionists had worked with the
family for about a year. The interventionists were a nurse from the local
health department and an early education teacher from a different agency,
who had tried to promote Jonah's language development and encourage more
adaptive behavior. These colleagues felt that they were not making enough
progress; they were "stuck." As an infant psychiatrist, I was called in to consult
on this difficult case. It was hoped that I might shed light on the diagnostic
picture of the boy, and particularly that some additional interventions might
help to improve Jonah's behavior and promote his development.

From the beginning of our team's involvement, Jonah's grandmother and
mother said that they had "tried everything" to curb Jonah's aggressiveness,
agitation, and constant hitting and slapping. Their interventions ranged
from giving him "time outs" to yelling and spankings. In turn, they complained, "Nothing has worked." They added that Jonah had a very difficult
time going to sleep and staying asleep and, consequently, they themselves
were quite sleep deprived.

I was familiar with the interventionists who requested my opinion, as we
had worked with previous cases in this collaborative fashion—when the

interventionists wondered if there was a more ominous diagnosis of the child and whether other interventions were necessary, in addition to those designed to help a toddler with inattentiveness and hyperactivity. After providing an opinion on the diagnosis and suggestions for intervention in such cases, I may or may not continue to be involved with the child/family in the long term.

## FAMILY CONSTELLATION

Jonah lived with his biological mother, Jeanette K., who was 32 years old and single, and his maternal grandmother, Roseanne K., who was 59 years old and retired. Also in the home lived Roseanne's 19-year-old son David, Jonah's uncle, who was described as autistic. David had no verbal language. He was a rather tall and strong young man, who was constantly active and had a number of behavioral peculiarities. He had to carry a shoe with him all the time, next to his face as though it were a security blanket or a transitional object. He moved from room to room throughout the day. His mother encouraged him to spend lots of time in his room playing with various shoes and stuffed animals. He had little interaction with the family members, including Jonah who seemed used to seeing his uncle go from room to room throughout the day.

In the first session, I saw Jonah at the home of his grandmother and mother. The teacher from the early intervention program and a nurse were also present. Also, a visiting professor from Chile accompanied me to this first consultation. The interventionists had specifically requested that even this first session take place in the family's home as they would "never accept to go to the mental health clinic" where I work. They explained that the family was very suspicious of mental health professionals and would not be willing to go to a clinic. They were accommodated, and all of the sessions took place in the home.

During the first session with me, Roseanne K. explained that she recently had "put out of the house" a 16-year-old daughter, Mary, because she was disobedient and was insistent on dating a man who was more than 20 years old. Mary was a sister to Jonah's mother, Jeanette. Roseanne verbalized that she felt so angry at the boyfriend that she had even threatened to shoot him if he ever came into the home again. She felt that her daughter had "made her choice" to continue dating this man, so she had to "kick her out" of the house.

Jonah's grandmother complained intensely about him. She took the lead in describing her frustration with him and "did most of the talking" consistently. She felt that Jonah was extremely "ornery," and said that he "does not want to sleep" and woke up at night several times, making them exhausted. Jonah's mother, Jeanette, took the "back seat" in the complaints and just endorsed what her mother said by nodding or adding confirmatory exclamations to her statements. She spent most of the time in front of a laptop. She explained that she was studying business administration in a distance education program. From time to time, she would answer telephone calls on her cellular phone: she might go to the next room and talk for a few minutes and then return.

From the start, Jonah's grandmother explained that she had a lot of experience with psychiatrists and with psychiatric medications. She explained that with her son David, she had taken him to be seen by several psychiatrists. She spoke fondly of a child psychiatrist, Dr. P., who had treated her son for a long time. In addition, she had worked as a psychiatric nurse's aid in a state hospital for many years.

From the start there was the suggestion that the "clients" here were the interventionists, perhaps rather than the child and the caregivers of the infant themselves. Grandmother presented herself as an expert. They expressed their frustration, but "would never attend a clinic," which suggests that they were less than convinced that a clinician could be helpful. I did not see this point clearly during the first interview.

## BACKGROUND INFORMATION

Roseanne, the grandmother, soon recounted the story of how Jonah had come into this world. She said that no one knew that Jeanette was pregnant until an hour before Jonah's birth. Jeanette confirmed this by nodding in agreement.

She then said that she never realized that she was pregnant at all. She just thought she was "getting fatter" during that time. She said that she always had been rather overweight, and her menstrual periods had always been irregular, so she did not think it was unusual not to have them for several consecutive months.

The day Jonah was born, Jeanette thought she just had some "cramps" and assumed she had a digestive problem. Finally, the pains were so intense that she and her mother went to the emergency room at the local general hospital. There, the diagnosis of the pregnancy and imminent delivery were made. Jeanette said she never thought she could be pregnant, as she felt nothing unusual in her body, like fetal movements or any changes in her appetite nor nausea. The baby was a term child and weighed about 7 pounds. He was considered healthy by the pediatrician.

Roseanne, the grandmother, said that she at first reacted very angrily to the news of the pregnancy and imminent birth, and had decided to "kick her daughter out of the house." She told Jeanette in the hospital that she could not come home again, and that she herself was not going to "take care of no child." She also was extremely disappointed and enraged that her daughter had a child without being married or having an ongoing relationship.

Roseanne added that she "cursed" her daughter many times during the delivery, and was very angry at the idea of having to help her take care of a newborn. She initially did not want to see her grandson, and was very disgusted with the whole idea of his birth. However, she said that "The Lord spoke to her" on the third day after the birth. God told her that she should take care of the baby, and that this was His gift to her. She thought this gift might be a compensation for the death of her own son, James, 3 years before. She realized then that this child came to fill her life and that she "should spoil him." At that time, she forgave her daughter and held the baby. She felt she loved him and that he was a very special child.

Roseanne then recounted that her son, James, had been taken away by God 3 years prior to Jonah's birth. This boy was Mary's twin brother. She said that this child was a very good boy, in contrast to his sister Mary. Roseanne said that the son was very special, very kind, and a very happy boy. The night he died, he had invited a friend to spend the night, and they were "playing with a hunting gun." The gun was accidentally shot and killed him immediately. Roseanne tried to contain her tears when she recounted the situation. She showed then a picture of her son on the wall where the teenage child is seen smiling. She seemed very uncomfortable and not willing to discuss this any further.

This account was rather surprising to all present. I thought that it was a good sign that the grandmother had been convinced that God had given her this child to assist in his care, and that this revealed that he had a very special status as a "compensation" or replacement child given her previous loss. We thought that given her reluctance, it was better not to insist in getting more details about the idea of replacement at this point, but to take up the thought at some point when the therapeutic alliance with the family had developed further. Obviously, an issue that remained unclear was "whose child is this?" the mother's or the grandmother's? These were questions that I also felt could be explored only later on.

On her part, Jeanette, Jonah's mother, explained that she had suffered from seizures, grand mal epilepsy, for many years. She had taken anticonvulsant medication for a long time, including during her pregnancy with Jonah. She had been taking two anticonvulsant medications: carbamazepine and valproic acid. These two medications are contraindicated during pregnancy, as they are known to cause teratogenic effects in the fetus. Specifically, both of these have been associated with causing a syndrome similar to autism. Jeanette said that she was mad that her pregnancy had not been discovered earlier so these medications could have been stopped. She knew they were "not supposed to be taken" during pregnancy, but did not know what specific effects they might have had. When asked, Jeanette seemed reluctant to talk about the Jonah's father. She said he was "about 40 years old," but he did not take responsibility for the baby. Jonah saw him occasionally (he came to the house), but he did "not really know how who he is." The grandmother did not like this man at all, referring to him as a "sperm donor."

I had the clear impression that Roseanne was a very strong personality and the dominant force in the family. She indicated very clearly her dislike for several people during this session, and the fact that she saw things in a very determined way and that if one "crossed her," she had little patience for that. It appeared that one had to try to be on her good side and agree with her as much as possible to be included in her circle of acceptable people. This gave me the clue that it would be best to try to first develop some sort of therapeutic alliance with the family, and particularly the child's grandmother, and to gain her confidence, perhaps by making things somewhat better with her grandson.

During this session, we agreed to try to understand the situation better and to make some suggestions about how Jonah might overcome his behavioral difficulties. I believed it was understood that this was to be an open-ended process of consultation with the child, family, and colleagues.

## CHARACTERISTICS OF THE INFANT

Jonah was a rather short and well-nourished boy. He had short hair and deep-set eyes, which appeared to be placed too close to each other. He made only fleeting eye contact. Jonah was extremely hyperactive and would go from person to person saying "Oh, shit," and then slapping or kicking each person with whom he came into contact, without being particularly angry, but almost as a way of relating. When he slapped his grandmother she yelled at him "Stop!", then Jonah appeared somewhat frightened, stopped, and moved back. Then he would resume his hitting or kicking the other people in the room. He seemed to "bluff" or try to scare other people by "puffing himself up" and appearing strong; later he would hit and push them.

When I attempted to contain Jonah by sitting him on my lap or beside me on a couch, Jonah would sit there for a few minutes and perhaps look briefly at a book with me. However, he quickly was ready to go on to something else and would struggle to release himself and start hitting me. At one point, as I attempted to engage him, he slapped me on the face several times without seeming angry. He would say "you nigger!" repeatedly as though he expected a reaction. His grandmother yelled at him to "stop that," and then he would cease for a few seconds. If Jonah's hands were held to prevent further slapping, he tried to kick and was very amused trying to manage to hit me somehow. This seemed a very surprising and baffling behavior, constant hitting without much anger, bluffing to "scare the other" and an intense counterreaction by the grandmother. Obviously he would have heard the words from family members or people around him. They presented his behavior as unexplained and unexplainable, as a sign of some sort of mysterious disturbance. I thought it would be good to focus on teaching the child other ways of relating, rather than hitting and "shocking people" with his language and actions.

Roseanne explained that Jonah had his own television and DVD player in the dining room, as well as a small computer where he could "play his computer games."

She said he had a lot of toys that she had bought so that he would learn a lot of things and be entertained. She said he had "seven Elmos." I asked her to show them to me to help me understand what she meant. The family produced seven very large red stuffed figures that would shake and make noises by pushing a button. When the seven Elmos were activated, they made conjointly a lot of noise. Jonah would just hit them, push on them, throw them around, and be very amused with all the noisiness that seemed (to me) overwhelming. Roseanne seemed proud to prove her point that she "spoiled" Jonah by buying him many toys, any toy he wanted in order to make him feel special.

Jonah seemed fairly unable to stop or modulate himself from the constant hyperactive running around the house and hitting people passing by. His mother and grandmother said this was how he was "all the time." They complained about his constant hitting and kicking, yelling, and saying bad words. They said they thought perhaps he had heard a relative say those words during visits to the house because they did not use those words routinely.

Jonah spoke very loudly. His mother said that he yelled constantly, but he had had his hearing evaluated before and it was concluded it was entirely normal. Jonah did not seem to be able to use language for ordinary communicative purposes. To communicate strong emotions he said "oh shit" or "nigger" to convey his anger quite loudly. He seemed unable to answer questions, to point to things in the room, or to name the most obvious objects, such as body parts. He did not respond to questions of this sort, nor did he utter any other words either spontaneously or by request. He did not seem to be able to point to things that he wanted. When I attempted to show him pictures in a children's book, he had very little interest, wanted to tear the book, get out of my lap, and resume his running around. His attention span seemed very short, and he was able to make only the briefest eye contact.

It was very difficult to engage Jonah in any sort of playful interaction, except at the level of the interaction with the body, such as tickling, moving him in the air, turning him around, and so forth. He took pleasure in these activities, but quickly became overaroused, agitated, and just started hitting, kicking, and wanted to be put down. His body seemed to seek constant touch and "crashing" with other people, hitting and slamming against others. There was no evidence of any symbolization in his play. The only circles of interaction managed with him involved mutual touching, tickling, and manipulating the other person's body in some way. Jonah seemed very reactive to any noises in the room. He would turn around to the slightest noise (there were many noises in the room with the Elmos, the television, his computer, etc.). He seemed hardly able to relax his body and to mold to anyone's body. Rather, when approached, he would quickly become "stiff" in his limbs and appeared hypertonic in his muscles. He kept on moving around and jumped to the floor as quickly as possible. He did not seem to want to be touched softly, but only brusquely and intensely. He maintained the focus of his eyes on any one object for a very short time, a few seconds.

Jonah seemed very intensely emotional and reacted quickly with anger, joy, and tears when things changed around him. If frustrated, he quickly would yell, hit, and run away. If unable to get something he wanted, he might readily cry and tearfully go to a corner or withdraw. At times he would quickly become overjoyed for a few minutes, then jump and dance with his whole body for several minutes.

## CAREGIVER–CHILD INTERACTION

As I entered the house, the grandmother was obviously watching television while the mother was alternating her attention between Jonah, her laptop computer, her cell phone calls, and discussing the situation at hand. Jonah would go from being in the room with us, hitting and jumping around, into the next room to look at his small computer, only to come back shortly and resume the hitting and saying "you nigger!" Jonah seemed to get attention mostly at those times, when his grandmother would say "stop!" or "don't hit!"

Roseanne took the center stage in talking, saying in her opinion Jonah was very spoiled. So on one hand she appeared very proud of the fact that she was "spoiling him" while at the same time she was concerned that his aggression was the result of being "spoiled" (i.e., not to respect other people). The first "spoiling" is a sign of love, and the second, of uncontrollable anger. She complained mostly about his poor sleep, and wished we could do something to help him go to sleep at night. From time to time, David, his uncle, would come into the room, holding a shoe close to his face, run around with it, and then disappear to another room. Roseanne explained that David has an "obsession with shoes." Jonah paid very little attention to David, and vice versa.

## HOME ENVIRONMENT

The house was fairly small, and most of the interactions took place in the living room. The grandmother said that she was very busy cooking, and said that she was making fried chicken for several church members she would see later on. She offered a plate to us. The offer was accepted as a plate "to go" as the time of the appointment was very shortly after the lunch hour. The noise level was fairly high, and I asked Roseanne if it would be possible to turn off the television, which she did quickly but her body language suggested she was somewhat annoyed. The request to turn off the television was presented as my need to concentrate on what the family would have to say. As to the fried chicken, it seemed obvious that Roseanne took great pride in her cooking, and I hoped that accepting her food would be a move to strengthen the possible therapeutic alliance. In all of these interactions, Roseanne always had the upper hand, except on the television issue. She complied with that request somewhat reluctantly. It must be said that in most home visits, families understand that the television being off may be necessary to be able to focus on the questions at hand. So this reaction seemed unusual.

When asked if there was a backyard, Roseanne said they had a large trampoline in the backyard as well as some other equipment, such as swings. However, she quickly added that Jeanette, the mother, would hardly ever take Jonah outside because she could not stand the feeling of air on her skin. This was confirmed by Jeanette who said she did not like to go outside. Roseanne said that she occasionally would take Jonah outside, when she was not so busy as today. I asked if we could see the backyard, and shortly after this, the grandmother, mother, Jonah, and I went outside. Jonah was put on the trampoline, and he readily jumped on it. The grandmother seemed a bit more involved in these sequences than the mother, who said she would prefer to go inside. She confirmed the notion that she did not like to be outside because it was difficult for her to feel the air on her face, her hair, and so forth, so she tended not go to outside as much as she could avoid it. One had the impression that the family saw these requests as somewhat unusual and unnecessary. They wanted mostly to focus on "how to make him go to sleep," and wanted some fairly immediate advice on that point. However, they gave me "a chance" by following those suggestions and requests.

## COURSE OF INTERVENTIONS

In the following pages, I will describe the visits with Jonah's family, the attempted interventions, and how they were received.

### First Session

In the first session, I had a feeling of being somewhat overwhelmed by Jonah's aggressiveness, almost total lack of positive engagement with others (including his family), and with the noise level and agitation in the house. After having obtained the history outlined previously, I reflected with the family on the fact that sometimes the exposure to those anticonvulsive medications in utero can create difficulties for a child in terms of the development of language and the ability to relate to others, as well as sleeping and impulse control problems. No "diagnosis" was mentioned, but I thought it was pertinent to suggest that the medications might have contributed to the present problems. I hoped that this intervention also would alleviate the common fears of parents or caregivers that one might "blame them" for the problems and aggression in their child. I took the nonjudgmental stance that, given that Jonah has these problems, it would be useful to find ways of helping him calm down, sleep, and engage in more pleasurable interactions with those around him.

Obviously, the grandmother and mother had presented the notion that they had "already tried everything" and "nothing has worked" from the beginning of the interview. This left me feeling that, in a manner of speaking, I was being challenged to prove that I could offer particularly helpful suggestions that had not been tried before.

Perhaps responding to this sense of being "tested," toward the end of the first session, I made a number of recommendations. I suggested they try to diminish the level of noise in the house, and that they limit the number of toys the child interacted with at one time. I suggested it would be wise to turn off the television more of the time as it dominated the ambiance during most of the day. I also suggested that they let Jonah use his computer and his DVD player only for finite periods of time, rather than having them on always. I advised mother and grandmother to give Jonah massage and deep pressure in the body as strategies to help him calm. This was demonstrated and practiced during the session, showing them how this might be done. We discussed the importance of helping Jonah focus a little more by engaging him in play with another person in two-way interactions, first in the ways he liked to play, such as tickling, but emphasizing turn-taking and not getting him too agitated. Jeanette, the mother, showed very little interest in this but said she would try the strategies. The grandmother said she would do all of this. The notion of taking him outside, for instance, to a park, was mentioned in terms of expending some of his apparently boundless energy, which might help with the level of agitation while inside the house. Lastly, I mentioned that they might prepare a brief diary of the sleeping problem, to keep a record of how much time he took to fall asleep and of his waking during the night. An appointment was made to come to the house the following week.

## Second Session

This session in the home was conducted during the morning; the nurse health visitor was there at the same time as she wished to be aware of further recommendations. At the beginning, the large living room television was on, as well as Jonah's own television. He was watching a soap opera in which one could see scenes of domestic violence taking place. Jonah was watching while hiding behind a chair as if frightened by the scene of the physical confrontation and the yelling, pushing, and hitting on television. The mother was sitting on the couch in front of her laptop computer and from time to time would excuse herself to talk on the cellular phone. She was polite, but only partially involved. The grandmother was again cooking, as she was preparing a dinner for that evening. She already had the table set for about 10 people. She said she liked to entertain people and "cook for others." The kitchen was very hot from all the baking and the things that were still being cooked. Roseanne, the grandmother, said that Jonah was not allowed to go in the kitchen. On the issue of his constant activity and aggression, Roseanne said that everything was the same if not worse. She and Jonah's mother said they were exhausted as they got little sleep due to his crying during the night or his wanting to play and roam around the house, and his reluctance to go back to sleep. Even when they managed to get him back to sleep, he would wake up in an hour or two and resume the loud play and running around the house, laughing, and throwing things. They said they were tired of his behavior and wished he would go to sleep and stay asleep.

This was a surprising outcome. Usually after recommendations like those described previously, the child should become a little calmer, more able to stay organized for longer periods of time, and so forth. Alternatively, the child may not get better, but usually the child would not be "worse." This raised in me the question of why the child was "worse" in every way. The question of the family defeating the therapist came into mind, but I tried to remain empathic to their experience of being disappointed and exhausted. On one level the family presented a simple outcome: everything was worse. On the other, there was a sense that there was no reason for things to be "worse" and for the family to be angry about it.

This clearly raised my anxiety and created a need to "do better." So I tried to give even "better" recommendations that would make things improve.

When asked if they had tried some of the recommendations to diminish the noise level, physical activity, the massage, and playing with him a little more one-on-one, they said summarily that they had "tried everything" and nothing had worked. I tried to get some details about when they had gone out with Jonah to the park, or when they had tried the massage, and so forth, and the answers were quite vague and dismissive. It was clear that Roseanne, in particular, would become angry with my questioning and my trying to elicit details.

Finally, the grandmother said, "Look, I know a lot about these things," because she already had an autistic son and because she had worked at the state hospital for years. She said that nothing had worked. She said that the most important thing was to get Jonah to sleep.

This seemed like a rather clear message to stop questioning them about the specifics of what they had attempted and to move on to the issue that worried them the most at the time. I tried then to focus on those issues that today seemed to take precedence over the hitting and the constant hyperactivity in the daytime. Given the level of frustration shown by the family, and the fact that "nothing had worked," I felt the need to make additional suggestions. Perhaps a medication might, at least initially, help the child go to sleep, and the family would then be more amenable to other interventions and more likely to really follow the recommendations outlined previously.

When some "sleep hygiene" strategies were suggested (such as giving Jonah a bath, engaging him in calm activities, the massage at bedtime, lying down with him at the onset of sleep, avoiding overstimulation in the evening, etc.), the grandmother said that they had already tried "all those things." Jeanette confirmed this by moving her head up and down. They said they were desperate for sleep. At this point, I suggested that perhaps a dose of an antihistaminic (ciproheptadine) could be tried, and gave them a prescription of 1 milligram of this medication in the form of a liquid. We discussed the fact the medication should induce sleepiness and help him stay asleep a little longer, but the other measures would also have to be attempted. The family agreed to do so. I also ordered an electrocardiogram (EKG) as this medicine might not help and another different one might need to be tried, which required evidence of normal heart functioning. The side effects of the medication were mentioned, but Jonah's grandmother interrupted saying that she "already knew all that."

Toward the end of the session, I engaged Jonah in some activities, giving him pressure in his limbs and trunk, and then looking at a book together. He seemed calmer and quieter despite all the reports of lack of sleep and worse behavior. The grandmother had been asked to turn off the television at the beginning of this session (which she again did reluctantly). Jonah was able to pay attention to several things being named consecutively in a book, to noises of animals shown there, and he seemed to focus a little more. However, after some minutes of calm activity, Jonah slapped me and said "oh shit." I took his hand and told him that if he slapped, that hurt. The action was repeated, and the child was surprised. He seemed to expect a scolding, and instead, I showed him how to "touch softly" my face, holding the child's hand. The point was to show him that if he slapped, the other person would hurt. Then his hand was placed softly on my face, and I whispered to Jonah "soft," suggesting that it was better if Jonah touched my face softly rather than slapping. Jonah found this amusing and touched the cheek softly several times. After this, he slapped again and laughed as though it were a game. The grandmother yelled at him not to slap, and he seemed afraid. She seemed very frustrated with her grandson and complained that she did most of the disciplining of Jonah, as his mother often is too busy with her schoolwork.

She hinted that her daughter did not do all she might be able to do for the child, and that consequently she had taken too much responsibility for her grandson. I sensed that the grandmother was impatient to have the visit be over to resume her cooking and to turn on the television again.

## Third Session

The third session also took place in the home. From the very beginning, Roseanne again said, "nothing had worked." If anything, the ciproheptadine made him more restless and overaroused at night. They had tried a higher dose and it was not helpful. The mother quickly went into another room, in order to work with her laptop, after having said that she agreed with her mother. I then asked Jeanette if it were possible for her to stay in the room and perhaps focus a little more on the conversation at hand because her point of view as the mother of the child was very important. Her facial expression hinted that she did not understand why this would be so, if Roseanne already was giving all of the information about the situation.

There was a sense of tension between the family and me. I felt they perceived me as making unusually high demands, and that I had too many expectations of them. They only wanted the child to behave and sleep better, and could not understand why this did not happen with the medication. We agreed that if the EKG was normal, and given that the blood pressure was normal, we would try a different medication (i.e., an alpha adrenergic medicine, clonidine, at a very small dose—0.025 milligrams), which would hopefully help Jonah go to sleep and stay asleep. I agreed to this trial, once the EKG was normal. We talked about trying to actually implement the techniques of one-on-one interaction mentioned before.

## Fourth Session

The session also took place in the home. The family continued to express much frustration with Jonah's sleep. Roseanne reported that Jonah was not sleeping at night, and that the new medication had not made any difference either; perhaps it might have "made him more aggressive" during the day-time. She then wondered if the medication was addictive and was reassured that this was not the case. The mother said she agreed with her mother and was frustrated that "nothing helps."

Given the focus on the immediate issues of medication and the fact that every-thing to this point had been counterproductive, I decided to shift the focus to issues of how Jonah was perceived and how he came about to be the way he is. I tried to explore further some of the background material, as it was obvious that the more "pharmacological" and behavioral approach was not helping. I suspected that in reality none of the recommended measures were being followed. The televisions appeared to be constantly on, there was still a high level of noise, and it was very doubtful that any massage or calming routines were being followed at all. I had the impression that the grandmother had taken Jonah to the park a few times, and he appeared to be a little calmer and more able to focus than before. He made more eye contact, and even pointed to some pictures on a book or exhibited some instances of joint atten-tion with me. I wondered why there was such a reluctance to consider the recommendations, and what might be fueling the resistance to trying different things. This was not mentioned to the family, but it seemed important to better understand their perception of Jonah and the points of view of mother and grandmother.

Jeanette was asked to reflect on the experiences during her pregnancy. She then got a telephone call and excused herself for a few minutes. In her absence, I tried to explore with the grandmother her belief that the Lord gave her this child to spoil. I noted that she at times appeared amused with his aggressiveness and bluffing behavior, as if she could hardly contain her smiles. At other times, she would yell at him in anger. She said that spoiling her grandson was "her privilege," just like her daughter Jeanette had been "spoiled by her own grandmother." When Jeanette returned, she confirmed that indeed this was "the way it is." Because Roseanne was very busy working outside the home during Jeanette's childhood, her own maternal grand-mother raised her and she "spoiled her a lot." She recognized that her mother now had the right to spoil Jonah, and there was nothing she could do. The term *spoiling* seemed to mean the idea of buying the child whatever he wanted, all of the toys in which he showed an interest and not containing his actions, except when he was "being mean." Jeanette was reluctant to talk about how she did not realize that she had been pregnant with Jonah. It was obvious that this matter was very sensitive, and that Jeanette was not in a position to trust me enough to talk about this in any depth.

I again suggested they try to keep the house quieter and use the relaxation techniques instead of any medicines, as they did not help. Roseanne then was angry. She said that this was her house, and she should have the chance to watch "all her shows" because she is now retired and she enjoys a number of shows in the morning and in the afternoon. We thus had to figure something else out because she was not going to keep the television off. Another appointment was set for the following week. She seemed as usual very firm on this point, and I felt it was better not to question this but to try to understand their point of view. They had felt that the recommendations had been contrary to their lifestyle, and that the questions had been perhaps too intrusive. We made another appointment for the next week.

Before that appointment could take place, Roseanne telephoned the office and asked to "talk to the supervisor." She complained that I was just giving Jonah medications to "keep him doped up," and claimed that I had taught the child to say "you nigger" and also to slap people on the face. She said that after the first visit, Jonah had started slapping people on the face, which he had not done before.

I had previously contacted Jonah's pediatrician, Dr. C., with whom the family had a long-standing collaborative relationship, to discuss the case (the family had given permission for this). Dr. C. felt that the grandmother was very dismissive of any mental health interventions, and that she was the "boss" in the house. He felt that often the family wants things to be solved, but not with their having to do things differently, but with medicines or some sort of immediate remedy. He conveyed that Roseanne was talking to him in a disparaging way about me.

A few days later, Roseanne called the office and asked that I not come to the house any longer. She announced that she was considering a lawsuit for the negative habits taught to her grandson and thought that I was "just a quack," who should not come to see her grandson any longer, and she was not considering any further appointments.

I contacted the risk management staff in my office to discuss whether I could, as I would have liked to do, talk with the family about their perceptions of how the child had been damaged. However, this staff advised against further contact even by telephone as Roseanne was so angry and clear about not wanting further interventions.

## FINAL REFLECTIONS

In retrospect, one of the main questions that seems not to have a good answer is "who is the client" or "who is interested in change." The two interventionists who requested the consultation were feeling "stuck," and thought that a different approach might be helpful in the situation at hand. On the face of it, it also seemed clear that the family had a series of concerns about Jonah, and that they would have liked it very much if he would sleep better, talk, not hit people, and mind them more, and so forth. However, it appears that the "cost" of the intervention was too high in the sense that it implied a number of changes in the family's routine that they were not willing to make at present.

The grandmother clearly took the lead in deciding what was done in the household and what was not, and she was very clear in her desire for a medication that might help her grandson but was also very ambivalent about it. I was left with a sense of defeat as all the interventions I suggested were dismissed. The family insisted that they had been tried before without success, were of no help now, or were even harmful and made the child worse.

In retrospect, it might have been better to explore further the desire for change and what the family perceived as the main problems, and to obtain further information about what they thought an acceptable course of action or what they could really attempt. I unwisely just "assumed" that if I was being called, there was a therapeutic alliance or a wish to change some things by the family. Neither of these things really materialized. Rather, I had a sense of being tested and failing miserably. The recommendations were seen as counterproductive, silly, naïve, or too unrealistic. It might have been better to attempt further exploration of what the child meant in the family, what it meant to be spoiled, and what was the motivation to change given this family tradition.

Perhaps I was led by a "wish to cure" that in this case really was a misreading of the situation. The urgency to "cure" was more in the mind of the therapist than in the agenda of the family. Perhaps the complaints were taken too literally, and it might have been better to listen to more of the implications of the complaints, dealing empathically with them and to work harder first on establishing a true therapeutic alliance before intervening in any way. Without such an alliance, the interventions felt like an intrusion and alien to the family, who quickly discarded them.

Another dynamic force is worth considering. I was "called in" to make some sort of "change" in this entrenched system. There was an internal pressure on the part of "the doctor" to make a difference when two other colleagues had felt "stuck." This led to a sort of messianic hope that somehow I—the doctor—would be able to offer something new. This was connected with the hope of finding some wonderful medication that might make things move along. Obviously, this was not the case.

There are other important dimensions to the case: one is the clash between "therapeutic cultures" of expectations.

Although it is very tempting to blame the family's resistance entirely for this therapeutic failure, it may be inaccurate to do so. Certainly there was great resistance to change, and a number of negative projections toward the child, the "gift from God," who had turned into more of a burden and was seen in quite negative terms by the grandmother and the mother. Also, the failure of the strategies recommended to help can be readily attributed to the mother's and grandmother's need to be victimized by the child, perhaps as a punishment in the psyche of the mother, and as a way to appear as a victim on the part of the grandmother. After all, she may have had many guilt feelings because of the death of her son, her failure to raise her daughters well, and the negative events in her life in general. This grandson appeared as a "replacement child" by which God compensated the grandmother.

However, the fact is that the grandmother and the mother appeared to accept the offer of the interventionists to bring in a third person, "a doctor," to help them solve the problems they themselves identified: restlessness, aggressive behavior, poor sleep, and poor language development. At this level, the family was at least accepting that there was a problem and were ostensibly accepting the offer for further help.

The "clash of therapeutic cultures" occurred between me—the psychiatrist—and the family. I tried to help at several levels. I offered medication to attempt to improve the most pressing problem—poor sleep. With many families, it is necessary to first establish relief of some symptoms and then develop a liaison with them and to start working on other, deeper issues. If the child had responded to the medication prescribed, it is possible that he would have been less sleep deprived in the day, less restless, and less aggressive. However, at least on the face of it, he responded in a counterproductive way. This is not unusual either. Many children with developmental disorders (like pervasive developmental disorder) respond in a paradoxical way to a number of pharmacological agents. What was unusual in this case was being "fired" so quickly after these therapeutic attempts, which, though unsuccessful, were reasonable and evidently sought by the family. Most families would either try a different medication or decline medications altogether given the poor results and try other approaches. In this family, this did not happen.

It appears that the family's definition of "helpful" was to "fix the child." This is, in principle, the same expectation of any other physician who attends a child who is sick. If one takes a child to a doctor for fever and cough, and the doctor prescribes medications that do not help, it is understandable that the family would become skeptical and perhaps seek another opinion from a different physician. It appears that the view of the family was that the child should have improved, and as this did not happen, they had lost trust in me.

Another issue that is also part of this therapeutic clash in this case is that all of the behavioral recommendations I gave were felt by the family to go against their practices and lifestyle. They also were in conflict with the need to "spoil" the child. I prescribed a quiet atmosphere, less noisy toys, less toys altogether at one time, massage, exercise in the outside, and engaging the child in two-way interactions in a one-on-one fashion. These suggestions appeared to the family as unreasonable or silly. The grandmother was retired, very tired, and felt entitled to her rest, her entertainment, and the freedom to enjoy her constant cooking and helping people from the church. This was essential to her role as a matriarch, who is also very experienced and knowledgeable about medical things. She had a severely autistic 19-year-old son who did not relate and did not talk. Her favorite child, her second son, was lost to her through a tragic act of violence. Her two daughters were unsatisfactory: one was out of the home because of her disobedience and the other got pregnant out of wedlock and was seen as handicapped (epilepsy) and quite limited. The grandmother was the sole person who "knows what to do." Perhaps she had never had anyone in her life who helped *her*. From the start, she was very skeptical of all the indications I suggested. She wanted concrete, noticeable, and obvious improvement in the boy, which did not happen. Her definition of improvement might have been "Jonah sleeps, is calmer, does not hit" without her having to change everyday practices—this is what she might have seen as helpful.

In a way, the grandmother did not want to know or theorize why her grandson is the way he is; she just saw him as a normal little boy who should know better and should be calmer and be able to sleep. The grandmother and I had two very different world views. I proposed seeing the child as having difficulties in self-regulation, relatedness, use of language, and needing external help, from people and medications, to improve. The grandmother saw the child as ornery, strong-willed, and needing a stronger hand to improve. She was willing to try the medications for sleep, but on seeing their failure, she became disappointed and frustrated.

It appears that I made the error of not thinking enough about the family's world view and their expectations of me and of their child. I responded literally to the request for immediate symptom relief and improved sleep, trying to provide this with the medications. In many cases, this would have been perceived as helpful and would have strengthened the therapeutic alliance, but this did not happen in this case. What should I have done next? Would it have been more helpful to resonate with the frustration of the grandmother and to empathize with her disappointment and the sense of burden she appeared to experience? She was in her own house, retired after decades of working, trying to cope with her autistic son, her dependent daughter, and a very highly demanding little boy. It might have been helpful to explore her feelings about these demands on her and about her daughter taking the "back seat" vis à vis the grandson. It might have been more helpful to explore further her belief that the child was a replacement of the dead son and to understand better the need for spoiling and showering him with gifts and expensive toys to convey how special he was. Also, it might have been better to reflect with the family on how Jonah might experience the world, his mother, his grandmother, and why he seemed to engage people through slapping and yelling. This approach might have elicited more compassionate feelings toward his difficulties and mobilized forces to support him in his attempts at self-regulation and engagement with others.

As it happened though, the therapeutic discourse was kept more along the lines of a "medical model." Given the unfortunate results, there was no time for further explorations or reflecting on what was going wrong. Usually, when there is a poor response in a case, the clinician can reflect on what might be interfering with improvement and allow time to "shift gears" and modify the therapeutic intervention. Here, my experience is perhaps similar to that of the younger daughter who was "thrown out of the house," being given but a few chances to help. Here the mistakes led to a cutoff and a threat. This aroused considerable frustration in me and a sense of inadequacy in the face of a complex multiproblem family.

## ACKNOWLEDGMENTS

I would like to thank Gonzalo Manzano Zayas, a family psychiatrist in Mexico City, who allowed me to sit in and taught me family therapy when I was a medical student in Mexico City. He conducted home visits at times and "took me under his wing" to learn strategies of intervention with families and children. I owe him much gratitude for having been initiated in this field when I was very young. He nurtured my interest and encouraged me to become a psychiatrist.

CHAPTER 11

# HELPLESS BEFORE GOD: A COMMENTARY ON "A GIFT FROM GOD"

*Toni Vaughn Heineman*

As a reader of Martin Maldonado-Durán's case report (chapter 10), I felt that I, like all of the characters in the story, was in the grip of some extraordinarily powerful, unstoppable force. This force propelled this family— those in its immediate orbit and those, like myself, far removed from the immediate situation—forward through almost unbearable psychic pain and daily reality. Jonah, Roseanne's "gift from God," began to feel more like one of the plagues that God allowed to be visited upon Job than a precious, loving gift from heaven. Additionally, as Maldonado-Durán discovers, Roseanne's suffering, like Job's, cannot be relieved by mere mortals.

Experience teaches us that psychic reality does not easily give way to common sense. We are willing to suffer for years—sometimes for generations— for real and imagined hurts, injustices, or misunderstandings for all manner of complex psychological reasons. Yet common sense tells us that we would feel better, lead more productive lives, and have more satisfying relationships if we could banish the "ghosts" from our psychic nurseries. When the ghosts have transformed themselves into persecutory demons, relief from suffering may simply not be possible. I would like to consider the tension between the incredible spoken and unspoken pressure to offer relief and the absolute insistence that no such thing is possible in Maldonado-Durán's presentation.

Both the rigidity of the family dynamics and the sense of urgency about this case are evident from the very beginning of Maldonado-Durán's learning of it. He is brought in because two other professionals are "stuck," not only in terms of being able to help the family in ways that they ostensibly want, but they are also stuck at home with them. The family will not leave home for a consultation; indeed Jonah's mother cannot bear the feel of the outside world on her skin.

We learn quickly that misfortune permeates Roseanne's world. Jeanette is seemingly unknowingly impregnated. One has the feeling that the doctors who discovered the pregnancy are somehow held responsible for both Jonah's birth and not magically knowing about the baby growing inside Jeanette. We are left wondering how Jeanette, who does not like to leave the house and appears to be connected to the outside world only by her cell phone and laptop, had the opportunity for even one sexual encounter.

Roseanne stands in the midst of children who, one way or another, have placed extraordinary burdens on her. Jeanette suffers from epilepsy, and at the age of 32 is still living at home, and has just delivered an unexpected grandchild into Roseanne's arms. David's autism leaves him locked in a world of his own, presumably beyond Roseanne's reach. The extensive chaos and overwhelming misfortunes of this family tempt us to simply accept the fact of David's profoundly debilitating condition and put aside thoughts of the burdens autism places on a parent. Surely, Roseanne, not only made the expectable rounds of child psychiatrists with numerous trials of medications and behavioral interventions, but also had to deal with bureaucratic tangles of special education programs and occupational and language therapies. While David is psychically lost, Roseanne has actually lost her beloved son, James, through a tragic accident and then his twin, Mary, through their inability to find a way of holding their relationship together in the midst of their stormy lives. Finally, Jonah arrives—first as a curse, then as a blessing. As he grows, he learns only how to curse and appears to be more blessed with toys than with love or attention.

However, like Maldonado-Durán, we barely have a chance to absorb the enormity of these tragedies or to reflect on the meaning of these events for the individuals or for the family together. Everything about their daily lives appears to be consciously or unconsciously constructed to avoid thinking—to mitigate any possibility of introspection or reflective thought. Although they cannot move outside of the house, inside they cannot stop moving. Ironically, David's transitional object is a shoe, which he holds against his face as he repetitively moves from one room to another, apparently oblivious to the activities of the family. Jeanette moves from laptop to cell phone and back again. Roseanne moves from her stove in the kitchen to her TV in the living room. Jonah is constantly on the move—morning, noon, and night—from seven noisy Elmos to his DVD to his computer to hitting and cursing and jumping and back again. It is painful to try to imagine the cacophony of sounds from the toys, the TV, the sizzling fried chicken, the ringing phones, the DVD player, and the curses and reprimands—all along with the changing flashes of light from the various electronic devices in this small house. We might wish to think of this family living in the eye of a tornado, but their lives offered no such relief. The eye of the storm offers some momentary peace between the terrifying swirls of the storm. In the eye of the storm the winds are quiet enough that one might have a chance—however brief—to consider one's own thoughts—to know the depths of terror and sadness that cannot be heard in the midst of a whirlwind.

In another interesting parallel to the Book of Job, the voice of God is said to come to Job "out of the whirlwind." In this case, I think we can see that Maldonado-Durán was swept up by the chaotic whirlwind of the family activities and the disorganized inner worlds that they effectively drowned out. The force of this maelstrom was so powerful that he was sucked into the family's primitive need for constant noise and activity as the only means they have of overriding the screams of their internal demons. During the first session, Maldonado-Durán suggests the following 11 interventions:

1. Diminishing the volume of noise in the house,

2. Turning the TV completely off some of the time,

3. Giving Jonah only one toy at a time,

4. Limiting Jonah's use of his DVD,

5. Limiting his access to his computer,

6. Giving him massage and deep pressure,

7. Engaging him in play,

8. Helping him to focus,

9. Getting him to take turns without getting him too agitated,

10. Taking him to the park, and

11. Keeping a diary of his sleeping problems!

Maldonado-Durán describes feeling under incredible pressure to find something that would work and to demonstrate his potential usefulness. Having been told that the family "had tried everything and nothing worked," I believe that he correctly understood that his true purpose was to perpetuate this family's being stuck. He complied with the unspoken demand that he make suggestions that were bound to fail because of their nature and number. He asked them to give up the very defenses—externalizing the internal chaos through unremitting noise and purposeless activity—that kept at bay the persecutory demons. Of course, they could not accept these suggestions, but Maldonado-Durán followed his directive to offer suggestions that they could not possibly accept in order that they and he successfully fail.

One element of the first visit deserves particular attention; namely, Roseanne's offering her visitors some of the fried chicken that she is preparing for church members who will be arriving later for dinner. We could see this simply as a generous offer from Roseanne to share something that is important to her and a statement of her wish to care for Maldonado-Durán as she cares for her children, members of her church, and previously her charges in her work as a psychiatric nurse's aide. Psychically, Roseanne is being "eaten alive" by her children and grandchild. There is no indication anywhere in the presentation that they offer her anything in return for her, albeit disturbed and disturbing, care. I think we might also consider the possibility that Roseanne's unconscious motivation for feeding the "god" who has arrived with his powerful potions and prescriptions is to keep him from destroying her (Ehrensaft, 2007). Roseanne makes him an offering of food—a "sacrificial lamb" that is, on a very primitive level, intended to protect the most precious of God's gifts—a child.

In thinking about Maldonado-Durán's case, I was reminded of a young man I worked with several years ago. He had been raised in a very strict religious home, and, as an adult, regular participation in church services and activities continued as an important part of his social life. His periodic transgressions into premarital sexual relationships or experimentation with recreational drugs did not cause him any particular moral anxieties, even though they were expressly forbidden by his chosen faith. However, he was continually and intensely tormented by the least temptation to take personal credit for even the smallest accomplishment in his work or personal life. If he worked hard to accomplish a goal at work, the merest hint of a sense of pride would bring on a wave of terror that he would be punished for taking credit that should be attributed to God's power. When he succumbed to the temptations of illicit sex or drugs, it was from his own weakness; when he resisted, it was because of God's intervention. Most frequently, the punishment he expected was that someone he loved would be taken from him or would be harmed. His belief in God's absolute power over the universe offered him little comfort because it conflicted with his own wishes to feel some control over his own life, aspirations, and sense of accomplishment. Fortunately, he was able, through psychotherapy and counseling from his minister, to forge an identity and world view that could accommodate a profound belief in God and an equally profound belief in the importance of maximizing his talents and determination. His religious beliefs then offered him a source of comfort, strength, support, and joy.

Sadly, there is little room for joy in Roseanne's internal or external life. We do not know why she feels that she is absolutely destined to suffer—only that she does. I do think that the clinical material suggests that she expects that she will have to endure yet more intolerable loss if she attempts to thwart the "will of the gods" or if she is forced to confront their demonic transformations in her internal world. Unlike my patient, who could think about the similarities and differences that joined and separated the gods that he had created and the God of his faith, Roseanne must hold separate her gift from God and the plagues that have been visited upon her. I can only conjecture that one of the difficulties in this extraordinarily complex case is Roseanne's terror at tempting the fates—at the very suggestion that she would have the audacity to try to mold or transform or tame a gift from God.

When a case falls apart, as this one, and the others described in this volume, so emphatically did, we understandably and rightly feel compelled to examine our contribution to its demise. Sometimes our mistakes are egregious; usually they are small and subtle, but of exquisite importance. Often they stem from our wish to be helpful and our assumption that help is wanted. We know that internal change is difficult and often excruciatingly slow. It is extraordinarily difficult for us to understand and truly accept that sometimes psychic change is simply not possible—even under the best of circumstances with the best of resources. Unlike my patient who could not accept his efficacy, we often have difficulty fully accepting both the limitations and power of our personal, theoretical, or technical impact. The unconscious is extraordinarily powerful—as is genetic loading—as is the impact of the family and community.

## REFERENCE

Ehrensaft, D. (2007, April). *A child is being eaten.* Paper presented at the Division 39 meeting of the American Psychological Association, Toronto, Ontario, Canada.

CHAPTER 12

# INFANT–PARENT PSYCHOTHERAPY
# MINUS ONE

*Toni Vaughn Heineman*

Infant–parent psychotherapy is based on the assumption that young children in emotional distress come to us in the company of a parent. Often we undertake the process of intervening in the infant–parent relationship when the parent either cannot hold the child in mind or holds a distorted picture of the child that, in large or small measure, threatens to interfere with the child's development of a cohesive sense of self. It is difficult for a mother suffering from depression to make space in her mind for her child; her own preoccupations consume all of her available psychic energy. The distortions of reality arising from psychosis or character disorders make it virtually impossible for a parent to create a reasonably accurate picture based on the cues the baby sends rather than the expectations and assumptions arising from the parent's own internal processes. Despite the enormous difficulties these situations pose for a clinician wanting to realign and strengthen the parent–child relationship through infant–parent psychotherapy, the clinician can come to know the mind of the parent, the mind of the child, and the ways in which they influence and alter each other.

This is very often not the case for the clinician undertaking psychotherapy with a very young child in foster care. That child has been separated from one or both parents, possibly at birth. He may have gone directly into the care of a single foster parent or he may have had a series of substitute caregivers who

225

may have very limited information about his background or his experiences in previous foster homes. The status of the child's future may be as murky as the details about his past. The agency responsible for his care is legally bound to work simultaneously toward his reunification with one or both parents, and arrange suitable, permanent, and substitute care should reunification fail.

The tasks of providing services to support reunification typically fall to the child's caseworker or a series of caseworkers, depending on the administrative structure of the foster care agency. The biological parents may be required to participate in a drug treatment program, psychotherapy, parenting classes, and other activities designed to ensure that they can provide a safe environment for their child. While the parents are working to regain custody of their child, they are usually required to have somewhat regular visits with their child, which may be supervised by a professional supervisor, a relative, or the child's foster parent. Alternatively, the visits may be part of the parent's treatment program or, particularly if reunification is progressing well, may not be supervised at all.

During this period, the caseworker(s) must also look for people who might be willing and able to raise the child, in the event that the parents voluntarily relinquish their parental rights or those rights are terminated by court order. This process involves the legally mandated search for relatives, ascertaining their interest, willingness, and suitability. Typically, relatives, even if they are not available to step forward as potential adoptive parents or guardians, want to visit with the child. Sometimes this visit takes place in the child's foster home; often it takes place in a neutral setting—a park or a playroom at the foster care agency.

Very often, particularly in highly contested or unusually complex cases, each of the parties will have legal representation—the governmental agency responsible for the care of the child, the child, and the parent. If there are siblings in foster care, they may all have different attorneys, and the same attorney typically does not represent both parents. If, as happens not infrequently, two or more relatives want to become guardians or adoptive parents, they will each have legal representation.

Finally, a pivotal player in the life of a young foster child is often the court appointed special advocate (CASA). This person is a trained volunteer from the community who is charged with developing a relationship with the child, gathering information, presenting it to the court, and advocating for the child's best interest with the court.

It is not surprising that in the foster care system the job of identifying the "parent" is rarely simple or straightforward. Sometimes there simply is no one who can give information about the child. At other times multiple people, with overlapping, ill-defined, or conflicting roles, rightly feel that they have some claim to the role of primary "caregiver." When adults are at odds over the "ownership" of a child, it is nearly impossible for them to create a unified and cohesive narrative about the child—each must construct a version of the child that supports his or her claim to primacy in the child's life.

This makes identifying the infant an even more difficult psychological task. The actual child, too young to create or hold his own story, may appear in the therapist's office accompanied by an adult who is a virtual stranger to him. That person is often merely delivering the physical being and has nothing in mind about the child except the appointment time and place or the contents of the case file. The file does not contain information about the way in which the child was held in mind during pregnancy, what kind of greeting the world offered at birth, or the nature of his relationships.

## THE JOYS OF INFANT–PARENT PSYCHOTHERAPY

This relational void is quite different from our contacts with children in a reasonably well-functioning parent–child relationship, in which the parent mediates all of the young child's relationships. The parent knows the important people in the child's life—relatives, neighbors, family friends, babysitters or day care providers, and playmates. The parent knows what each of these people brings to the child and what each expects in return. It is the job of the parent to hold all of these people in mind and to help the child gradually come to know each of them—which grandparent expects good manners but is generous with cookies, which neighbor sounds frighteningly gruff but will answer endless numbers of questions, or which playmate is likely accidentally to break a fragile toy but will happily share every plaything he owns. In these cases, the clinician can reasonably assume that the parent can and will give a clear and coherent picture of the child, her likes and dislikes, and the nature of her relationship with these important people. In the event that the therapist had reason to meet any of these people, it is unlikely that they would be markedly different from the expectations created in the clinician's mind by the parent. In this way, the clinician's experience mirrors the child's experience. The "good-enough" parent gives the child information that is reasonably accurate, complete, and developmentally appropriate about the important people in the child's life, along with the information that the parent conveys to the child about herself, including that she is loved.[1]

Through this process, she learns about relationships and the ways in which people value and care for each other. Clearly, communicating important information about relationships is not simply a recitation of facts. Parents convey their excitement about visiting some people and their hesitancy about seeing others. They may be angry about the intrusiveness or emotional distance of a relative, disappointed when the director of the day care center retires, or excited when an old friend moves into the neighborhood.

If a clinician is called upon to intercede in this kind of a parent–infant relationship, it is most likely because of an event or situation that has stressed the relationship beyond its usual functional capacity. Patricia and Andrew illustrate this kind of situation. Patricia sought consultation following her brother's diagnosis of a terminal illness that threatened to claim his life in a matter of weeks. She worried enormously about the impact this would have on her young son, Andrew, whom she expected to be inconsolable and to suffer lasting harm from the loss of his favorite uncle. Patricia was fond of her brother, but not very close to him, describing him as somewhat emotionally

---

1 When Benjamin's father died suddenly, one of the routines that comforted this not-yet-3-year-old at bedtime was a recitation with his mother of "everyone who loves Benjamin." Foster parents may not have the slightest information about the people who love the young child who has been placed in their care, and the child may not know either (Heineman, 2000).

distant. She could not imagine how she would explain death to a toddler and could not figure out how to have the necessary phone calls with relatives and medical personnel without having Andrew overhear them. The daily decisions about whether to leave him playing alone so that he would not see her crying on the phone or to keep her close to him, even if it might be upsetting to him, seemed impossible. Patricia's sense of enjoying a close relationship with Andrew was echoed by her husband who was confused by her sudden loss of confidence in herself as a parent. He did not entirely understand her absolute conviction that she would be unable to soothe her son. As the consultation progressed, Patricia talked more about her unhappiness at the approach of Andrew's third birthday and her guilt over not feeling excited about this milestone in his life. She felt that he had been more distant than usual and worried that her grief was driving him away. Andrew's outbursts of temper and enormous sadness in the face of disappointment or frustration seemed to her to be more frequent and intense. She worried that he would become uncontrollable. Gradually it became clear that, for Patricia, the anticipation of her brother's death coincided too closely with Andrew's developmentally appropriate bids for autonomy. Previously, she had been able to help Andrew manage the intense feelings that are an integral part of the life of a toddler (Lieberman, 1993). However, with the unexpected news of her brother's impending death, Patricia felt overwhelmed and undone by her own grief and the sadness she felt for her mother as she faced the loss of her child. Understandably, she could not be as emotionally available or reliable for Andrew as he had come to expect. Equally understandably, he became more unpredictable—sometimes withdrawing from his mother's sadness and sometimes becoming more demanding of her attention. Just as he was learning to manage the intensity of his own feelings, he was confronted with the unexpected force of his mother's grief. The relationship that had been a predictable source of pleasure and mutual regulation was becoming derailed by an unexpected, tragic external event. Fortunately, Patricia recognized very quickly that her distress was threatening to overwhelm her and her relationship to Andrew. In this case, the parent–infant therapist did not actually see Patricia and Andrew together. He felt that he could know the relationship and Andrew through Patricia, and that the most important step was to help reestablish Patricia's confidence in her capacity to parent successfully, even under difficult circumstances. Andrew did not need the help of a professional to resume his positive developmental trajectory. He needed to regain his mother and her sense of parental authority in order to learn that they and their relationship would not only survive the intensity of their feelings but could also draw strength and grow from their shared experience of grief and loss.

This is the kind of case that our dreams are made of—a psychologically minded parent, a child who is developmentally on track, a single non–life-threatening event, and adequate social and financial resources. Patricia's confrontation with the premature death of her brother was relatively uncomplicated. Because it did not raise the ghosts of past traumatic losses, she had the luxury of dealing with it for what it was—a loss that made no sense and came too soon. With the therapist's help, she recognized relatively quickly that her identification with her mother was causing her to merge and confuse her own expectable and normal feelings of loss in the face of Andrew's developmentally appropriate separation with her mother's anticipatory mourning for a child she was about to lose forever. With this awareness, she could reclaim her dual roles: first, as the parent of a little boy who needed her help in the emotional process of separating from and returning to her, and second, as the daughter of a mother who needed her help in the process of separating from a child who would not ever return to her.

Grief is an underappreciated luxury. People who have the opportunity to mourn the loss of a loved one without the intrusions triggered by previous unresolved traumas often do so simply with the help of family and friends. When they do ask for professional help, like Patricia, they often make quick and good use of what we have to offer. Although their lives may have not been without turmoil or trouble, typically they have enjoyed enough satisfying relationships based on mutual value and respect to expect more of the same. These cases make it easy for us to be helpful and give the best of what we have to offer.

## THE PAINS OF INFANT–PARENT PSYCHOTHERAPY

However, the cases that make up the reality of our day-to-day working lives infrequently offer simple satisfaction, gratification, or opportunity to enjoy a sense of professional competence and confidence. More often, the children and parents who come to us for help are beset with multiple current and past stressors that continually threaten the stability and coherence of their internal and external worlds. The difficulties they bring to us endanger our sense of clinical identity and well-being. Because they have rarely enjoyed a preponderance of satisfying relationships, based on mutual value and respect, they do not look for or expect to find them. When they do—and relationships form the foundation of what we have to offer—they either do not know what to do with them or feel an almost overwhelming need to destroy them in order to preserve reality as they have come to know it.

One of the gravest difficulties facing therapists working in foster care is that it is a system that, despite the rhetoric, fundamentally does not value relationships. Because relationships stand at the core of our beliefs and our insistence that they are essential for children's healthy development, we will at some point find ourselves at odds with the system charged with the child's care. In some cases, this conflict will destroy the treatment; in other cases, the disagreement may be barely noticed. The toll on the therapist is particularly onerous when "the system," which often feels like a disembodied, uncontainable force with power far greater than the sum of the players in it, purports to support relationships while steadfastly interfering with the child's opportunities to build important, consistent connections to nurturing adults. In these situations, I have often had the feeling that even if I devoted every waking minute to my therapeutic charge, I could never possibly protect her from the misery that will be inflicted upon her by a system whose supposed task is to rescue her.

This certainly characterized my work with Christina. Indeed, the CASA who volunteered with Christina and her older brother and I both frequently wondered whether, even together, we could sustain the energy and resources needed to keep the lives of these young children from spinning completely out of control, let alone help them overcome the effects of the tragic events that had brought them into the foster care system.

Christina and her brother, Jack, entered foster care when she was 2 years old and he was 4. They were delivered to the foster care office by an elderly great aunt who had tried to care for them following the death of their mother some months earlier from a drug overdose. At the time of their mother's death, the children were living in a single room of a residential hotel with their parents. Following her death, their father's drug use continued unabated. Their great aunt took them to her home when she found them unkempt and the room without food.

The aunt was frail and in poor health. She explained to the intake worker that she could not manage two young children whose behavior was totally uncontrollable and unpredictable. In addition, their father, Harry, frequently came to her home angrily insisting that if she did not let him see his children, he would report her for kidnapping. He also raged at her, demanding money and food before he would leave. The aunt had been a foster parent as a younger woman, and was extremely reluctant to have these children placed in foster care. She had tried to prevail on her own daughter to take the children, but she refused to do anything that might bring her own family into contact with Harry, who had stolen money from her in the past. As a working parent with a marginal income, she felt that she and her husband could barely take care of her own children. She worried that she might lose her job any time she had to take time off work to attend a doctor's appointment or meet with the school counselor. Christina and Jack simply had too many problems, and she had too few resources.

When they entered the foster care system, both children suffered from chronic diarrhea. Jack had severe tooth decay; Christina had a bilateral ear infection. Neither child slept well—they had trouble falling asleep and woke frequently with nightmares. Christina wailed almost incessantly—everything seemed to frighten her and nothing seemed to soothe her; she seemed immobilized by fear. In contrast, Jack could not hold still. He ran, he jumped, he screamed, he fought. Both children had seemingly insatiable appetites. Their foster mother felt as if they would eat "until they exploded." She worried that Jack would make himself sick by eating the food he tried to forage from the garbage or hurt himself while climbing to reach food on the kitchen shelves.

Christina and Jack, who spoke only English, spent their first month in an emergency foster home with a very caring, experienced Spanish-speaking foster mother because there were no other homes available. However, they did begin to calm down, and their physical health began to improve in that foster mother's care. In the next foster home, where they were to spend the next 3 years while the legal system moved with inexorable slowness toward what was supposed to be a permanent plan, they again had the good fortune of having a patient and experienced foster mother. Maria had two adult children and a grandchild who visited frequently. Her daughter helped her with the day care center she ran in her home. Most days there were six preschool children in the home during the day who were joined by Maria's grandson between the end of school and the dinner hour. At the time of this move, the children's case was transferred to another social worker as a matter of routine practice.

Their social worker was concerned that Maria might not be able to keep the children in her home because of Jack's behavior. She referred him for therapy about 6 months after he entered the foster care system because he was so out of control that Maria feared for both his safety and that of the other children in her care. He recklessly climbed to high places, and frequently lashed out at other children when his wishes or will were thwarted. Jack also grabbed anxiously at his crotch throughout the day, gyrated in a sexualized way when he was being dressed or bathed, and liked to sneak into the bathroom to watch other children on the toilet. Maria was also worried about Christina's continual inconsolable sadness, but the social worker felt that she was too young for psychotherapy. When they had been in foster care for about 9 months, Maria discovered Jack in Christina's crib. Her diaper was off, and Christina was in tears and appeared to be frightened.

At that point the social worker asked for a psychological evaluation of Christina, fearing that Jack had molested her. She also began to worry that Jack might have been sexually abused while in the care of his parents. At the time of these events, Jack was approaching 5 and Christina was 3 months shy of her third birthday. The evaluation to establish sexual abuse was inconclusive in regard to Jack. However, the therapist who saw him in individual therapy felt that his play strongly suggested that he had either been engaged in or witnessed explicit sexual behavior. The evaluator found no evidence in Christina's play or behavior to warrant concern about sexual abuse or exposure. However, she did refer Christina for therapy because of her extreme sadness, rote and repetitive play, and propensity to make indiscriminate attachments. She noted that during the course of an evaluation that stretched over several weeks, Christina had made overtures to every adult in the clinic—therapists, secretaries, and adults sitting in the waiting room. She showed little interest in the other children at the clinic.

Christina was referred to me for therapy. Her social worker scheduled and brought her to her first therapy appointment because the foster mother was unable to leave the other children at her day care center and did not drive. Maria felt very strongly that Christina should have therapy because of "the things had had happened to her." However, she was adamant that she did not have the time to take Christina to appointments, could not take time away from the children in her day care center to take part in home visits, and did not feel that she had any reason to participate in Christina's therapy. She explained to the social worker that she would be happy to speak with the therapist by phone at anytime and would gladly pass along important information about events in Christina's life and any changes in her behavior. She felt that her relationship with the little girl in her care was good, that Christina's troubles had started long before they met, and that Christina had only improved since coming to live with her. Of course, all of that was true, but it also aptly demonstrated the limits of Maria's attachment to Christina. She truly cared very much about this little girl—perhaps even loved her; Christina often said that Mama Maria loved her. However, she saw herself as a substitute and temporary caregiver. In the 3 years I worked with Christina, I never met her foster mother. During this time, the court ordered two additional evaluations of this child, and neither of the other psychologists met her foster mother—the adult who had primary responsibility for her day-to-day care.

When I was asked to see Christina, I was told that this would most likely be a brief intervention to help her with an expected move into a permanent placement with relatives in another part of the state. The social worker explained that she had tried desperately to find a therapist who saw young children on the list of approved therapists; there were very few and they had no time. The clinics had waiting lists and generally were not taking new patients because it was at the end of the training year. My schedule was very full at that time, and it was with more than a little reluctance that I agreed to see this little girl, but I expected that I could make time during the summer months and that she would be settled in her new home and with a long-term therapist when I returned from vacation. Like Maria, I saw myself as a substitute and temporary caregiver.

As I write this, I am again confused, horrified, outraged, embarrassed, and exhausted by the thought that I treated a young child for 3 years without ever having met her primary caregiver. When we started, it didn't seem to matter so much—this was to be a short-term relationship. Maria and I both saw ourselves as transitional folks in Christina's life, charged with helping her move on with as little disruption as possible. Then we just continued as we had begun. Perhaps we did not meet because of force of habit, inertia, or denial of the reality of our relationship to Christina or some form of acting out our resentment of being expected to deliver far more than we had promised, or all of the above and more. The fact that both evaluators also neglected to meet with Maria suggests another possibility that is a frequent aspect of the transference/countertransference paradigm in our work with foster children—we "forget" about the other adults in the child's life. The immediacy of the child's emotional needs in combination with tenuous attachments to caregivers who can be replaced without warning can make it easy for us to set them aside or to overlook their importance.[2]

---

2 I think it is important to remember this when we find ourselves overlooked or forgotten, for example, when meetings or hearings are scheduled or plans for the child's future are made without regard for our input. Such oversight may reflect a general disregard for psychotherapy, but it may also indicate an unconscious recognition that unlike parents, we—along with foster parents and caseworkers—are temporary figures in the child's life.

The neglect of this important person also, of course, reflects Christina's reality—there was no parent available for infant–parent psychotherapy.

We spoke by phone with some frequency. Maria readily called me when there was information that she thought would be helpful to me. She never asked for advice or for suggestions about how she might help Christina. Periodically, I would plan to call to see if I could arrange to visit on a weekend, when she would be free from her child care duties. These good intentions briefly assuaged my guilt and temporarily covered the swells of outrage, resentment, and sorrow that frequently overwhelmed me as I helplessly watched and participated in a system, in this instance, so consumed with meeting the letter of the law that the spirit of the law intended to protect the best interests of the children was continually overrun.

When I returned from vacation, Christina was still with Maria. The relatives who were supposed to materialize had withdrawn their offer to care for the children. There were no alternatives on the immediate horizon. Their father was in a drug rehab program, and was demanding reunification services and visits. His program was expressly designed for drug abusing parents with the intent of bringing families back together. His continuing in the program—which contributed to their funding—required that he have increasingly greater time with them, and that the children would eventually live with him at the center during the latter phases of his treatment.

So Christina and I continued to see each other on a somewhat regular basis. We talked and played. She especially liked the dollhouse, from which the dolls came and went in an unpredictable and haphazard way. I was never sure who would bring Christina to her appointments. Sometimes it was her social worker; sometimes it was one of several drivers. Christina and I had our two favorites of this group—they brought her on time, picked her up on time, chatted with me, and had running jokes and stories with her. Things could seem almost normal—it could seem as if a parent was looking after her and that I was delivering her back into the hands of someone who knew and cared about her.

During one stretch of several weeks, for reasons that I could never understand, the transportation became wildly erratic. Christina probably had seven or eight different people driving her to and from therapy sessions. Sometimes she arrived just as her appointment was scheduled to end. Sometimes I had to reschedule the appointment of the patient who followed her because the driver was so late. During these times I often found myself drawn toward anxiously joining Christina in her vigil at the window. One day, as our wait was approaching an hour, I was stunned by the fear on Christina's face. I then recognized the anger in my voice as I was leaving a message for her social worker. When the driver had not arrived, I had called Maria, only to discover that she had rushed to a doctor's appointment because of an urgent medical problem. Her daughter could not fetch Christina because she had to mind the children in the day care center. I had called the social worker, who was not in. I had then tried the transportation office, only to receive a recorded message instructing me to call the emergency number. At the emergency number, another recorded message greeted me, explaining that the machine was full and that I should call back at a later time. That prompted my help-lessly enraged message to the social worker, which was interrupted only by the look on Christina's face. I tried to remind myself that we needed a least one person in the room to act like an adult. I seemed a more likely candidate than Christina. Perhaps the truism that children need parents most when they are least available extends to therapists.

Christina and I had been left stranded, helpless, and, for that moment, alone in the world together. This wait, that lasted a little more than an hour, provided me an intense, affective glimpse into Christina's world. Even though I knew better, when I could pull my rational self together, I felt as if we had been totally and completely abandoned—*forever*. My calls for help went unan-swered. No one cared. No one even knew I needed help. It was past lunchtime. I had not brought my lunch that day. Should I leave with Christina to go for food? What if the driver came while we were gone? What if someone called while we were out? What if no one ever called? What if the driver had actually forgotten about us? We were hungry, scared, and confused, and our resources were diminishing rapidly. Maybe that is what if feels like to be stranded on a desert island. Maybe that is what it feels like to be a foster child. There was no one to call.

Indeed, during much of the time that I worked with Christina I alternated between feeling that there was no one to call and that I had to call everyone all the time or all would be lost. Fortunately, as a volunteer member of A Home Within, I had the wise and supportive counsel of the clinicians in my consultation group. Through A Home Within, clinicians, like myself, volunteer to see a current or former foster child in weekly pro bono psychotherapy, and senior clinicians offer pro bono group consultation. At the time I began seeing Christina, I was leading a consultation group; when her funding ran out, I continued with her on a volunteer basis and brought her story to the group.

It is difficult for me to imagine how I would have been able to manage all of the feelings—particularly the sense of despair—without the group's help. Our talking together made it possible for me to maintain some capacity to think when the facts of this child's life made a state of blissful ignorance seductive.

The 3 months that I expected to see Christina stretched to 3 years. Over the course of this time, I developed a deep affection for this little girl and a profound feeling of sadness about the limitations—both internally and externally imposed—on my capacity to help her. Christina had a beautiful, engaging smile and a delightful sense of humor. She flourished in the care of Maria, and became one of those children who seemed always to get the best that people have to offer—within limits. Maria did not want to raise another family; she had agreed to take Jack and Christina on a short-term basis, not to consider adoption or legal guardianship. After protracted legal battles and additional evaluations and reviews of evaluations, Christina and Jack went to live with the relatives who had initially come forward and then withdrawn. Unfortunately, after about a year that "placement failed," and these children were returned to the county that held jurisdiction, but not to the mother with whom Christina had spent more of her life than any other. Christina been "sent back," but she had not returned home. Maria was out of the foster care and day care business. Christina was distraught—her overwhelming sadness and confusion showed in angry temper tantrums and massive regression. When she left her relatives, she had expected to return to the one adult she felt loved her and whose love she could count on.

## BEYOND INFANT-PARENT PSYCHOTHERAPY

When I again saw Christina she was 7 years old. She entered my office hesitantly and stopped to inspect the dollhouse. In a quiet voice she offered, "It's been a long time since I've seen you." I agreed and said that I was glad to see her. She responded, "No one in that place liked me." Fighting back tears, I told her that I was so sorry and that I had heard that it had been very, very difficult. She began to explore the office tentatively, commenting on what was new and what she remembered from our previous life together.

What made me want to cry? Everything about this child's life and our therapeutic life together. I had to take care of her, and I could not take care of her. I had battled the system for 3 years and had been defeated; I did not want to resume that fight, but I had no choice. My relationship with her was not only just about psychotherapy; it was also a battle about emotional life and death and one that I stood a very good chance of losing. I knew the players in this drama, and I had enough experience with the tragedy of foster care to predict that we were moving Christina inexorably toward life in long-term foster care. Christina was a beautiful child whose sweetness and charm masked an emptiness that could make an hour with her feel like an eternity. It was often tempting just to go through the motions of psychotherapy because fighting to stay psychically alive and connected to her was so difficult. It was equally tempting to go through the motions of psychotherapy in relation to the foster care system because fighting for Christina to have a chance to stay psychically alive and connected was just so difficult. I wanted to cry because when Christina walked through my door, I instantly knew that there was no turning back, and that I had just put my sanity on the line.

Despite my split-second recognition that I had already implicitly agreed to resume psychotherapy with Christina, I behaved as if the question was still open and a matter of rationally weighing the pros and cons of an argument. Christina's return came at a particularly busy time in my professional life. Because of other commitments, I knew that I would have a very difficult time maintaining a regular schedule for this child for whom any disruption was overwhelming.[3] I knew that my schedule would not allow me to attend all of the meetings that would determine Christina's future, and it was essential that her therapist be present. Christina's distress was threatening her placement; she really needed to have therapy two or three times a week, at least until her overpowering feelings could be contained. I did not have that kind of time. Every bit of logic argued for my transferring Christina to a new therapist. However, this was not about logic.

In one sense, this phase of my work was the most clearly defined in any of the time I have known Christina, yet it also caused me the greatest ambivalence about my relationship to her. The recurring message from all of the many players in Christina's life at the time she returned was that I had to "stabilize the placement." Christina was in very grave danger of being moved to yet another home, which would have been absolutely disastrous for her. Because her disruptive behavior clearly had psychological origins, everyone was expecting therapy to accomplish this task and, fundamentally, really did not care whether that job fell to me or someone else. I felt that on the most basic human level, I had no choice about resuming my therapeutic relationship with Christina. I had to see her. However, I also knew that my schedule would not allow me to give her the time and attention that she needed and deserved. What if I failed, and she lost both her current foster family and me as a result? I wondered if it would be better if I referred her to someone who could be more available while I stepped into a role more like a special friend. So often this is the dilemma facing the therapist working with young children in foster care—which is the least bad of the available choices.

---

3 Christina was not my child. Christina was not Maria's child. When their children are in overwhelming distress, as Christina was, parents drop everything. They rearrange their schedules; they put their busy lives on hold. No one in Christina's life had that connection to her.

With the help of my consultation group, I struggled with the limited options facing me. Fortunately, in the process of sorting through them time and time again, I had the opportunity to talk with Jeree Pawl about this case. With her usual wisdom, Jeree redefined my task. She counseled that my job was to "want" Christina. This cogent advice eased the anxious burden of "stabilizing the placement" that had been defined by the foster care agency. I had to reconnect with Christina. I did want her, but I did not want full responsibility for her emotional well-being. If I could want her, others could want her as well. My wanting her would allow her to become a "wantable," loveable child.

At this writing, Christina and I are meeting on a regular basis. Her new foster mother is loving and experienced, and she or a member of her family brings Christina to her appointments. The legal process that will decide her future has resumed. A new evaluation is in process that includes a review of the evaluation that was done when Christina was living with her relatives, along with the two evaluations that took place when she lived with Maria. When she comes to my office, we talk and play in old and new ways. She likes to go through the office and remember what is old and discover what is new. In a recent session, her eyes lit up when she found a toy that I had bought at a craft fair. She exclaimed, "I made this for you and it's still here. Do you remember when I made this for you?" I really did not know what to say.

Much of the time in my work with Christina, I really did not know what to say because I did not really know what my job was. Obviously, she has passed through the age of infant–parent psychotherapy, but in a very profound way we are still at the point where we started—without any clear idea of who the parent is in this parent–child relationship. When Christina first moved into her current foster home, I included her foster mother in some of the sessions in order to help her understand and manage Christina's anger, confusion, and grief about not being with Mama Maria as she had so fervently wished and reasonably expected. After a while, Christina protested having to share her time. Her relationships at home and school were beginning to offer her pleasure, and her foster mother was increasingly confident about her ability to understand and respond to the full range of Christina's behavior and feelings.

## REFLECTIONS

It is not unusual for therapists working with young children in foster care to feel that the full weight of the child's life is on their shoulders. In a system that is geared toward action as the solution to most problems, this overwhelming feeling is often concretized into plans for action. Particularly for young and inexperienced therapists, it often manifests itself as a wish to adopt the child (Birch, 2000; Heineman, 2001). In other instances—perhaps with older, more experienced therapists or with clinicians working with adolescents or older children who do not as easily pull on our heartstrings as potential adoptees—it may manifest itself in a wish or attempt to take charge of the myriad players in the child's life (Weston, 2006). In either case, I believe that these concrete solutions can best be understood as a profoundly experienced need to create a parental mind to watch over a child. We know that there are no babies without mothers.

When we are confronted with the vacuum of maternal care that engulfs children in foster care it surely stirs a primitive panic in us. We know that a child simply must exist in someone's mind—always and completely. When faced with the absence of a parental mind, we imagine filling the void permanently with adoption or, at least, completely by gathering and ordering the fragments of information and responsibility that are held by the many people in a foster child's life. However, when we, as therapists, step into the void—because a child must be held in mind—we may inadvertently preclude another from filling that psychic space. When we feel or act as if we are the child's parent, we may not leave room for a real parent to begin to hold the child in mind. We frequently see this played out in relation to foster parents, who are given sole responsibility for a child's care, but often not allowed to voice an opinion about how best to meet a child's needs. We ask them to assume parental responsibility without conveying parental authority.

I believe that my contribution to the crisis that we narrowly averted when Christina returned from the relatives who did not want her was my sense that I had to step into the parental void—not by adoption or becoming her foster parent—but by pulling all of the pieces and players together and holding them in mind for and with her. It was a job I had no hope of doing successfully and in the face of this formidable task, I felt hopeless and anxiously overwhelmed. Having psychically put myself into the center of the melee, everyone understandably looked to me to solve the problem. They themselves became anxious when they recognized that the limitations on my time, energy, and psychic space would make me fall short. When I found the freedom to step back and simply "want" Christina, her life began to shift subtly, but remarkably quickly. With more space to assume the parenting role, her foster mother introduced more structure. With my help, she began to act more independently and to solve problems at home without continually asking for advice from the caseworker, which only made both of them worried that she could not handle Christina. As Christina calmed down, the caseworker turned to other, more demanding situations, which, in turn, created more space for her foster mother to parent.

Psychotherapeutic work in any system or culture imposes particular pressures and expectations that create unique psychological dangers. In some instances, the culture creates a pressure to politicize the therapy; in others, it creates an enchantment with the life of the mind that can undermine the work of true introspection. In the foster care system, the pressure to act often and profoundly endangers the therapist's capacity to think. It is very difficult to make time and psychological space to think with and about a child when there is no one to join in that process—when there is no one with whom to have a "meeting of the minds."

I was in danger of succumbing to the pressure to act—of accepting the charge to "stabilize the placement," rather than thinking about what Christina needed from me and what I had to offer her. Stabilizing the placement really translates into asking children and foster parents to change behavior that is symptomatic of a difficulty in the relationship before there is time to understand the relationship or the difficulties it poses for each of them. When I was free to want Christina, and not to measure that desire by the number of hours I had for her or the speed with which I could calm the reverberations her behavior was sending through the system, I regained my capacity to think. Although it seems painfully obvious from this distance, at the time it was not so clear to me that "wanting" was at the core of the problems in the relationship between Christina and her foster mother. Christina did not want her; she wanted Maria who did not want her. Her new foster mother had initially wanted Christina, but her attachment to Christina was too tenuous to withstand Christina's not wanting her. With this in mind, I could help Christina and her foster mother think alone and together about what they wanted and the disappointments attendant to not being able to have what we often want so desperately that we believe we cannot live without it.

## CONCLUSION

The placement was indeed stabilized—not because of any particular action, but because a shift in my understanding of my role restored my capacity to think and to bring my understanding of relationships to bear on this child and the adults in her life. At least temporarily, we have prevented more disruptions in this child's life. I was able to help Christina and her foster mother find ways of wanting each other. However, my next task may be helping them face the disappointment and grief over losing what they now want. The legally required search for potential adoptive parents among relatives has resumed. It may succeed. Christina's father may recover enough from his addiction that he would prevail in an action to terminate his parental rights. Christina's present foster mother may become her legal guardian—a tie that might not withstand the storms of adolescence.

Christina's life is not easy, and probably never will be. She is impulsive and prone to hitting other children. It is exceedingly difficult for her to take any kind of responsibility for her actions. She has the kind of charm that pulls people in and then leaves them feeling angry and cheated at the shallowness of the connection that Christina offers. She is only 7—she has time. She is already 7—she does not have much time.

I fully expect that Christina will spend the next 11 years of her life in foster care. I hope that she will be able to stay in the same foster home, and that she will have good and frequent contact with Jack and her father. I could hope that her father would relinquish his parental rights and allow for an open adoption, but at this juncture I am not prepared to face the disappointment that that particular hope would almost surely bring. I hope that Christina and I will stay together, and that she and I will both have the energy to keep that connection alive and enlivening. I hope that my wanting her will help her to want relationships with others who truly want her.

## ACKNOWLEDGMENTS

In more than two decades of professional work, I have enjoyed far more than my share of support and encouragement from teachers, colleagues, students, patients, friends, and family. I have also had the good fortune of being associated with many forward-thinking institutions and organizations that have had a profound influence, not only on those in their immediate sphere, but also on the ways in which both professionals and the public have come to understand and address mental health and illness. My fellowship through the Leadership Development Initiative offered by ZERO TO THREE brought me into contact with an incredible range of thoughtful, experienced, and knowledgeable people with an irrepressible dedication to making the world a better place for babies and their families. My association with ZERO TO THREE has had a profound impact on my professional life, as well as creating opportunities for new and important friendships. I am deeply grateful for the support of the people at ZERO TO THREE who helped to shape the work and thinking of this chapter.

## REFERENCES

Birch, M. (2000, April). *Love in the countertransference: Attachment issues in the treatment of a motherless child.* Paper presented at the 20th Annual Spring Meeting, Division 39, American Psychological Association, San Francisco, CA.

Heineman, T. V. (2000). Beginning to say goodbye: A two-year-old confronts the death of his father. *Journal of Infant, Child & Adolescent Psychotherapy, 1*, 1–22.

Heineman, T. V. (2001). Hunger pangs: Transference and countertransference in the treatment of foster children. *Journal of Applied Psychoanalytic Studies, 3*(1), 5–16.

Lieberman, A. F. (1993). *The emotional life of the toddler.* New York: Free Press.

Weston, R. B. (2006). In search of the fuzzy green pillow: Fragmented selves, fragmented institutions. In T. V. Heineman & D. Ehrensaft (Eds.), *Building a home within: Meeting the emotional needs of children and youth in foster care* (pp. 43–74). Baltimore: Brookes.

# CHAPTER 13

# THE NEED TO FILL IN THE HOLE: DISCUSSION OF TONI VAUGHN HEINEMAN'S CASE

*Susan Sklan*

In Toni Vaughn Heineman's chapter (chapter 12), she movingly highlights the complex undertaking of a therapist working with a little girl in the foster care system in the worst-case scenario of a young child for whom no parent can be found. While the therapist works with Christina, the foster care system is unable to locate a committed parent for her, such that Christina continues to be abandoned and unwanted by a series of substitute foster parents and serial caseworkers. Heineman's account of her work with Christina addresses the heart of the anguish of the therapist. In thinking about the countertransference issues, I recognize Heineman's gravitational pull to both jump in and fill in the hole of overwhelming needs and also to feel pulled into a hole herself of overwhelming feelings in response to the overwhelming needs and feelings of the young child.

## THE NEED TO FILL IN THE HOLE

The need to fill in the hole for the young child with no parent is a predictable path with its own minefields for the parent–child therapist. The therapist feels an impulse to become a reparative parental figure. The impulse is elicited by the absence of a parent for the young child. Heineman refered to "a profoundly experienced need to create a parental mind to watch over the child," a

247

particular legacy of the infant mental health field. The "parental mind" is aware of everything pertaining to the child, both currently and over time, and actively helps the infant or child integrate with meaning the multiple layers of her own experiences. In the absence of a stable parental figure or a vulnerable parent figure that needs support, the therapist feels an intense pressure to be at the center of the infant's or child's world, a huge responsibility. This carries with it complicated implications of relational meaning for both the therapist and the infant or child. The infant or child needs to develop a deep emotional bond with the parent or parent substitute, not a therapist. It is not unknown for therapists working in the protective care field to adopt children they come across in their work. This speaks to the intense and compelling pressure in our field to provide restitution even if this means that in order to fix a child's life the relationship with the therapist becomes a permanent component of the child's life.

With a fragmented family and a changing procession of foster parents and caseworkers, Heineman felt compelled to hold together for Christina a sense of her life with relationships over time. A vital continuous thread is lost for a young child at moments of significant transition, such as a scheduled therapy appointment or being sent to live in a new foster home, when no adult caregiver holds in mind the child's "before," "now," and "after." Someone should know and keep her past story and use this knowledge to help Christina understand herself. The therapist wanted to protect for Christina her life narrative and the meaning of her story. I recognize that impulse in myself as I took photos and made little photo albums for Julia and Miguel (chapter 2).

Returning after a failed attempt at a preadoptive placement with relatives, both Christina and Heineman grappled with loss and how to reconnect. Everything seemed so tenuous, and the feeling that everything could fall apart and disappear was the "elephant in the room." How moving and painful it is to sit with Christina's longing. How much could Christina count on her therapist? Christina shows what she needs by sharing her fantasy that her therapist is the person who would keep and implicitly value something Christina made for her when she was younger. Christina wants to acknowledge that they have a relationship and that it has a past. Christina's yearning for some links to her own past were acted out each visit by Christina commenting on what was there and what had changed over time. Heineman's presence and the therapy room provided the only stable stage for Christina to mark her own growth and emotional changes.

## TO FEEL PULLED INTO THE HOLE

The lack of institutional supports also places the therapist in a hole in which there are overwhelming needs and overwhelming feelings of her own. Christina begins therapy with the intense needs of a young child with disordered attachment and multiple layers of pain and loss. Christina has suffered at a very early age the death of her mother, profound physical neglect by both mother and father, and possible sexual abuse. We can only imagine what emotional abuse Christina suffered and witnessed at a preverbal age with her biological parents. Christina needs to be loved by an adult who is committed and responsible for her. It is difficult, even impossible, in these situations to engage the child in the relational treatment needed if there is no suitable parent substitute ready and willing to be a loving parent. Heineman alludes to failures in the child protective system's attempts to find a caring; relationship from Christina's family; an aunt who returns Christina after a year and a father who is in a drug rehabilitation program and who has so far not shown the capacity to parent. Heineman feels quite isolated and overwhelmed in her relationship with Christina; she mentions the court appointed special advocate's role, but it is not clear how supportive that was.

## THE COST OF THE HEART

As parent–infant and parent–child therapists, we are painfully aware of the needs of the infant or child. We are professional and caring. However, there is that edge of "hate in the countertransference" (Winnicott, 1947/1975), an ambivalence that we as therapists are paid to care, yet the payment for doing this work does not absolve us from intense negative feelings. What happens after sessions or when the driver does not show up to collect the child?

What do we do with our panic, our uncertainty, our lack of professional confidence, our fears, our resentment, our anger, and our sense of failure, and even betrayal, for this child? As infant–parent psychotherapists, we know this is not enough for the child to whom we provide our services. The child needs not just services, but truly also needs to be loved. We are well aware that our role in the child's life is temporary (Tessman, 1978). Our shortcomings are painful as we take on the huge task of activating and sustaining a child's psychic life. How do you work with a child with an attachment disorder if there is no reparative substitute parental attachment relationship in place? Heineman refers to the huge energy required by the therapist to help Christina with the effects of the tragic events that led her into foster care, as well as her attempt to keep Christina's life from spinning out of control and meaning. The impact of the trauma is shared, and there is a parallel process within the therapist as we struggle to make sense of it. The therapist is motivated by the presence of an infant or a young child to push to integrate the material and make for healthy relationships. It was Christina's presence that helped the therapist to collect herself and not outwardly express her full fury and fear when the driver did not appear to collect Christina. Both the therapist and Christina were abandoned at that moment, and Heineman felt it along with Christina or perhaps for her. "Maybe that is what it feels like to be a foster child. There was no one to call." (p. 238)

One aspect of the countertransference for the therapist, as a result of taking on the "parental mind," is feeling isolated. Heineman writes clearly of feeling "totally and completely abandoned—*forever*" (p. 237) in caring for Christina. She felt there was no one else who was really committed to Christina, no one who would drop everything for her in a crisis as a parent does. That feeling of isolation in the work is underscored by the system that often forgets or overlooks the therapist or the foster parent who is also not included in conferences to process the needs of the foster child. The therapist as well as the foster parent is regarded as transitory and therefore not taken seriously by the foster system. Heineman makes an important point that, as professionals in the work, especially charged with the care of a vulnerable child, we also often forget that other adults are involved. The feelings of urgency and fear propel us into a mental vortex.

Heineman acknowledges that she felt sick with anxiety when she signed on again to continue to see Christina, after Christina was returned after a year at a preadoptive home. Heineman anticipated failure and further grief in her own advocacy role on behalf of Christina with the institutions that were responsible for foster care. The system itself is toxic and crazy-making for therapists who are committed to supporting and enhancing the positive nurturing relationships for the young child. The protective care system has its own contradictions, dilemmas, and tensions. It is required by law to simultaneously give the biological parent a chance to repair him- or herself and the relationship with the child, as well as to identify a parent substitute for the child who is meanwhile in need of a relationship with emotional commitment. Heineman's experience leads her to conclude that the foster care system fundamentally does not value relationships, as it often interferes with a child's opportunities to build an important nurturing relationship with a parent figure. She sees the therapist as helpless to protect a child from further misery when all caregivers see themselves as temporary and transitional figures in a child's life. Separations can be abrupt and arbitrary in nature.

It is too easy to project our fears and hate onto other players who are not "holding" or supporting us in our parent–child relationship work. The therapist's own internal negative feelings are likely to be more pronounced in a foster care case. Here the therapist is often asked to "fix" or "stabilize" a child's distressing behavior with no caring "parent" figure in sight. This is a weighty responsibility for a therapist working alone in a fragmented foster care system. If the child is not fixed, then the child will be less lovable and less likely to be even eligible for adoption, let alone be ready to receive and give love in a caring relationship. Heineman writes of her fears of seeing Christina settling permanently into the foster care system. What do we do when we lose our vision because it is emptied of faith?

A significant shift in the work occurred with the insight of good supervision. Heineman was able to reduce her role to just simply wanting Christina.

Rather than feel she had to hold everything and satisfy all Christina's needs, the therapist released her grip and allowed space for others such as the new foster parent to move in and claim parental roles for Christina. The therapist no longer had to undertake what she could not manage. The supervisor's wise counsel allowed Heineman simultaneously to no longer feel so alone and to not be overwhelmed by overwhelming needs.

## ACTING ON OUR COUNTERTRANSFERENCE FEELINGS

The "perfect attunement" is not able to tolerate hate and rupture. It is a sign of the maturing in professional development in an individual therapist as well as the maturing of the field of infant mental health to be able to look at aspects of the work that feel unbearable. Just as the mother, as described by Winnicott (1947/1975), is able to walk the line of ambivalence of the love and the hate, the ability to contain the hate is the ability to acknowledge it.

Stress is a motivator for developmental change. Creative changes to impact services at a policy and structural level can be seen in a program such as Minding the Baby, an inner city home visitation program to support parent–infant relationships. This program design addresses the need both to have the pieces held together for a vulnerable parent–infant and parent–child dyad, and to address the needs of the therapists to be supported and not isolated in the face of overwhelming needs (Slade, Sadler, & Mayes, 2005). This program uses a multidisciplinary team. Slade noted the importance of the integration and holding of the team as a necessary component for a model of working with families whose basic and psychological needs are overwhelming. The working team provided not only collaboration, timeliness, and efficiency in the provision of services, but also important support for the individual staff who could so easily feel drained. If we are able to identify that this work can lead the therapist to feel isolated and overwhelmed, then we can create ways to address this for the therapist. On a deeper level, the team in the Minding the Baby program provided sensitive responses to the family needs, integration, and a holding on a deeper level for these very troubled families with vulnerable infants.

This discussion would not be complete without a reference and appreciation to the pioneering work of Heineman as a founding member of A Home Within, an organization that provides support to therapists who commit to seeing children within the foster care system "for as long as it takes," at no charge. This commitment addresses the need a child has for a stable, lasting relationship within the foster care system at a structural and policy level. It elevates the therapist to the status of a long-term, not merely transitory, relationship. Volunteer therapists also have ongoing free consultation with senior clinicians in small groups for as long as the treatment lasts. A Home Within is now a nationwide nonprofit organization that is focused on the emotional needs of foster children and youths (Heineman & Ehrensaft, 2005).

## REFERENCES

Heineman, T. V., & Ehrensaft, D. (Eds.). (2005). *Building a home within: Meeting the emotional needs of children and youth in foster care*. Baltimore: Brookes.

Slade, A., Sadler, L. S., & Mayes, L. C. (2005). Minding the baby: Enhancing parental reflective functioning in a nursing/mental health home visiting program. In L. J. Berlin (Ed.), *Enhancing early attachments* (pp. 152–177). New York: Guilford Press.

Tessman, L. H. (1978). *Children of parting parents*. New York: Jason Aronson.

Winnicott, D. W. (1975). Hate in the countertransference. In D. W. Winnicott, *Through paediatrics to psychoanalysis*, (pp. 194–203). New York: Basic Books. (Original work published in 1947)

# CHAPTER 14

## RADICAL HOPE AND INFANT–PARENT PSYCHOTHERAPY

*Marian Birch*

If what I say has truth in it, this will already have been dealt with by the world's poets, but the flashes of insight that come in poetry cannot absolve us from our painful task of getting step by step away from ignorance towards our goal. (Winnicott, 1963/1989, p. 87)

The cases in this book were offered to the editor in response to an invitation to write about a case that "that broke your heart and what you think went wrong." In the preceding chapters, we have come to know six families, six therapists, and their shared experiences that are self-identified by the therapist as "heartbreaking failures." No other parameters were suggested, so it is interesting how many qualities these cases do share. It may be useful to look at the shared characteristics of these families whose treatment experiences failed to set their children on a positive developmental trajectory.

In this final chapter, drawing on what we have learned in the preceding chapters from the six heart-wrenching and courageous case reports and discussions, we address two central questions that run through all of these cases:

The first question is: Where are the limits of a supportive, strengths-based approach? Is it when parental projections onto the child are extremely toxic? When the child's caregiver appears unable to metabolize the "support" that is offered? When the child is in (how much?) emotional peril? Does more severe psychopathology in child or parent call for additional services, skills, or techniques? What are the alternatives and how can we make them acceptable to severely troubled families? How can we combine the "outreach" that has always been a piece of infant mental health services with a better understanding of and respect for a family's right to refuse treatment? What are the minimal requirements for a therapeutic alliance that make psychotherapeutic intervention with infants and their families possible? Without our giving up outreach, are there formalized "contracting" and assessment procedures that would make it more likely that we and our clients had the same idea of what we were working on, and that it might not always feel good or be easy?

The second central question that runs through these case histories is, what is it, in work with infants, that makes us so partial to being supportive and makes it so difficult to tolerate, metabolize, and use therapeutically the intense countertransference feelings that are evoked when we see children suffering and we cannot stop it? Is there a special kind of "parental countertransference" that such cases evoke? How can we support and cultivate the skills, equanimity, and fortitude necessary for this kind of work?

## COMMON THREADS: GHOSTS THAT DO NOT GO AWAY

There are eight issues that seem germane to all or most of these cases that may bear closer examination as we try to learn from our "failures":

1. Unresolved trauma

2. The absence of angels: Families that lack social support, including community resources

3. Issues of race, class, and culture

4. Intervention with older toddlers with symptoms that are not relationship specific

5. Isolation of therapist

6. Choices about inclusion and exclusion

7. Abrupt, unplanned termination

8. Disorganized families/disorganized transference–countertransference patterns; who is keeping baby in mind?

Unfortunately, we cannot offer a method or an insight that teaches us how to turn these tragic failures into happy endings. On the contrary, the goal of this book is to help us learn to do better at managing failures by understanding more clearly the limits of our tools and the psychological dangers of the work. In this final chapter, we look at how these eight issues are manifested in each of our six cases, and conclude with reflections on how our practice as infant mental health professionals might be able to adapt to them. We seek the infant mental health equivalent of Freud's (1955) wonderfully mature statement of the goal of psychoanalysis, which is "to replace hysteric misery with common human unhappiness" (p. 305).

## Unresolved Trauma

It is no coincidence that these six families share an extraordinarily high incidence of what Felitti (Felitti et al., 1998) and his colleagues referred to as "adverse childhood events." This study, using a largely middle-class sample of 15,000 patients in a health maintenance organization, examined the relationship between a wide range of severe and chronic medical and psychiatric conditions of adulthood, to such adverse childhood events as the absence of a parent, physical and psychological abuse, neglect, familial substance abuse, mental illness, and criminality. The research found that those patients who reported four or more adverse childhood events had a four- to twelvefold increased likelihood of alcoholism, drug abuse, depression, and suicide attempts, as well as a two- to fourfold increased likelihood of smoking (including smoking by age 14 and chronic smoking as adults) and sexually transmitted diseases. They also had significantly elevated risk for a wide variety of potentially lethal medical conditions.

It is important to keep in mind that trauma in infancy and early childhood is particularly toxic and devastating because of its impact on the rapidly developing and organizing brain, particularly the neurological systems for regulation and integration.

The families we have come to know in these pages are simply off the charts for adverse childhood events, as Table 1, which only reports if an event has occurred, not how often it occurred, illustrates.

As Harris, Lieberman, and Marans (2007) have pointed out, the Adverse Childhood Events (ACE) study is designed in such a way that it underestimates the incidence of traumatic events, as it simply records whether such an event occurred, not how often, over how long a period of time, and with what, if any, sources of support. This caveat certainly seems to apply to the families discussed in this book. Just to take the case of Ben, the 2-year-old adoptee I worked with in his adoptive home, it is reasonable to think that he was exposed to physical and psychological neglect, substance abuse, and parental mental illness daily for his first 19 months. Domestic violence between his parents was frequent and severe enough to occasion several hospitalizations. It is also reasonable to assume that he had no alternative caregivers to offer him an alternative template for his emergent sense of self and other.

### Trauma and Disorganized Attachment

Contemporary neurodevelopmental research strongly suggests that individuals reared in chronically severely toxic, and traumatic physical and psychological environments literally suffer brain damage (Perry, 1997). Although a young child retains a high level of neurological plasticity, a young brain subjected to these kinds of assaults and deprivations can never be what it might have been given a more nurturing medium for development. There is also considerable overlap between the populations of individuals with histories of early trauma and individuals with disorganized attachment (Lyons-Ruth & Jacovitz, 1999). Lieberman and Harris (2006) described these concerns as follows:

> There is now incontrovertible evidence that children's responses to trauma can render them simultaneously over-reactive, helpless and immobilized—whether as victims of abuse, witnesses to domestic and

Table 1. Adverse Childhood Events (ACE)

| ACE | Sklan | Birch | Ruth | Stone | Maldonado-Durán | Heineman |
|---|---|---|---|---|---|---|
| Violence against mother | Child Mother | Child | | Child | | |
| Absence of a parent | Child × 2 Mother × 2 | Child × 2 | Children × 5 Mother Grandmother? | Child | Child Mother | Child × 2 |
| Physical abuse | Mother | ? | Children × 5 | Child Mother | Mother? | |
| Psychological abuse | Mother | Child | Children × 5 | Child | Child Mother | Child |
| Sexual abuse | Mother | ? | Not known, suspected with Khadija | Child? Mother? | | Child? |
| Physical neglect | Mother | Child | Children × 5 | | | Child |
| Psychological neglect | Mother Child | Child | ? | Child | Child Mother | Child |
| Subsance abusers in household | | Child | ? | Child | | Child |
| Mentally ill in household | Mother Child | | | | Child Mother | Child (father was in and out of mental hospitals) |
| Felon in household | | | ? | | | |

[1]Not mentioned in case report. Source: Personal communication with author.

community violence, or survivors of natural and man-made disasters. The experience of overwhelming and often unanticipated danger triggers a traumatic dysregulation of neurobiological, cognitive, social and affective processes that has different behavioral manifestations depending on the child's developmental stage, but is usually expressed through problems of relating and learning in the forms of aggression, hyperarousal, emotional withdrawal, attentional problems, and psychiatric disturbances (Pynoos, Steinberg, & Piacentini, 1999; van der Kolk, 1994). These problems can have an enduring impact on development and may substantially alter a child's biological makeup through long-lasting changes in brain anatomy and physiology, particularly when the traumatic circumstances are chronic and sources of support are inadequate (Carrion, 2006; DeBellis et al., 1999a, 1999b). As a result, the unaddressed consequences of trauma not only have an adverse impact on individual children through-out their lives, but also affect the lives of those around them and can ulti-mately mar the healthy development of their own children. (p. 2)

These brutal truths about the enduring impact of trauma must be kept in mind, not only with regard to the infants with whom we work but also with regard to their parents. Our access to the details of parents' early histories is often limited, but what we do know makes it reasonable to suppose that they too were once infants and toddlers who suffered chronically traumatic circumstances without emotional support that may have been neurologically damaging and may have left them without coherent strategies for meeting their attachment needs.

## The Absence of Angels

On the other hand, and perhaps even more troubling, there is little evidence in these six case histories of the presence of what Lieberman, Padron, Van Horn, and Harris (2005) called "angels in the nursery." In contrast to the "ghosts" that Fraiberg, Adelson, and Shapiro (1975) described as the psychic residue of painful experiences with the caregivers of the parents' childhood, Lieberman et al. described "angels" as the psychological sequelae of

Care-receiving experiences characterized by intense shared affect between parent and child in which the child feels nearly perfectly understood, accepted, and loved . . . that provide the child with a core sense of security and self-worth that can be drawn upon when the child becomes a parent to interrupt the cycle of maltreatment. (p. 504)

My experience as a clinician is consistent with the authors' contention that it is extraordinarily difficult, if not impossible, to establish a positive and trusting therapeutic relationship when a parent cannot draw on *any* previous experiences of being understood and valued by a beloved caregiver. Sometimes these angels have been forgotten and sometimes their presence in the child's life was truly minimal. I am reminded of a client telling me that she had spent her whole life trying to be like the stranger who reprimanded her mother for beating her in a department store, but it is on the shoulders of such angels that we stand as therapists. Without them, our task is like that of Sisyphus, the mythological Greek who was condemned to push a boulder up a hill over and over only to have it roll back each time down to the bottom again.

### Absent and Violent Fathers

A related absence—the absence of fathers and the impoverished or abusive sexual and intimate relationship patterns of the various mothers and grand-mothers in our families—is either ignored or treated very marginally as if irrel-evant to the parenting issues. Over and over, the women in these pages involve themselves with sexual partners who are utterly negligent, brutally violent, or both. There are well-known parallels between adult relationship patterns and parent–child relationship patterns (Sperling & Berman, 1994). Furthermore, a mother who is unable to meet her needs for emotional and sexual intimacy with another adult is liable to place inappropriate burdens on her child. When mothers lack supportive partners, it becomes extremely challenging to muster the social support that makes "the motherhood constellation" (Stern, 1995) possible.

None of the children described in these pages has a biological father who is actively involved in his or her life. All of them have fathers, but only Ben's adoptive father is playing an active role in caring for his child. In addition, the fathers of Miguel, Ben, and Jay have been violently abusive to the children's mothers. Therapeutic efforts to involve the fathers, or to address their absence in their children's lives in treatment, are either nonexistent or minimal. To what degree does infant mental health inadvertently collude with a worldview that sees fathers either as hopelessly disordered and dangerous or as unnecessary as participants in a child's life? Contrast the active outreach that pursues and encourages even very marginal mothers with the very common total absence of any effort of outreach to fathers. A noteworthy exception to this neglect of fathers is The Child Trauma Project in San Francisco directed by Alicia Lieberman, a treatment program that integrates intensive efforts to preserve and heal the violent father's connection to his child with rigorous attention to issues of safety.

While the clinical and logistical challenges involved in trying to engage with absent or violent fathers are immense, their absence from our clinical narratives is an elephant in the living room that we ignore at our peril. We have not worked out how to consider simultaneously a young child's need for a father and the frequent violence between fathers and mothers. What is most important for the child: a father, or a mother who is safe? Faced with this impossible choice, we have preferred to, and perhaps are less frightened to, work with the victimized parent, usually a mother, rather than the violent parent, usually a father.

Here our field, more often than not, mirrors a cultural phenomenon in which increasing numbers of children lack any consistent relationship with a male caregiver.

### Who's Holding the Environment? (Birch, 1994)

Finally, social support comprises not only personal bonds of family and friendship, but also community resources such as health care and education, social policy, and economic realities. Many would argue that verbal and reflective therapies have limited if any impact when the patient is actively abusing drugs or alcohol, or when he or she is in a chronic, unrelieved state of danger, deprivation, or severe pain (van der Kolk, 1994).

Program design and policy often reflect this; for example, many chemical dependency treatment programs for mothers allow the children to join the mother at the treatment center only *after* she has demonstrated some minimal capacity to engage in treatment in good faith. Programs working with victims and perpetrators of domestic violence typically advocate or require that families commit to specific "safety plans" to minimize the ongoing risk of violence during treatment.

However, it must be acknowledged that we are rarely in a position to make treatment conditional on stable housing, safe neighborhoods, financial security, cultural integrity, and educational opportunity. Yet in the absence of these, there may be realistic limits to what reflective therapies can achieve (Lieberman & Harris, 2007). This is especially true when such community hazards and deficits reinforce and validate a hostile/helpless stance toward others that is rooted in attachment disorganization.

## Issues of Race, Class, and Culture

> Every single encounter in the United States between a White man and Black people is alive with potential to be intensely complicated, and charged, in ways that are difficult to capture and impossible to evade— clinical encounters especially so. Whether the White participant is thoughtless or thoughtful, unaware or conscious, a lifelong battler against racism or someone proud of their prejudices, the ghosts of the victims *and the perpetrators* of the Middle Passage, slavery, and segregation are right there with us. If we are therapists, then these ghosts supervise our work— silently, like wise old supervisors who hold us to the task of thinking through. (Ruth, this volume p. 118; italics added)

There are numerous limits to what society is presently willing to offer to impoverished and deprived, traumatized new mothers. The dominant culture in the United States is very afraid of "creating dependency" and tends to think that everybody "should" be able to be on their own, in their own apartment, and somehow find happiness in that isolation and lack of support from other people. It would require a much more ambitious social commitment to reach the many mothers who find themselves trapped being the only source of support and satisfaction to their baby in very difficult conditions and having themselves received so little. (Maldonado-Durán, this volume, p. 191)

Our families are also affected by larger scale issues of race (two are African American), class (all are poor, except for Ben's adoptive parents), and culture (two are African American, one is Hispanic [born in the Dominican Republic], and three are not specified). The poverty into which all of these children were born is the single most significant risk factor for future dysfunction, and one that infant–parent psychotherapy can do nothing whatsoever about.

The fact that we therapists are all middle-class professionals earning at least a living wage for providing therapy for families that lack such an economic foundation is enormously significant. Seligman and Pawl (1984) pointed this out in their paper on impediments to the therapeutic alliance in infant–parent psychotherapy occasioned by families' and communities' histories of exploitive, discriminatory, and abusive relationships with representatives of mainstream culture and institutions—typically European American, White, and middle class. Because of this history, the poor and minority populations who have been the prime consumers of infant mental health services in the United States are often legitimately suspicious of middle-class professionals offering "help." Even beyond this suspiciousness, important and valid questions exist about the usefulness of such intervention, or why this kind of help is available (though rarely) and other, more concrete help—child care, for example—is often not. Lieberman and Harris (2006) cautioned:

The training of mental health providers and the structure of medical and mental health institutions may predispose towards a solely clinical bias in choosing interventions that may address (a child's) needs, but clinical

experience also teaches us that mental health intervention, while necessary, is not sufficient to help (a child). Safe neighborhoods, appropriate
housing, adequate sources of employment and family support, remedial
education, external limits and consequences, and reliable access to medical care need to form the backdrop for any mental health intervention
that would otherwise be ineffective on its own. (p. 14)

These cautions remain important and valid in each of the cases described
in this volume. Such cultural and socioeconomic impediments to trust are
only compounded and made more intransigent when they are added to the
propensity to view all relationships as inherently dangerous, painful, and
untrustworthy that is characteristic of traumatized individuals with disorganized states of mind with regard to relationships. Paradoxically, being honest
and humble with families about the needs we cannot fill makes them more,
not less, likely to engage with us.

## Treating Toddlers With Relationship-Independent Symptoms

Although much of infant–parent intervention is *preventive* (Fonagy, 1998)—
that is, engages with high-risk families with the goal of facilitating secure
attachment and heading off the development of mental health disorder in
the infant—only one of our six cases (Julia and Miguel, Sklan, chapter 2)
can be so described. Sklan engaged with her 16-year-old client in the third
trimester of her pregnancy, before any relationally mediated disorder could
have occurred in the infant (this would not rule out, obviously, social and
emotional challenges attributable to genetic defect or complications of
pregnancy and fetal development).

All of the other children we meet in this volume enter treatment with very
significant histories of adverse events and severe symptoms and disorders,
and Sklan's Julia is, herself, a child with a significant history of trauma and
severe symptoms.

These children and their families are no longer candidates for prevention.
It is also arguable that, in these families, treatment of the parent–infant

relationship, even when desirable, is not necessarily the first or best treatment one would offer in a world with adequate mental health resources for young families. In every case except Sklan's, there was a significant disorder not merely in the parent–child relationship but in the child (i.e., not relationship specific, but present no matter with whom the child is interacting). In Sklan's case, the mother was a child with a significant mental health disorder.

Certainly such discrete disorders impact and are affected by caregiving relationships. However, that does not mean that they are either entirely caused by or entirely curable by relational means alone. This issue is clearest when a disordered child (like Ben, Christina, or the Muhammad children [chapters 4, 12, and 6]) is placed in a new, more nurturing environment, but it also needs to be kept in mind when the child remains with his birth family, as did Miguel, Jay, and Jonah (chapters 2, 8, and 10).

In preventive work, the therapist is able to ally herself with the healthy, undamaged attachment behaviors of the infant to draw the parent out of her historically determined defensive cocoon into interactions with the infant that are inherently rewarding. This is what Fraiberg (1980) described as "having God on your side." The children described in this volume are by and large not easy to be with, not experienced as rewarding. They need not "good-enough parenting" but therapeutic parenting.

If we use the identical methods for the prevention of disordered infant–parent relationships, as we do for the repair of disordered infant–parent relationships with families whose children have such relatively stable disorders, we may inadvertently be acting in a fashion that echoes Winnicott's (1963/1989) wonderful description of psychiatric illness as a condition in which the individual organizes his or her whole existence to prevent something that has already happened.

Another important distinction between preventive work with infants and reparative work with toddlers is that toddlers are far more active, willful participants in meetings, whose presence normally makes it challenging for adults to have an adult conversation in their presence (Lieberman, 1993). Understanding and responding meaningfully to toddlers' and preschoolers' expressive gestures and actions so as to include them are fairly specialized therapeutic skills.

## Isolation of the Therapist

Only one of our six contributors (Heineman) had regular reflective and supportive consultation while working with these very difficult families. Those who worked with a team, Stone and Maldonado-Durán, did so in a supervisory capacity, providing support for others. Heineman participated in a consultation group sponsored by A Home Within, a foundation that provides long-term therapy free of charge to children in foster care, and provides its volunteer therapists with free-of-charge consultation. However, it is worth noting that Heineman is the founder of A Home Within, so it is reasonable to wonder if she too was in more of a leadership/role model relationship with her group, as opposed to receiving supportive, reflective guidance from it.

In addition, five of the six authors experienced significant challenges and frustration in attempting to collaborate with other providers and agencies to integrate and coordinate the services the family received. These difficulties can be attributed, in part, to an inadequate social safety net that places all providers under stress and leads to competitive turf battles in lieu of collaboration. However, on another level, all providers working with such traumatized and disorganized families are subject to the same countertransference pressures faced by therapists, but often lack the conceptual tools to recognize or process them. All of us experience the contagiousness of the helpless/hostile state of mind that is so characteristic of these families and that impedes their and our capacity to allow others to help.

Although reflective supervision has long been valued in our field, it has perhaps not been emphasized enough that because of the intense emotional pressures that work with massively traumatized and disorganized family systems places on the therapist—especially when done in the client's environment—

such a consulting "container" is critical even for the most experienced and skilled practitioners.

No amount of skill or experience can protect one from countertransference responses to such families, and a safe emotional space for reflection is essential to permit such responses to be metabolized and used to inform the intervention, instead of being acted upon. Often even that is not sufficient to prevent errors of over- or underestimating and reacting to need, pathology, and danger.

## Choices About Inclusion and Exclusion

Fraiberg et al. (1975) and Stern (1995) have led the way in defining "the patient" in infant–parent psychotherapy as the infant's relationship to the caregiving environment. In each treatment, choices have to be made about which aspects of that environment we try to engage. These decisions are typically made with a combination of theoretical (e.g., mothers are important, mothers need support, and children need experiences of calm containment and acceptance) and pragmatic (e.g., who will actually talk to us and how much time do we have) considerations. Yet those people and institutions that we do not include—elements that we define as "external" to the treatment (e.g., legal, financial, parties not included, like foster parents, and birth parents)—affect the family in each case, and militate against therapy's potential benefits, like the excluded fairy who cursed Sleeping Beauty.

To the extent that choices about inclusion or exclusion are made on theoretical grounds, they are influenced by the theoretical orientation of the therapist. Our six cases also show the range of techniques and concepts found in infant mental health. Perhaps Sklan comes closest to Fraiberg et al.'s (1975) original model of therapy in the kitchen, combining concrete support, developmental guidance, and psychoanalytically informed insight, and focusing on the infant–parent relationship as the patient.

Both Ruth and Stone are strongly influenced by the object relations and middle schools of psychoanalytic thinking (Bick, 1968/2003; Bion, 1979;

Winnicott, 1980), schools that conceptualized the developing mind of the
infant and a model of working with infants in their families independently
of Fraiberg et al. (1975) and attachment theory. After decades of mutual disdain, these schools are now mutually informed and respectful of one another
(Alvarez, 1999; Lieberman, 1997). At the heart of work with infants in the
object relations tradition, drawing on Bion (1979), is the concept of "containment" (p. 31). Winnicott's (1960/1980) discussion of "the holding environment" (p. 49) provided by mothers for infants and analysts for patients is a
closely related idea. The concept of containment is applied by Ruth to allowing the fractured Jones/Muhammad family a physical and emotional space with
him in his office to be and to be seen as a family. Stone, on the other hand,
focuses on engaging with little Jay's mind directly, endeavoring to give him
the emotional space to "go-on-being" even while his mother insists that he
is incapable of relating and is openly irritated and offended by Stone's efforts.

Maldonado-Durán describes his work with Jonah's family as being consistent with a medical model, in which a consulting expert—here, an infant
psychiatrist—makes observations and recommendations in response to family concerns. As he notes, such a model requires a basic capacity to accept
help that is absent in this family.

Heineman, having no family to work with, offers Christina a traditional
psychoanalytically informed play therapy, wrapped in a most exceptional
level of case management by the therapist. My own case is also fairly close to
the classic infant–parent psychotherapy model, improvising adaptations to
accommodate the fact that the working models of relationship in Ben and his
adoptive parents are, in the beginning, unrelated to one another. As Ben
grew older, his treatment came increasingly to resemble play therapy.

Another critical factor influencing who and what was the object of intervention is the fact that all of these therapies were authorized/funded by agencies;
these agencies' commitment to families was *not* ever "for as long as it takes."
Whether a public health service (Maldonado-Durán and Stone), child protective services (Birch, Heineman, and Ruth), or grant-dependent social
service agency (Sklan), each of these systems is an often-unacknowledged

ghost in the therapy. Perhaps our relational model, with its emphasis on the importance of the therapist offering sensitivity, attunement, and reliability in her demeanor and exchanges with the family, is inclined to deny, or at best "contain without confronting" (Ruth, p. 132) the real limits in our availability to families. As one of my clients brutally pointed out: "You're paid to care, and when the money runs out you will too." Often our families need our caring presence so desperately that they avoid confronting us this way—and perhaps they often avoid consciously *knowing* this about us as well. We, in our eagerness to connect with them, to be useful to them, and, often, to advocate for their interests with these very agencies, may not pay enough attention to the ambiguities and complexities of our own roles as employees of the system and thus may offer, and want to offer, more than we are in a position to deliver.

Julie Stone gently and teasingly remarks, in her discussion of Ruth's case report, that Ms. Jones, the family matriarch, was a "strengths-based grandmother" whose focus on the abilities of her daughter and grandchildren comprised an apparent inability to even remember or consider events and behaviors that suggested their limitations. How do we know when we, like grandmother Jones, are "containing without confronting" these kind of deep denials in our therapeutic relationships? Consider in this light Sklan's omitting to challenge Julia's dream that Miguel would always love and never leave her, Birch and the Doyle family's minimizing of the scars left by Ben's traumatic gestation and infancy, Stone's hope that 1 hour of weekly attunement could be "held" by Jay in the other 171 hours per week he was needed to absorb his mother's negative attributions, Maldonado-Durán's stalwart offerings of rational solutions to a flagrantly mad family, and Heineman's sense of omnipotent responsibility in a situation in which she had remarkably little power or control.

In addition, it may be even more difficult for us to own and expose the darker side of our own involvement rather than clinging comfortably to our "strengths": our passionate concern, exquisitely subtle understanding of developmental dynamics, sensitivity, empathy, and so forth.

Even our sense of guilt and responsibility when we are not able to help is somewhat flattering—look how much we care! We *do* care, we *are* skilled, and we *are* gifted. However, we must also give ourselves permission to invite families to see and process with us that we are also paid professionals whose allegiances are not wholly altruistic and pure and whose availability has real limits that may be utterly unrelated to the families' needs. Paradoxically, such openness about our limits often facilitates trust, and helps us avoid falling into the omnipotent rescuer mode.

To do this kind of painful work, we ourselves must have the sturdiness to acknowledge that we are unwilling to give up our professionalism and the boundaries it places on our availability, and we must do this without either masochistic self-reproach or defensive disapproval of the overwhelming nature of our clients' needs.

## Abrupt, Unplanned Termination

In the words of Ruth, "time ran out" on each of these cases. Only Christina remains in treatment (with Heineman), a treatment that has already been interrupted once by a change of placement and that remains vulnerable to similar disruption in the future. (As this book went to press, Heineman told me that Christina has been moved to "long-term foster care" in another county—this is termed an "indefinite placement" as distinct from a "permanent placement"—and she will no longer be able to come to therapy.) None of the therapies ended with a shared agreement that the work was complete. In some cases, there was some time and some willingness to discuss the ending of the work; in others, in which the therapist was "fired," such a discussion never occurred. It is interesting and painful to reconsider these firings and premature endings in the light of these families' repeated experiences of abrupt and arbitrary termination of relationships with care providers in the past. Thus, tragically and inadvertently, each of these therapeutic relationships recapitulated the families' traumatic experiences of abandonment by those on whom they depended, by those they loved. As Stone (chapter 7) reflects in her discussion of Ruth's case:

> Precipitous endings are all too common in work with families entangled in a child protective system—sustained, effective, complex logistics much less so. It is more amazing that Ruth managed to see this family for so long than that this therapy ended so abruptly. (p. 155)

This kind of arbitrary foreclosure is more the rule than the exception in the health care climate of our time and our nation, even for the middle class. Would it soften its impact somewhat if we anticipated it with families early in our work and sturdily tolerated the appropriate anger and outrage that gets stirred up in our clients when they are told they can only have so much, no matter how great their need?

## DISORGANIZED FAMILIES/DISORGANIZED TRANSFERENCE–COUNTERTRANSFERENCE PATTERNS: WHO IS KEEPING BABY IN MIND?

A clinical encounter is not a research situation in which attachment disorganization is formally assessed, and we often have only limited early history for parents. Sometimes, we have little history for children who are in foster care. However, any historical or current trauma should alert the clinician to the possibility that significant disorganization is present in the family system. The toxic combination of unresolved trauma, typically at the hands of intimates, and the absence of positive loving experiences of intimacy during infancy, is a formula for producing attachment disorganization. Lyons-Ruth and her colleagues (Lyons-Ruth, Bronfman, & Atwood 1999) have described "hostile-helpless states of mind" with respect to relationship as characteristic of attachment disorganization. Furthermore, it is a formula for producing stable neurophysiological malfunctions of the stress response system. These factors have significant ramifications for the therapeutic alliance.

When no "parental mind" has ever existed that holds the details of the child's being and history, the child is in the attachment equivalent of free fall. This has extraordinarily powerful effects on any adults that interact with him. For most of those adults, these effects will remain unconscious and will be acted out. The challenge for us as infant mental health professionals is to experience, contain, and learn from what is stirred up in us, rather than springing into frantic activity to make it stop.

## OUR CASES REVISITED

In the following pages, I will revisit each of the six cases discussed in chapters 2–13. I will examine how the common threads described above: unresolved trauma; the absence of angels; issues of race, class, and culture; intervention with older toddlers whose symptoms are not relationship-specific; therapist isolation; choices about inclusion and exclusion; and abrupt, unplanned termination play out in each case. Finally, I will look at the ways that each treatment was affected by disorganized transference and countertransference patterns.

### Miguel and Julia

In chapter 2, Susan Sklan described her work with an adolescent mother from shortly before her son's birth until around his second birthday. At the heart of the case was Sklan's struggle to offer a "corrective attachment experience" to a child–mother who had been repeatedly and traumatically abandoned and abused by her own family, a pattern that continued during the treatment. Sklan, caught between the rock of the mother's violent and painful internal world and the hard place of inadequate and poorly coordinated support services in the community, found herself "wanting to leap in and put out all the fires around them."

### *Unresolved trauma:*

Julia, Miguel's 16-year-old mother, was left in the Dominican Republic with relatives when her parents immigrated to the United States when she was 5. At age 9, she was sexually assaulted, an event she claimed not to remember. At 10, she left the Dominican Republic to rejoin her parents. Her parents' relationship was intensely conflictual and violent. At 13, she was sent to live with an aunt, whose boyfriend raped her. She became pregnant and was forced by her family to have an abortion. The family was furious at Julia for "causing trouble." Returning to her parents' home just in time for their separation, she became "unmanageable" and was placed in foster care when her parents were separating, fighting violently, and unable to care for her. While in foster care, she became involved with a brutally violent man 20 years her senior. He impregnated her, and thus Miguel came into the world. When we bear in mind that Julia was only 16, this relentless stream of trauma cannot really be thought of as ghosts. This was Julia's present reality, and these were monsters or demons that were very much alive. Sklan wrote:

> Each week I could count on another crisis: an eviction, a court date, the baby may be blind, Julia's belief that no one in her family wants her or her baby, CPS wants to have Miguel adopted, her uncle was just shot in front of Julia's grandmother in Santiago. (p. 36)

During the 2 years of treatment, Julia was abandoned repeatedly by her mother, father, and foster mother. Miraculously, given this maternal history, Miguel reached age 2 without any traumatic separations from his mother except for the couple of days when she ran away from their foster home shortly before his first birthday. Nor, to our knowledge, was he exposed to violence, except when Julia and her mother fought when he was 4 months old—a conflict that ended with Julia and Miguel going to foster care. He did experience two major relocations, with the loss of familiar, though not primary, caregivers: his grandmother, his aunt, and Julia's foster mother. He was notably depressed and low-keyed following each move.

### Absence of angels and social support:

None of the adults charged with responsibility for Julia's care had been able to protect her, and, in many cases, they were overtly abusive and violent toward her. In addition, her family showed a tendency to blame Julia when she caused trouble and a shocking readiness to discard her. Despite the evident charm and appeal that connected her so powerfully with Sklan, she was not effectively able to enlist either her mother, her foster mother, the protective services caseworker, or the staff at the residential shelter as her advocates. Nor had Julia been able to benefit from her experiences with previous therapists.

### Issues of race, class, and culture:

Julia was a bicultural teen, whose family members were first generation immigrants to the United States and retained extensive family ties in the Dominican Republic. Her adolescent immersion in a culture different from that in which her parents grew up may have compounded the more "psychological" reasons for her estrangement from them and their anger and bewilderment with her. Her therapy was conducted in English, which was not her first language. Possibly a therapy conducted in Spanish, her mother tongue, would have more readily accessed the parts of Julia that made her so "difficult" for her mother and other caregivers. Alternatively, as bilingual coauthor Richard Ruth suggested to me, the other possibility is that therapy in Spanish would have had the potential to put her in touch with primitive feelings too intense for her to handle. She may have preferred or have been better served by using English, a language in which emotions could have been safely kept at arm's length.

### Age and symptoms:

Sklan began her work with Julia in the third trimester of her pregnancy and continued into Miguel's third year. Perhaps, in large part, because of this early involvement and Sklan's guidance and support, Miguel remained relatively symptom-free as an infant. As he entered his third year, he was showing signs of increasing anxiety. However, these symptoms still appeared to be specific adaptations to his relationship with his increasingly distraught and distracted mother, and were not yet solidified into free-standing maladaptive patterns.

## Isolation of therapist:

Sklan's program was falling apart as she did this work, resulting in the loss of supervision and consultation, layoffs of her team, and the chronic threat of the termination of her position. These circumstances left her feeling alone and overwhelmed.

## Choices about inclusion and exclusion:

Sklan was not consistently able to involve Julia's mother or foster mother or shelter staff, despite her openness to the potential value of their participation. Because she took the initiative, she did have ongoing contact with protective services and tried with some success to advocate for Julia and Miguel. However, in parallel to Julia's paucity of angels, there appears to have been no individual or agency that truly collaborated with Sklan and shared the commitment she showed to this dyad.

## Abrupt, unplanned termination:

Sklan continued to see Julia and Miguel probably far beyond the parameters set by her agency, following her to a foster home "several towns away," and then to a residential treatment center whose therapy staff appears to have treated Sklan as a kind of fifth wheel. She ended the treatment only when her own position ended, and even then, she was beset with fantasies of continuing, somehow, to be available. Yet despite these truly heroic efforts to continue the work, powers beyond her control made it impossible for her to avoid repeating the abandonment theme that ran through Julia's life. The saving grace was that, unlike previous abandoners, Sklan made time for a mutual leave-taking and made explicit her own treasuring of the relationship and her grief at its end.

> Julia's presentation was a good camouflage of someone who lives in a dangerous, chaotic world. When she did share some of her pain, when I asked her how she was feeling, she said, "I don't feel anything. I must move on and not let it get me down." As I got to know more of Julia, I perceived an

anger that could erupt anytime, and I was aware of a deep sorrow. (Sklan, p. 39)

### *Disorganized families/disorganized transference–countertransference: Keeping baby in (whose) mind?:*

Sixteen-year-old Julia's immaturity, her lack of a secure and stable living situation, and her massive backlog of unresolved trauma combined with a paucity of community resources to make it impossible and perhaps unwise for her to address her trauma issues. Her resolutions to "be strong" and not to let herself "care" were both prudent (given how close to the surface is psychotic disorganization for her), and discouraging for enduring therapeutic "progress." Her incoherent outpouring to Sklan at the point when she had been formally disowned by her family, had started running away from her foster home, and was about to be placed in a residential treatment program gave us a glimpse of the chaos and horror that lay just beneath that strong and well-behaved mask:

> She saw Miguel laughing in his crib, reminding her of his father and the hatred she felt for him. "I want to control myself and my anger. I just can't." She talked of her rape at age 9 years. "I used to lock it in a box and put it away. I am taking it out now; I want to open it up and I want to fix it. I don't want to endanger Miguel. I wanted this baby so much. Babies always love their mothers, no matter what. Everything fell apart. My perfect life is breaking to pieces and nothing is there. I was so rapt in this man. I was blind until the last Sunday we were together. Someone cut my heart to pieces. 'If you truly love me our love will last,' he told me. The father of my son is leaving. Something happened to me. I am here with Miguel but not really here with him. I am not making it right. My mother got up and left. Something happened to me in Santiago. She told me it was my father or one of my uncles. I can't function the way I used to. I was an adorable child. No one wants to tell me what happened to me in Santiago. (pp. 47–48)

If we imagine the best future we can for 16-year-old Julia, does it include raising Miguel all alone—a child who is the result of a sexual encounter of this vulnerable girl child with a brutally abusive and abandoning older man?

If we imagine the best future we can for Miguel, does it include a severely traumatized, culturally dislocated, homeless, abandoned teenaged mother with limited education and few resources?

Sklan, whose mission it was to support and encourage Julia to be a mother, was faced with Julia's passionate love for her baby and her outrage at others who had suggested adoption. This made it difficult, if not impossible, for her to ask if it was in anyone's best interest for Julia to be Miguel's primary caregiver.

The relationship between Sklan and Julia, Miguel's mother, was very warm, supportive, and caring. However, as presented in these pages, it did not appear to have included any direct discussion either of the factors in Julia's history that would have made it almost impossible for her to trust Sklan as much as she appeared to or of the reality factors that limited what Sklan could offer her to far less than what Julia wanted and needed. This was a strengths-based relationship in both directions: Sklan focused on and reinforced the positive elements in Julia's mothering. Julia was grateful. Sklan reports:

> Julia told me how much she had felt the support and care and how much she now understood about Miguel. She shared with me that when she first had Miguel as an infant, she was afraid she would not be able to be a parent. "Yet you believed I could be a parent and that helped me." (p. 56)

Julia refused transfer to another therapist. Yet, as I suggested in my discussion of Sklan's case, in addition to the good side of her feelings about Sklan, whom she, realistically, experienced as kind, reliable, enlivening, and safe, there *had to be* a darker side, less conscious and less acceptable, that hypervigilantly monitored the therapist's every move, anticipating that she, like the mother, the aunt, the grandparents, and the foster mother, would allow her (which in a child's magical thinking is the same as to cause) to be raped again.

## Ben

Chapter 4 followed a 2-year-old boy whom I saw in his adoptive home for 2 years and in my own office for another 2 years. In my work with Ben, I focused on fostering an emotional attachment between a numb and frozen child and his adoptive parents. Despite Ben's history of extreme neglect and trauma, he made rapid progress in attachment, language, and emotional expressiveness. However, the adoption of his newborn biological sister threw him into a malignant regression. Ben seemed locked into treating both parents and therapist as his abusers, and the therapy was unable to relieve this.

### Unresolved trauma:

Ben had experienced extensive trauma and neglect, and had lost both his birth parents and his shelter care family by the time he was 19 months old. He was born premature and addicted to cocaine and heroin, following an episode of domestic violence which sent his mother to the hospital. An overloaded city hospital discharged this infant to "home," where Ben's parents continued to use drugs and batter each other until his mother passed out in a shopping mall with Ben in her arms. He was taken into protective custody at 19 months. After a brief stay in a shelter care home, he was placed in a pre-adoptive home. For the next 14 months, he continued to have visits with his birth parents despite their failure to engage in any reunification services. After 2 years in his adoptive home, Ben was precipitously presented with his biological baby sister, who was removed from his birth parents' custody at birth and placed with his family on extremely short notice.

### Absence of angels and social support:

Ben's adoptive family, the Doyles, was a working-class family with supportive friends, grandparents, aunts, and uncles living close by. They had been married for 10 years, and had an evidently loving and mutually supportive relationship. The Doyles had a steady income and secure employment, although their choices to have Peggy be a full-time mother, and, later, to send Ben to a private school with small classes and a nurturing atmosphere, caused considerable financial pressure.

However, Ben lived his first 19 months in a terrifyingly neglectful world. His parents, in the grip of drug addiction, domestic violence, and mental illness, evidently did not even feed him adequately. Born multiply addicted and premature, following an incident of domestic violence, Ben was also the victim of a health care system that discharged such an infant to home with no follow-up, and that had no mechanism for following up on the diagnosis of "failure to thrive" that was given at his only known doctor's visit as an infant. The safety net of social services also failed Ben by taking almost 2 years to end visits with his noncompliant birth parents, and by giving his adoptive family only a week to assimilate the information that Ben had a newborn biological sister and to decide whether to adopt her.

### Issues of race, class, and culture:

These factors were relatively insignificant in this case, with the important exception that Ben was born into poverty. His adoptive family was solidly working class (father belonged to and was active in his union) with steady if modest income. Ben, the Doyles, and I "matched" ethnically and culturally.

### Age and symptoms:

Ben was 26 months old when treatment began, and exhibited severe delays in language as well as very atypical social and emotional behavior. At the time of his treatment, far less was known about the enduring neurophysiological effects of being, what Perry (1997) in his trenchant phrase, called "incubated in terror" (p. 124). Thus, while Ben was able, with the provision of consistent sensitivity and protection by his adoptive parents, to relinquish his defensive numbing and inhibition, he retained significant impairments in his capacity to self-regulate that included a vulnerability to explosive rage states. Given his prenatal drug exposure, as well as his severe and constant traumatization, these impairments may have included neurodevelopmental deficits in brain function, not readily remediated by environmental changes.

### Isolation of therapist:

I saw Ben and his family in my private practice. I saw him at a stage in my career when I had recently emerged from years of intensive supervision and, mistakenly if understandably, relished my "independence." Although I had access to some of the best and most generous mentors in our field, I used them far too begrudgingly. When I did, I was too eager to impress them to fully disclose how baffled and troubled I felt.

Communication with Ben's social workers, visitation supervisors, and, later, teachers did occur, but not frequently enough to create any sense of a team working with this family. Ultimately, the child psychiatric service that I turned to for consultation recommended to the family that my services be replaced by its own, and made no effort to communicate or collaborate with me.

### Abrupt, unplanned termination:

The ending of Ben's therapy was neither abrupt nor unplanned. Yet neither was it the result of a mutual agreement that our work was satisfactorily finished. Rather, it reflected a paucity of financial and human resources that made it necessary for Ben's parents to choose between continuing with me and trying a new approach. Despite the frustration we all felt with Ben's persistent unhappiness, anger, and destructiveness, the Doyles and I valued my long relationship with them and with Ben. They were unhappy about having to make such a choice. I was perhaps too discouraged and self-disparaging of my work with Ben to appreciate fully the sadness for him of losing me.

### Choices about inclusion and exclusion:

In retrospect, I second-guess my choice not to include the birth parents in my work with Ben. Their ongoing contact with Ben and their possession of his history were factors that received inadequate attention. I began with the assumption that the warm and sensitive Doyles could function as co-therapists, and that I need not concern myself with their ghosts, who promised to be manageable and well-behaved. Here I underestimated the degree to which a severely traumatized child can evoke shockingly troublesome feelings in even the best parents (and therapists). Later, I acquiesced as financial and logistical considerations resulted in, first, a reduction in therapeutic frequency and, second, the ending of therapy.

### Disorganized family/disorganized transference–countertransference: Keeping baby in (whose) mind?

The Doyles signed on to rescue Ben, then a mute and numb little boy. They had no way to anticipate the dark and frightening places in themselves that Ben would stir up. In fact, their very willingness and availability to rescue such a wounded child may have depended upon their being the kind of people who, in the words of Peggy Doyle, "never knew I had a dark side." For his part, Ben engaged with both me and the Doyles in ways that, on the one hand, powerfully activated in us the "omnipotent rescuer" mode of parental attachment behavior (the kind that enables mothers to stop locomotives when their babies are on the tracks), and, on the other hand, stirred up in all of us the buried pockets of unresolved trauma, loss, insecurity, and disorganization that everyone contains. Maybe, inside, we each felt like a baby facing an oncoming train, and mobilized to get ourselves off the tracks by any means possible.

If we imagine the best future we can for the Doyles as they adopt, does it take the form of a severely delayed and psychologically impaired little boy with unmanageable rage states?

How can we imagine (but we can, I myself did) that an infant like Ben, who experiences almost 2 years of unrelieved terror and deprivation, can form a "secure attachment" and that his intruding ghosts will depart?

The relationship between this writer and Ben and the Doyles is quite one-sided—strengths-based to a fault. I engaged with them as if there were and could be no open questions about their desire to parent and their emotional availability to Ben. When I was startled by their decision to adopt Julie without even mentioning it to me until it was a fait accompli, I failed to address this as an issue in the therapeutic relationship that needed to be explored. Paralleling my efforts to be warm and supportive with a hateful, provocative Ben, I attempted to reassure the Doyles when they expressed worry about how enraged they felt with Ben, rather than signaling my ability to tolerate knowing about and dwelling with their rage, Ben's rage, and my own. Ruth eloquently described this omission:

> We cannot operate as caring professionals other than on the assumption that children have parents, protection, provision, love, and at least a grounding modicum of safety; therapy, in a sense, structures itself on the assumptions that something in the essential context of life has gone wrong and needs to and can be repaired. The clinical experience of work with severely traumatized and brutally neglected/abused children, however, involves a confrontation with realities that such children can be thrust into this world without any of this—that there is no context, for such children, against which to react and work at repair. When we do our work, we come to know this impossible reality not from the outside but from the inside. The child re-creates it in our presence, projects it into us, and depends on us to experience it. We have no good choices. In a way more like shamans than like surgeons, we have to either experience the horror and try to survive (first) and then make sense or reject what the child needs us to come to know. Either way, we find ourselves in a life or death struggle with hate, the deepest and most primitive kind of hate, the hate of life, or the possibility of life for death. To be very specific, I think my colleague had to face, and try to overcome, not just hatred for what Ben was doing, but hatred for who he was. (Ruth, pp. 111–112)

## Jacques, Akil, Khadijah, Mahmoud, and Abdul

In Richard Ruth's work with a family referred by child welfare, his office became the de facto home for a three-generation family whose five children were living in three separate foster homes. The children's mother and several of the children had been diagnosed as developmentally delayed. Time was a central theme in the case: the time involved in establishing an atmosphere of

safety and trust in which therapeutic work could occur, the time of the inexorable development of children, and the time of the legal system in which
the family was entangled and that first supported and then terminated the
therapy. Support was abruptly and irreversibly withdrawn, and the family was
legally dismantled in what appears to be a profound breakdown of communication between therapist, service providers, and family.

### Unresolved traumas:

All five children had experienced significant neglect while in their mother's
care, and had suffered the trauma of separation from their mother, grandmother, and siblings.

### Absence of angels:

The five children were said to have three fathers; all were absent and some
were unknown. We heard nothing of additional family, friends, or community
involvements such as church (Ruth asked if they are Muslim, because of the
children's Arabic names, but never received a clear answer). While it is not
uncommon for foster parents to mentor biological families when they are as
cooperative and nonthreatening as Ms. Jones and Ms. Muhammad appeared
to be, this did not happen here. We have reason to suspect that the twins'
foster family held the birth family in disdain. The family's growing attachment
to and trust of Ruth appeared to be a unique and a surprising development
for people with long histories of disappointment in "helpers."

### Issues of race, class, and culture:

Ruth addressed the possible impact of his Whiteness, as well as of his being a
middle-class male professional for this matriarchal family in which adult men
were as scarce as hens' teeth, and in which there had never been enough
money to do more than just barely get by.

With regard to the Jones/Muhammad family, Ruth eloquently summed up
this quandary as follows:

> They met me with a sense—communicated by Ms. Jones, primarily, but
> reflected in the others—that life could be good, and they wanted life to
> be good for them. They also communicated a sense that life was not good,
> and might never be good for them. There was no escaping that. No run-
> ning out. (p. 122)

Ruth was clear and sturdily sorrowful about the relative deprivation with
which the family lived in contrast to his own privileged middle-class existence, including, regarding their shared therapeutic endeavor, that he has
"the luxury of reflection." He also never lost sight of "the ghosts of the
Middle Passage" who were inevitably present in the therapy. Perhaps his cultural competence led him to be, appropriately, gentler and less confrontive
than an African American therapist might have been able to be.

### Age and symptoms:

All five of the Jones/Muhammad children had developmental and behavioral
difficulties of sufficient concern to warrant special education and mental
health services. In the public sector, these services are so stringently "managed" that when they are made available it is usually a very significant red
flag. However, such public-sector assessments are rarely fine tuned enough to
distinguish between delays due to organic impairment and those that result
from trauma or environmental deprivation. The youngest child, Abdul, was
more than 2 years old when treatment began. He had been in foster care his
whole life. The older children, ranging in age from 4 to 8, had been in foster
care for more than 2 years, and continued to be symptomatic.

### Isolation of therapist:

Ruth saw the Jones/Muhammad family in his private practice. Ruth wrote:

> I can tally my burdens of stress, confusion, and pain, as I did this work, and
> they are all too high and probably intruded in ways beyond what I hold
> in present awareness. I would be reluctant to take on a case like this in

private practice again, at least without more regular consultation and more peer support than I had while I was working with this family. (p. 150)

### Choices about inclusion and exclusion:

Ruth chose to treat the Jones/Muhammad family as a family, doing family therapy in his private practice office. He accepted the preference of the foster parents to be uninvolved in the therapy. Ruth accepted the task of helping the mother and grandmother with understanding and planning responses to the demands of the systems—educational and legal—with which they and their children were involved. Although he did some advocacy for the continuation of the therapy, and wondered if he should have done more, he was committed to giving this family something close to the protected, contained experience of family therapy that a middle-class, intact family could expect. He was perhaps the clearest of our six therapists in his assertion of the value of such an experience, even for families with screaming "real life" needs.

His efforts at collaboration were consistently thwarted. The developmental assessments he recommended never happened. The change of therapist he requested for Khadijah did not take place. The foster parents were uninterested in meeting with him, and the social worker was not sympathetic to the idea of involving them.

Ruth did maintain communication with protective services staff, and the therapy was initiated and both paid for and made logistically possible (i.e., transportation services) by them. Yet he was not given critical information, information that was withheld both by the family and by the protective services system, which led him to underestimate the severity of the neglect experienced by the children in their mother's care.

### Abrupt, unplanned termination:

After more than 2 years of treatment that felt, on the whole, productive, time ran out for this work when the court determined that Ms. Muhammad had not made adequate progress toward being able to be reunited with her children, and that the children should be freed for adoption. Ruth felt shocked and betrayed by this sudden withdrawal of support and by the enormous loss this represented for all seven members of the family. He did not address the question of time running out as it pertained to these five children growing up without the security offered by permanence. He was allowed two sessions to process both the ending of therapy and, simultaneously, the official decision to permanently disband the family. Even had he been willing to continue to see them pro bono, the logistical difficulties of bringing the family together without either transportation services or the involvement of the foster parents were insurmountable.

### Disorganized families/disorganized transference–countertransference: Keeping baby in (whose) mind?

Stone commented in chapter 7 on the curious ways that Ruth joined with Ms. Jones and Ms. Muhammad in "not knowing" and "not seeing." She wrote the following:

> Despite Ruth's effort to include all members of the family in his writing, I find it very difficult to grasp what Ms. Muhammad ever really felt or thought. I am struck by the passivity and at times seeming emptiness that he describes in her. I am intrigued by Ruth's wondering whether Abdul, Ms. Muhammad's youngest, might have fetal alcohol syndrome. He leaves the question hanging. There is no other mention of Ms. Muhammad's possible substance abuse.

> Is this one of the horror stories that is being sanitised? I wonder what blocked Ruth's exploration of this important possibility in the family story? He writes that Ms. Jones "was raising her adult daughter . . . something she would have done naturally and willing but now was doing by court order" (p. 119). However, there is a whole chunk of history missing. What was Ms. Jones's place in the family when each of Ms. Muhammad's five children was born? What communication did she maintain with her daughter? When Ruth discovers, only after being deeply involved with this family and nearly 2 years into the therapy, some of the details about the evidence of 3-year-old Mahmoud's extreme neglect at the time he was

taken into foster care, Ruth writes, "It was outrageous that my social work colleague had painted a distorted picture of the family at the outset" (p. 140). Was it? How could it be otherwise? (p. 157–158)

Ruth, like Ms. Jones and Ms. Muhammad and the five children, was outraged with protective services for its refusal to reunite the family or to continue to support therapy, and he listed the "help" that had been promised and not provided to the family. For very sound clinical and cultural reasons, Ruth did not interrogate or investigate mother and grandmother, but contained and mirrored their way of seeing things instead. Yet as a result, he may have been a prisoner of the family's own limitations in what they were able and willing to "know." He did not tell us, and we do not know if he knew:

- What else the children's mother was expected to do to regain custody of her children and whether she had done it?

- Whether Ms. Jones had been rejected as an alternative placement for the children (and if so, on what grounds), or whether she had declined that role (and if so, why)?

- What the children's actual experiences in Ms. Muhammad's custody had been (other than the single graphic description of neglect that Ruth belatedly received), and whether either mother or grandmother could really acknowledge and take responsibility for these experiences?

- What was the nature and quality of the children's attachments to their respective foster parents, at least some of whom were interested in adoption?

From the outset, Ruth felt torn internally between his compassion and affection for the family, his sensitivity to their need for nonjudgmental acceptance to do therapeutic work, and his awareness that much was being left unsaid, perhaps unthought. He felt strains between his desire to offer them containment "without memory or desire" (Bion, 1967) and his concern about hidden "horror stories." He commented, "I felt guilty for thinking such thoughts, and naïve when, in moments, I tried not to think them" (p. 123).

Although the work "in the moment" consistently felt productive and meaningful, the family seemed unable to hold onto it; gains seemed to run out like sand through a sieve. Ruth wrote:

A pattern became recognizable in which Ms. Jones and Ms. Muhammad would ask for and receive information (e.g., about a child's developmental needs or the purpose and status of a particular service or court process). We would discuss the information thoroughly and establish through clear feedback that we were understanding each other; then, in a following session, it would seem that both Ms. Jones and Ms. Muhammad had forgotten not just what we had said, but that the conversation had ever happened. It was as if either their ability to contain the informational contents of our conversation had become, in the moment or perhaps even over time, inadequate, or that the contents of the conversation were somehow experienced as so unbearable that they could not be held and metabolized. (p. 131)

It is not clear in Ruth's account of his work with the Jones/Muhammad family the degree to which his conversation with them encompassed the reflections he shared with us about the ways that their shared therapeutic space was both precious and yet unable—not the right instrument—to address the family's very real concrete and practical needs. Ms. Muhammad's taciturnity may reflect her own sense that other needs were too pressing for her to fully engage here. Ms. Jones graciousness and compliance may have contained the same message in a more sophisticated, socially graceful form.

The case illustrated beautifully how difficult it is to provide simultaneously a respectful, affirming container for a fractured family while keeping eyes wide open to its actual wounds and their ongoing capacity for wounding one another. As Stone pointed out in her discussion of the case,

Radical acceptance is important, as is trying to hold the differences between the family's way of construing reality and our own way of construing reality—what we see as their distortions. How we build on the foundations of respect and courtesy to challenge the entrenched positions or beliefs of our patients, in ways that do not shut down thinking, is the challenge in our work. How do we hold the horror stories and keep the hope for transformation in thinking and feeling alive, in ourselves and in the work? (p. 158)

## Jay

Julie Stone wrote of her work with a young mother who determinedly insisted that her young son was "autistic." The mother doggedly sought professional confirmation of her "diagnosis"—her representation of her son—from one professional after another, obtaining eight evaluations in his first 2 years. She denied that her son's experience of domestic violence and emotional abuse by her and by her male partners had any impact on little Jay, whom she saw as being "not there" emotionally. Stone and her colleagues worked hard to soften these projections and to give the little boy space to "go on being" his unique self. Stone wrote as follows:

> My clinical practice, influenced by the work of Serge Lebovici in France and Ann Morgan, Campbell Paul, Frances Thomson-Salo, and others in Australia, has, at its heart, working directly with the infant and offering a meeting with him in his own right. That the infant has a mind and seeks to make sense of his world through interaction with the minds of others informs all of my clinical work. Charlene's need for attention and narcissistic bolstering made it seemingly impossible for her to put Jay's experience and his imperiled development at the center of the treatment. (p. 163)

To the dismay of Stone and her team, their efforts were abruptly ended when they were "fired" by the frustrated mother and replaced with a more "cooperative" professional who agreed with the mother that the child was autistic.

### Unresolved trauma:

Both Jay and Charlene had experienced domestic violence both at the hands of Jay's biological father and of Charlene's next partner. We do not know if Charlene experienced violence in her family of origin, but her choice of two violent partners in succession, and her joining with her partner, Al, in abusing Jay, make it probable that she did. She was abandoned by her father at the age of 2. Maldonado-Durán comments, in his discussion of this case (chapter 9), as follows:

In a sense she is also "autistic" in that that she is in her own world, her own space, and not so much thinking about the mind of her child. Her world seems "closed" to the beneficial effect of therapists and counseling. She is inside herself, perhaps mistrustful, scared, and "refractory" to outside interventions. This must be so for very good reasons. A thick protective shell has to form in children who are exposed to frequent disappointments, betrayals, and maltreatment. This is not easily permeable by the mere presence of a "helper." Her inner world cannot be easily reopened, and the invitation to do so may be quite painful. Therefore, the need to escape. (pp. 190–191)

Jay had already lost two father figures, Errol and Al. Errol was an intravenous methamphetamine abuser, and Al was a drinker. Finally, between the initial consultation and the beginning of treatment, Charlene had a miscarriage, possibly due to domestic violence.

### Absence of angels and social support:

Charlene was very isolated. Her mother was mentioned as confirming her view that Jay was autistic. If true, this suggested that grandmother was equally unable to see or respond to the sadness and distress that others saw in this little boy. Charlene's father left the family when she was 2. Neither Errol nor Charlene seems to have seen Jay as worthy of emotional investment, and Charlene showed a pattern of disrupting any relationship he formed with adults who saw him as likeable or loveable. Charlene's perseverance in pursuit of professional help was remarkable, both for its persistence and for her inability to accept help unless it exactly confirmed what she already thought.

### Issues of race, class, and culture:

Issues of race, class, and culture were not raised in the case report. However, in Maldonado-Durán's discussion of the case, he pointed to the clash of expectations and values, that he believes are illustrated by the case, between a struggling single mother with many concrete needs and an intervention that values reflection and thinking about painful things.

### Age and symptoms:

Jay was 26 months old when he was first brought to Stone's clinic, and just over 3 years old when treatment began.

Although I accept that Stone was correct in saying that he was *not* autistic, despite his mother's insistence that he was, Jay's language, social, and emotional development were very atypical. He was intermittently lifelessly immobile and hyperkinetically out of control. He avoided eye contact. His language, functional emotional level, and communicative gestures were significantly delayed. His mother reported that he was irritable and that he ate and slept poorly since birth. Jay had been variously described as "depressed," "sad and withdrawn," "very anxious," and possibly suffering "posttraumatic stress symptoms." These concerns remained, despite some improvement in therapy.

Stone did not so much disagree with Charlene that Jay was autistic as she disagreed about *why* he was autistic. For her, his autistic behaviors were actions, and *autistic* was an adjective. She commented:

> I wondered if Jay was dissociating or if his disconnection was evidence of a protective shell, as described by Tustin (1990), grown to ward off the traumatic attacks he had experienced in his short life. Tustin suggested when the mother, for whatever reason, is unable to protect the infant from frightening experiences that impinge upon him and threaten him, some infants "originate their own protective covering" (p. 82) by wrapping themselves in their own bodily sensations. They become preoccupied with their own sensations and so can "ignore their dependence on others." This pathological self-sufficiency is what Tustin saw as at the core of the autistic child's difficulties in engaging with the world; their protective shell is their defense against the terror of annihilation and also their barrier to the world of relationship with others. (pp. 173–174)

For Charlene, these "autistic" behaviors reflected a child who was fundamentally defective, lacking the human capacity to relate and love. For her, *autistic* was a noun.

### Isolation of therapist:

Although Stone was part of a team, and worked with a cotherapist, something about the work with Jay and his mother functioned to undermine collaboration and mutual support, to the extent that the cotherapist actually concealed her knowledge that the mother was actively seeking other services. She wrote:

> We did not spend enough time together thinking about these splits or the implications of them. Nor did Vicki and I engage fully with thinking about the difficulty we had in thinking together about this family. It was much more difficult than usual to come together to share our thoughts and reflect upon the therapy and how it was progressing. In our effort to heal the splits in the family relationships, we fell into them and seemed unable to breach them or to think about them. Reflective supervision with the team did not bring enlightenment either. Perhaps they too had become divided in a way that stopped us thinking creatively. (pp. 178–179)

### Choices about inclusion and exclusion:

Stone's mode of working prized direct work with the infant, and this was what she did with Jay. Jay's mother Charlene saw another therapist, Vicki, and there were also joint sessions including mother, son, and both therapists. Charlene was openly dismissive of Stone's inclusion of Jay as a person in his own right, scoffing, " 'Oh don't worry, Jay does not understand anything of what is happening around him. He is "not there",' she said, pointing to her head" (p. 166).

Neither the grandmother with whom the dyad lived nor Charlene's male partners were contacted.

Regarding her decision to work individually with Jay, Stone stated:

> Our hope was for Jay to become more alive to himself and to relationship through our psychotherapy, and that this, in turn, would enliven his relationship with his mother, who we assumed would be relieved and delighted by her son's increased liveliness. Looking back, they seem ambitious and

somewhat grandiose plans. However, as Thomson-Salo and Paul (2004) noted, "Most parents, if they present with a distressed infant, want help for their infant and welcome the therapist's direct intervention" (p. 14). This was certainly our most frequent experience. Thomson-Salo and Paul stated that "working with the parents was seen [by those who do not work directly with the infant] to affirm them as parents and not to exacerbate guilt or envy" (p. 33). Not working with Jay directly may have avoided Charlene's envy, and yet I think that Jay would have missed out on an important experience. In families in which the mother's guilty or rivalrous feelings are stirred up in the therapy, perhaps it would be more helpful for both mother and infant if we could find ways to think about such feelings and work with them rather than avoiding them. Sadly, we did not manage to do this in our work with Jay and Charlene.

Although the therapeutic plans were discussed with Charlene and she appeared to accept them, we failed to appreciate how fervently she continued to hold onto the idea that Jay had autism or to understand why this was so important to her. Her goal of ultimately receiving this diagnosis for him was at odds with the one we had identified for him and thought we were working toward together. (p. 176)

### Abrupt, unplanned termination:

Charlene ended therapy with a phone call, with no previous notice to Stone, although the co-therapist apparently had some idea that this termination was imminent. Despite repeated invitations, Charlene refused to return in order to say good-bye or to allow Jay to say good-bye. She let the dismissed therapists know she had finally found "proper help" from a team that agreed with her that Jay was autistic. She had refused to allow this new team to speak to or obtain records from Stone's group.

### Disorganized families/disorganized transference–countertransference: Keeping baby in (whose) mind?

Charlene's repeated involvement with violently abusive men, and her collusion with them in victimizing her son, Jay, were extremely worrisome and prognistically discouraging, as was her preintervention history of "diagnosis shopping." Both suggest a frightening inability to see her son except as the object of her own projections. Her relationships with Jay and with her therapist seem severely narcissistic and preoccupied with her own needs and feelings. Jay's withdrawal and delayed development made him need more than "good-enough parenting" to grow and thrive.

Yet Stone seemed to have found it unbearable to think about the true bleakness of this situation. She commented:

> Now reflecting on this case, many years later, I wonder what stopped me from further exploring the protective concerns that I had about Jay's safety in the care of his mother or from thinking more clearly and courageously about the limits to this young mother's capacity to provide Jay with a good-enough emotional environment in which to grow and develop. Was I seduced by this mother's seeming eagerness for help, and so rendered unable to think the terrible thought that Charlene really might not be able find to in herself a sustained and genuine longing for Jay to be happy? Maybe Jay's delayed and stunted development might be meeting a need in her, and, maybe, in turn, Jay's distorted behaviour had become his most potent and effective means of engaging his mother and so, in its way, it came to serve him too? (pp. 170–171)

The difficulty Stone and her co-therapist had with their divergent views of Charlene and Jay highlight the inevitable distortions of perspective inherent in both individual and relationship-based therapy. Charlene's therapist empathized with her perspective, and felt that what was best for Charlene was to manage Jay, while it may be fair to say that Stone strongly identified with Jay and focused instead on managing Charlene. Each therapist saw, identified with, and advocated for her own client's "strengths" in a kind of zero sum game in which one's strengths pointed to the partner's "deficits." Stone could not bear to think about the possibility that Charlene was simply not able or willing to see Jay as fully human and capable of loving and being loved. She had powerful emotions in response to the child: "I felt a longing for things to be different for this boy, and I was aware of an intense sense of loss and sadness" (p. 175).

On the other hand, Stone reacted viscerally to Charlene's insistence on Jay's so-called autism: "I felt wiped out by Charlene's comments, negated, dismissed. I wondered if this was an echo of how Jay might experience his mother" (p. 166).

Later, at the end of the first meeting, when Charlene briefly brightened with maternal pleasure when Jay said "bye-bye," Stone was again repelled:

> His mother was delighted, saying proudly that she had just taught him to wave good-bye. My heart sank. Charlene's claim to the one meaningful communication that Jay offered in our first meeting was an ominous indication that perhaps she experienced his accomplishments only in terms of their narcissistic value to her as an accomplished mother and not in terms of any empathic understanding of Jay's experience or wish to communicate. (p. 167)

Stone seemed to respond to Charlene much as Charlene responded to Jay and, in the face of her intense aversive feelings, she tried harder and harder to plead little Jay's case to his mother, despite the envy and fear that this stirred up in Charlene. Perhaps, as Ruth commented about my feelings for Ben, Stone had to face not hatred for what Charlene was doing, but hatred for who she was.

Stone and her team continued to assume, in their work with Charlene and Jay, that Charlene would feel relieved and supported by their belief in Jay's potential and their efforts to realize it. They drew on extensive fruitful clinical experience to validate this hope. Charlene, however, felt infantilized and disrespected.

Stone's team was unable to integrate the treatment of mother and child. The communication breakdown between the therapists mirrored that within the dyad. The therapists with whom the mother replaced them accepted Charlene's refusal to allow them to access previous treatment providers or records, leading to a kind of virtual erasure of the experience from history.

## Jonah

Martin Maldonado-Durán's case, like Ruth's, also involved a three-generation family. This little boy, Jonah, was caught up in what appeared to be extraor-

dinarily malignant and bizarre projections by his grandmother, who simultaneously saw him as "a gift from God," whom it is her right to "spoil," and
as an unmanageable terror who was spoiling her hard-earned retirement.
Maldonado-Durán, called in as a consulting psychiatrist, felt insistently pressured to confirm and validate the grandmother's mutually contradictory
projections of Jonah as special and deserving to "be spoiled," in the sense of
given whatever he wanted, and as "spoiled" in the sense of intolerably badly
behaved. Maldonado-Durán's own efforts to explore and understand the complex family dynamics were responded to in a frankly paranoid fashion, and he
was accused of making little Jonah worse.

### Unresolved trauma:

As Heineman pointed out in her discussion (chapter 11), Jonah's family had
sustained tragedy after tragedy. Two of his grandmother Roseanne's children
were severely disabled (epilepsy and autism), a third (Mary) was rebellious
and self-destructive, and the only "good" child had died of a gunshot wound
while playing with a gun. This gun or another may still have been in the
house, as Roseanne reported threatening to shoot Mary's boyfriend in one of
her first conversations with the psychiatrist. Jonah's birth was experienced as
another trauma, the shameful result of an out-of-wedlock pregnancy that
went unnoticed by anyone in the family, including his mother (who continued to take anticonvulsant medication throughout) until the labor pains
began. Truly, the God that gave Roseanne Jonah as a "gift" was not the
kindly benevolent patriarch of Sunday school bromides.

### Absence of angels and support:

Jonah's grandmother, Roseanne, conveyed the impression that no one in her
life had ever done anything to help or support her. At best, others gratefully
accepted what she did for them, like the members of her church group for
whom she cooked enormous meals. At worst, others ungratefully spurned her
efforts to care for them (like her daughter, Mary), or they made things worse,

more difficult, like the doctors at the hospital where she worked. Jonah's father still visited as a guest in the house, although apparently no one liked him. He was not recognized as a family member and may not have known he was a parent. We are given no indication about who was the father of Jeanette, David, James, and Mary. There were no "angels" in sight for three generations, with the intriguing exception of Dr. P., a psychiatrist who treated the autistic uncle, David, and of whom grandmother spoke "fondly." What did Dr. P. do? Despite this fondness, the grandmother was described as "very suspicious of mental health professionals and would not be willing to go to a clinic." Although the grandmother was very involved in her church, hers was a God who took away her favorite child and replaced him with an illegitimate and extremely unrewarding grandson.

### Issues of race, class, and culture:

We are told that Jonah's family is African American, and Maldonado-Durán is Mexican. He is a psychiatrist; Jonah's grandmother worked as an aide in a psychiatric hospital. Issues of race, class, and culture, given this constellation, would be significant for any therapist and family. When the family was as profoundly distrustful as Jonah's was, these tensions are compounded. Maldonado-Durán described in detail the clash of therapeutic expectations between himself and this working-class grandmother. Yet his sensitivity to these issues was so exquisite, that it seems likely that a less disturbed client would have been able to resolve these concerns, or at least raise this "clash" directly with him.

### Age and symptoms:

Jonah, a 20-month-old toddler when we meet him, was already exhibiting rather severe and worrisome delays and atypical behaviors. He was not able to sleep through the night. He was capable of only fleeting eye contact. His language was very delayed and peculiar (i.e., consisting entirely of expletives). Jonah was very active, disorganized, and aggressive, constantly moving around the house, hitting others, and not able to engage in any sustained play. He was hypertonic, and his functional emotional level was extremely delayed. Jonah appeared incapable of either sustained attention or reciprocal circles of inter-action with another. None of these symptoms were relationship specific, but all were exhibited with all his social partners. They made him a difficult and unrewarding child to be with. He had already been receiving early interven-tion services, apparently with little success, for a year prior to Maldonado-Durán's intervention.

### Isolation of therapist:

Maldonado-Durán was not isolated in his work with Jonah's family. He had been called in by a team he had worked with often, who had become "stuck" in their efforts to help this family. We are not told of the nature of the pre-ceding discussion among the team members about this "stuckness" and its probable causes. What is striking here is that Maldonado-Durán seemed to be in an authority position, a leadership role in this team, and to feel pressured to help the family and succeed where the team members had not. They served as an audience for his efforts, as did the "colleague from Chile" who accompanied him on the first home visit. There was no one who could func-tion as a container for Maldonado-Durán in metabolizing the extremely disturbing experience of being with this family.

### Choices about inclusion and exclusion:

As Maldonado-Durán commented, "In retrospect, one of the main questions that seems not to have a good answer is 'who is the client' or 'who is inter-ested in change' " (p. 212).

On the whole, Maldonado-Durán accepted the grandmother's presentation of herself as the spokesperson and commander of this family and accepted her claim to "ownership" of Jonah, who was hers to spoil. Like Stone and her team with Charlene (chapter 8), Maldonado-Durán assumed that she wanted her grandson to get better. He made several efforts to engage Jonah's mother, Jeanette, who was fairly unresponsive and disengaged; she seemed to accept her subsidiary role of endorsing whatever her mother said, and one has little sense of her emotional investment, if any, in her son. In view of the grandmother's frankly paranoid response to the psychiatrist, it is notable and remarkable that the public health nurse and early education specialist on the team had managed to be allowed to continue to visit for a whole year. We are not told whether they worked directly with Jonah, with Jonah and his grandmother, with Jonah and his mother, or some combination of these. Neither do we know the process by which Maldonado-Durán's own "inclusion" in Jonah's treatment was presented to or discussed with the family by the team, and to what degree the family may have felt that he was being forced on them.

### Abrupt, unplanned termination:

Maldonado-Durán was "fired" after four visits, and the grandmother complained to the hospital administration that he had made Jonah worse, had made him dopey with medication, and had taught him to curse, to hit, and so forth. She called him a "quack" and threatened a lawsuit. None of these complaints were directly expressed to him, and he was advised by the risk management people at his clinic not to seek to communicate further with the family to resolve these accusations.

### Disorganized families/disorganized transference–countertransference: Keeping baby in (whose) mind?

In his first moments with Jonah's family, Maldonado-Durán was put on notice about their characteristic way of construing relationships. He heard about the grandmother's throwing her daughter out of the house and threatening her boyfriend with a gun. He was told about the mother's "anger" that no one had magically detected the pregnancy of which she herself was unaware in order to prevent her from endangering the fetus with her medication. He heard of a God who gives unwanted, illegitimate, difficult children as gifts. Sensing that they must tread carefully to avoid being thrown out themselves, Maldonado-Durán's team felt they had no permission to address the symptoms of mental illness in the adults in Jonah's family. From the outset, the visiting psychiatrist was walking in a minefield, aware that the potential for catastrophic mistakes was both everywhere and unpredictable. In other words, the family made him immediately hypervigilant. As the intervention progressed, it gradually became clear that he could do nothing right in the family's eyes.

Roseanne's anger, suspiciousness, and unresolved trauma and Jeanette's apparent emotional detachment and passivity expressed powerful resistances to professional help. Jonah's aggressiveness, hyperactivity, and delayed development rendered him an unrewarding gift who was a perpetual trial and burden to his caregivers. As Maldonado-Durán noted, there was a virtual absence in Jonah's caregivers of the kind of reflective function that sees such problems as the outcome of cognitive or emotional misattunements and misunderstandings. Although this was to some extent due to cultural and educational factors, its intensity may have warranted a more ominous interpretation. Heineman commented:

> Everything about their daily lives appears to be consciously or unconsciously constructed to avoid thinking—to mitigate any possibility of introspection or reflective thought. (p. 221)

Furthermore she commented as follows:

> Maldonado-Durán was swept up by the chaotic whirlwind of the family activities and the disorganized inner worlds that they effectively drowned out. The force of this maelstrom was so powerful that he was sucked into the family's primitive need for constant noise and activity as the only means they have of overriding the screams of their internal demons. (p. 221)

In his encounter with the family of Jonah, Maldonado-Durán was guided by a wish to be concretely helpful to them and to be sensitive to their worldview, in the belief, well founded in extensive clinical experience, that such practical help and courteous respect would enable them to let down the barriers of mistrust that were so much in evidence. Yet here his efforts were counterproductive and appear to have infuriated instead of placated Jonah's grandmother. Heineman commented:

> Experience teaches us that psychic reality does not easily give way to common sense. We are willing to suffer for years—sometimes for generations—for real and imagined hurts, injustices, or misunderstandings for all manner of complex psychological reasons. Yet common sense tells us that we would feel better, lead more productive lives, and have more satisfying relationships if we could banish the "ghosts" from our psychic nurseries. When the ghosts have transformed themselves into persecutory demons, relief from suffering may simply not be possible. I would like to consider the tension between the incredible spoken and unspoken pressure to offer relief and the absolute insistence that no such thing is possible in Maldonado-Durán's presentation. (p. 219)

Time and again in the case report, Maldonado-Durán wrote that he noted many, if not all, of these concerns but chose to defer addressing them until the therapeutic alliance was stronger. Instead he chose to try harder and harder to offer something—a gift of some kind—to relieve the unbearable chaos and tension of the family. Paradoxically, these efforts seem to have enraged the grandmother and to have aroused her to experience his offerings as literally toxic.

It is noteworthy that Maldonado-Durán, in his reflections on the case, maintained that the family's agenda was "to fix the child," while Heineman, in her discussion, gave him credit for unconsciously understanding that its agenda was, in reality, that he *fail* to fix the child. Perhaps his feelings, combining helplessness with increasingly urgent efforts to offer something—anything—that the family could use, in some way paralleled those of little Jonah, the gift from God who was experienced as a curse.

### Christina

In chapter 12, Toni Vaughn Heineman described her ongoing work with a little girl in foster care whom nobody wanted. Lost in the limbo of the foster care system, experiencing repeated, inexplicable, and abrupt changes of placement, and with no one but the therapist to provide a "parental mind" to hold her story, this case report powerfully raised the question of what kind of therapy makes sense or is possible for a very young child who has no stable attachment figures at all, not even dysfunctional ones.

### Unresolved trauma:

When Christina began treatment, she had already been exposed to two substance-abusing parents, one of whom had died. She was a veteran of neglect, possibly of sexual abuse, and had been moved repeatedly: from her birth parents' care, to the care of her great aunt, and on to two (subsequently three) foster homes.

### Absence of angels and social support:

If we define "angel" as Lieberman and her colleagues (2005) did, as

> care-receiving experiences characterized by intense shared affect between parent and child in which the child feels nearly perfectly understood, accepted, and loved . . . that provide the child with a core sense of security and self-worth that can be drawn upon when the child becomes a parent to interrupt the cycle of maltreatment (p. 504)

it is difficult to identify anyone who played this role in Christina's life until Heineman began to do so. Her mother was dead; her father was an untreated substance abuser whose own family refused to care for Christina because it would entail contact with him. Her first foster parent did not speak her language and the second, though kind and caring, had many other obligations and saw Christina as a temporary charge.

### Age and symptoms:

Christina was older than 2 years when she entered foster care and nearly 3 when she began work with Heineman. She had spent those critical early months of life utterly without the kind of care that entrains a child's nervous system toward competent self-regulation, and that teaches confident expectation that help and support can be obtained. As noted previously, she had experienced a number of traumas that would be overwhelming for any infant. On entering foster care at 2, Christina wailed almost incessantly—everything seemed to frighten her and nothing seemed to soothe her; she seemed immobilized by fear. A psychological evaluation described her extreme sadness, rote and repetitive play, and propensity to make indiscriminate attachments. In addition, Heineman noted a kind of "emptiness" in Christina beneath her surface charm and appeal that was subtly off-putting. These symptoms were not relationship specific (nor was there a relationship to which they could be specific).

### Isolation of therapist:

Heineman, like Ruth and I, was working in a private practice setting. She described herself as overextended to the point that she only accepted the case reluctantly, on the mistaken assumption that it would be a brief involvement. Heineman was left feeling isolated and overwhelmed as the treatment stretched over months and then years with no change in the underlying uncertainty of Christina's predicament and no one with whom to form a therapeutic alliance on her behalf. She did meet regularly with her consultation group from A Home Within, the foundation founded by Heineman that offers therapists free consultation in return for offering a foster child psychotherapy for "as long as it takes." Christina's therapy was pro bono after the first few months, and Heineman credited her consultation group with keeping her from "completely losing my mind" (personal communication, July 22, 2007). However, it should be noted that as the organization's founder, and the leader of the consultation group, Heineman, like Maldonado-Durán, may have felt more supportive of than supported by the group members. It is notable that her single individual consultation (with Jeree Pawl) helped her to make a breakthrough in being able to conceptualize this therapy as a manageable undertaking.

### Choices about inclusion and exclusion:

There were both too many "care providers" to include and yet also none at all who had Christina at the center of their minds. Making choices in the ad hoc, improvisatory way that is typical of most of us in these complex and chaotic cases, Heineman involved those who wanted to be involved enough to make some effort. Yet this often meant that no one else was involved much. Heineman involved foster parents minimally; she did not work with the biological father. We do not know if Christina's brother Jack had a therapist, and, if so, whether Heineman was in contact with her. She apparently did not have contact with Jack's foster parents. She consulted when possible with the court appointed special advocate and the social worker(s) but not in the consistent, mutually supportive fashion that can happen with treatment teams.

### Abrupt, unplanned termination:

Therapy had already been interrupted once because Christina was moved to a potential adoptive home with relatives. When this placement failed, Christina was not able to return to her former foster home. She was able to return to see the same therapist only because Heineman ignored the reality of her full practice and her other professional obligations in the grips of a countertransferential moral imperative that she must take Christina back. Yet no one else in this system recognized this moral imperative, and the therapy could have ended again at a moment's notice if Christina was sent to join her father in a treatment program, was placed in another inconveniently located adoptive home, or the transportation had become unmanageable for the foster mother.

### Disorganized families/disorganized transference–countertransference: Keeping baby in (whose) mind?

Christina was a child in a chronically unstable and undependable environment, in which everything, including her therapy, depended on the whims of the dependency court. Was therapy possible? What kind of therapy was it when the therapist had no consistent adult partner with whom she could engage on the child's behalf, and the child was in a perpetual relational limbo? Heineman described very intense feelings stirred up by her work with this child: feelings of being overwhelmed, abandoned, and enraged. She wondered whether these feelings were telling her what it felt like to be a child in Christina's predicament. She felt intense pressure to act, to do more. It was as if, even if she had devoted every waking hour to trying to make Christina's situation bearable, it would not have been enough. In other words, she felt that Christina's situation was unbearable, and it took all her strength to follow Sally Provence's classic advice to "stop doing something, and just stand there." It was consultation with a treasured mentor that helped Heineman recover from her manic hyperactivity and learn to bear "just wanting" Christina.

## RADICAL HOPE AND INFANT-PARENT PSYCHOTHERAPY

> In trying to think about my experience with the Jones/Muhammad family, I have been listening to the blues—a genre rising from the African American experience of trying to find meaning by somehow making pattern or sense out of the complexities, impossibilities, absurdities, and horrors of life in a world in which the odds are impossibly stacked against them.
>
> Many blues songs talk about what happens at the crossroads—places, metaphorical and real, in which major lines of development reach choice points, and subsequent events can play out one way or a very different way. (Ruth, p. 117)

The psychoanalyst and philosopher Jonathan Lear (2006) defined the concept of *radical hope* as a faith in and commitment to "a goodness that transcended one's current understanding of the good" (p. 92). He illustrated this concept with the patriarch Abraham's response to the divine command to sacrifice his son.

Radical hope reflects an extraordinary tolerance for what Keats (1970) called *negative capability*, the capacity to bear and sustain states of not knowing. "Man is capable of being in uncertainties, mysteries, doubts, without any irritable reaching after fact and reason" (Keats, 1970, p. 43).

Lear (2006) used as his central illustration of radical hope the life and memoirs of a late-nineteenth century Native American Crow chieftain, Plenty Coups, who inspired and led his people in a period of history when their traditional way of life was rapidly and inexorably disintegrating. The relevance and meaning of their traditional values and beliefs about the nature of the universe and the place of human beings within it were also slipping away. Plenty Coups was inspired by a vision in which he was instructed to "become a chickadee" in order to save his people from the coming storm that would "knock down all trees in the forest but one." The chickadee was a creature, in Crow tradition, associated with remarkable capacities to listen to and to learn from everyone and everything, including its enemies. The chickadee was seen as a very powerful being, and its capacity to listen, to miss nothing, and to learn even from enemies, danger, and threat led to miraculous results. In being like the chickadee, the Crow avoided the twin perils of angry but hopeless resistance, on the one hand, and craven assimilation and repudiation of their unique culture and identity on the other. Under Plenty Coups's leadership, they held instead to a difficult middle path of courageous openness to the unknown and unfamiliar, and to a faith that a new way of being Crow, not currently imaginable, was possible. In other words, radical hope is the capacity to believe in the possibility of growth and healing, even when the mental tools at one's disposal cannot imagine what that would look like. Lear (2006) specifically links this capacity for radical hope to infancy:

> We are born into the world *longingly*. We instinctively reach out to parental figures for emotional and nutritional sustenance that, in the moment, we lack the resources to understand. This is the archaic prototype of radical hope: in infancy we are reaching out for sustenance from a source of goodness even though we as yet lack the concepts with which to understand what we are reaching out for. Let us leave to one side the misfires and tragedies of human upbringing and consider the case in which the parenting is "good enough." And by parenting I do not merely mean the acts of the biological parents but all the nurturing acts of all the nurturing figures in a nurturing environment. Part of the sustenance our parenting figures will give us is the concepts with which we can at least begin

> to understand what we are longing *for*. This is a crucial aspect of acquiring a natural language: inheriting a culture's set of concepts through which we can understand ourselves as desiring, wishing, and hoping for certain things. (p. 122)

Infant mental health, with its traditional confidence that "God is on our side" when we harness our work to the powerful *hopefulness and longing* of human infants, is a natural home for radical hope.

Cases such as those described here challenge our confidence in the goodness of our work, because they transcend our current ways of conceptualizing "goodness" and "success." The lives of the 10 children we have met in these pages (11 if we count the 16-year-old mother, Julia) are almost unbearably painful, and our efforts have not relieved their pain. Furthermore, some combination of our clients, our agencies, our communities, and our own guilt combines to tell us our work was rubbish, not what was needed, incompetent, or inadequate. Here I suggest that we learn to see our distress as evidence that we are being, like chickadees, unafraid to listen, even to the most terrifying and dire tales.

## LEARNING FROM THE DISORGANIZED COUNTERTRANSFERENCE

> How do we build on the foundations of respect and courtesy to challenge the entrenched positions or beliefs of our patients, in ways that do not shut down thinking, is the challenge in our work. How do we hold the horror stories and keep the hope for transformation in thinking and feeling alive, in ourselves and in the work? (Stone, p. 158)

We asked at the start of this chapter what it is in work with infants that makes us so partial to being supportive and makes it so difficult to tolerate, metabolize, and use therapeutically the intense countertransference feelings that are evoked when we see children suffering and we cannot stop it. Is there a special kind of "parental countertransference" that such cases evoke?

How can we support and cultivate the skills and fortitude necessary to this kind of work?

During the planning stages for this book, one of the questions raised by those who reviewed the proposal was whether readers could bear to read such a volume. The painfulness of "being with" families like the ones described here is indeed daunting. My own experience as a clinician, teacher, and supervisor persuades me that this pain drives many young practitioners to other "safer" domains of practice, and leads others to limit themselves to less intimate psychoeducational interventions. The deep pleasure and satisfaction we experience when we can help a child successfully elicit and connect with nurturing aspects of their caregivers is in stark contrast to the pain and distress that our failures often cause us.

In recent years, insights from the study of early parent–infant interaction by investigators such as Beebe and Lachmann (2002), Stern (1985), Lyons-Ruth (1998), Main and Hesse (1990), Sorce, Emde, Campos, and Klinnert (1985), Tronick (1998), and many others have had a major impact on current views about the nature of therapeutic change and therapeutic relationships in therapeutic work with adults (Bromberg, 1998; Mitchell, 2000; Schore, 2001a, 2001b, 2004; Siegel, 1999; Siegel & Hartzell, 2003). Increasingly the vehicle of change is conceptualized as an attunement, or entrainment, between the brains and neuroendocrine systems of patient and therapist that fosters increased self-awareness, affect regulation, and warm, stable relatedness. Although therapist and patient still converse verbally, much more attention is focused on the prosody of the dialogue—its music, as it were—and the dyad's movements in and out of harmony and dissonance (Trevarthen, 2001). In this work, much attention has been paid to the importance (and inevitability) of therapist misattunements and reparative efforts, again paralleling infant research (Beebe & Lachmann, 2002) on parental misattunements and repair.

The adult psychoanalytic literature uses the language of countertransference in this discussion. In other words, therapists sometimes respond in unempathic, misattuned ways because their own ghosts in the nursery have been awakened and are, transiently, it is to be hoped, clouding the therapist's ability to fully see and contain what the patient is presenting.

For example, a 60-year-old client of mine, talking about the anxiety she felt between sessions, told me that she had learned from a mutual acquaintance that I had had breast cancer and that she worried about a recurrence. My own response was initially strongly colored by my own anxiety about a recurrence and my anger that something personal I had shared in confidence with our mutual friend, to support her as she went through a cancer scare, had been passed along to others. These responses triggered an aspect of my personality, rooted in my childhood as the compulsive caretaker of a severely depressed and borderline mother, that deeply resents having to focus on others' needs at the expense of my own. I certainly communicated, through my voice and body language, that I *did not like* my patient talking about this. This was not therapeutic. However, my reflections with the patient, about my unsympathetic response and how it left her feeling, were extremely rich.

In infant mental health, we deal with, discuss, and respond to such misattunement and repair sequences between mother and baby as the bread and butter of our work. On the other hand, the discussion of *our* countertransference, or the primitive feelings, impulses, and actions evoked by the therapy in the therapist, is all but nonexistent in infant mental health.

Here our goal is to contribute to understanding how the complex and flawed humanity of the therapist may be activated in the crucible of relationship with a dyad (or with a child with no identifiable primary caregiver) whose attachment behavioral systems are highly disorganized and distressed.

## IMPEDIMENTS TO THE WORKING ALLIANCE REVISITED

The more disorganized the family is with respect to relationships, the more difficult it will be to establish a genuinely trusting therapeutic relationship and the more the clinician will be exposed to intense and disturbing countertransference feelings and thoughts (Slade, 2007). The presence of such feelings and thoughts should itself alert the clinician to the possible role of attachment disorganization in impeding therapeutic connection and progress.

As Heineman said in chapter 12,

> More often, the children and parents who come to us for help are beset with multiple current and past stressors that continually threaten the stability and coherence of their internal and external worlds. The difficulties they bring to us endanger our sense of clinical identity and well-being. Because they have rarely enjoyed a preponderance of satisfying relationships, based on mutual value and respect, they do not look for or expect to find them. When they do—and relationships form the foundation of what we have to offer—they either do not know what to do with them or feel an almost overwhelming need to destroy them in order to preserve reality as they have come to know it. (p. 231)

When such a need to destroy relationship is operative, our redoubled efforts to connect helpfully can have the paradoxical result of driving the client deeper into their self-protective destructiveness. Our best chance for connection may entail the dampening of our own eagerness and urgency to "help." When we seem to push them away, or when we reduce the intensity of our efforts, we must know how to process our own anxiety about the dire straits in which infants in such families live. We must be able to call on other services, such as child protection services, that have tools we lack. Without becoming complacent or numb, we must learn to bear the shortcomings of our own methods and those of these other systems.

Unlike mental health professionals, protective service workers live daily with "negative transference," with being demonized by clients, the community, and, all too often, by mental health professionals like ourselves. I believe that our profession has much to learn (as I personally have learned much) from the practice of the best of these protective service social workers. A skilled protective service worker knows how to tell parents things they do not want to hear with respect and compassion, but also with directness and a certain toughness about being perceived as mean, heartless, and destructive. She can go on feeling and being compassionate in the face of the client's rageful certainty that she is hateful. She is comfortable with not being "nice," comfortable with not being perceived as a rescuer, a comforter, or an angel. The service worker feels deep in her bones the truth that protecting a parent's children from his or her destructive behavior is the most compassionate act possible toward an abusive or neglectful parent. She always operates in conscious awareness that children do not always have parents, protection, provision, love, and at least a grounding modicum of safety, and that parents cannot always rise to meet their children's needs.

As therapists, we too must get better at integrating the setting of limits into our model of strengths-based, relational intervention. That includes learning to tolerate—even to welcome and to invite—taking the heat for the client's resulting feeling of anger and betrayal. This is very difficult; possibly it cannot be done without reflective consultation. As Stone commented in chapter 8:

> In child protection work, hateful acts are not uncommon, yet it remains extremely difficult to think, unflinchingly, about hate. As therapists working with young children and their parents, how do we find a place of compassion in ourselves that allows us to think simultaneously about the parent and the painful history that typically sets the stage for enactments of parental hate, *and* to see clearly the force of the hate in such acts and its impact upon the infant and young child? . . . [Do we] get caught in the pursuit of "not blaming" rather than thinking about what appears to be blameful[?]. Do we, and did I, flinch from thinking about hate because I was afraid of my own hate and destructive potential? Fearful perhaps that I too might be hateful were I unable to find and nourish the place of possibility for change within this troubled infant–parent relationship? (p. 171)

Perhaps there is a parallel between the infant–parent psychotherapist's tenuous clinging to the dyad and the battered spouse's clinging to the "strengths" (e.g., remorse, intense concern, protection from extrafamilial dangers) of the batterer. At times, we continue to admire a struggling caregiver's strengths, often exercising great ingenuity and creativity to find them, while containing without confronting harmful attitudes and behaviors. For instance, a therapist might not address the caregiver's constant yelling at the baby or leaving the baby alone for hours in a dark room out of fear that saying what he or she really thinks will result in being "thrown out of the house" and hence unavailable to the baby. When, for example, Maldonado-Durán commented in chapter 10 that "the question of the family defeating the therapist came into mind, but I tried to remain empathic to their experience of being disappointed and exhausted" (p. 207), it is implied that these are mutually exclusive positions. Would it not be possible and, perhaps, productive, to communicate both an observation that the parent seems to need or wish to show the therapist how useless he is and an empathic concern for how disappointed and exhausted the parent is feeling?

## "Mental Health" or "Public "Health": Who's Holding the Environment?

At the beginning of this chapter we asked where the limits are of a supportive strengths-based approach when a child is in emotional peril. What are the alternatives and how can we make them acceptable to severely troubled families?

In mental health, as in medicine, every intervention has a limited range of efficacy. Aspirin is good for headaches, bad for an upset stomach. Radiation therapy kills cancer cells but damages healthy tissue. Fluids and antidiarrheal medication cure gastrointestinal maladies, but only if the patient has access to clean drinking water. Cognitive–behavioral therapies are extremely helpful to clients who are able to trust a therapist enough to follow her prescriptions and less helpful to those whose entrenched fears and negative beliefs about authority figures impede their capacity to learn.

Infant–parent psychotherapy has its limits too. To say this is in no way intended to cast doubts on the very real and transformative impact that this form of intervention has on many, many struggling families. That positive impact is well documented in both clinical studies and empirical research. The exploration of limits, it is hoped, serves instead to make intervention more focused and effective. On the one hand, better understanding of the limits of effectiveness helps us as clinicians to make better informed choices about whom to treat and for how long. On the other hand, a clearer understanding about limits may help clinicians to avoid burnout, to preserve a belief in the value of their work, and to metabolize the often deeply painful situations into which they enter as participant observers.

Looking at the question of limits from a slightly different angle, every therapy and every theory both focuses and organizes the clinician's vision to heighten her sensitivity to and awareness of the phenomena of interest. At the same time, by virtue of doing just that (very helpful, worthwhile, and valuable) thing, every therapy and every theory make other phenomena less visible.

Our model, as well as our method, shines a brilliant and revelatory light on the infant's early movements toward relatedness and toward a relationship-embedded representation of self (Stern, 1985, 1995). Our lens also illuminates how the caregiving environment responds to these moves and reveals how the caregivers' state of mind with regard to relationship is communicated to the infant. Gestures, facial expressions, vocalizations, gaze, absence, and presence are then reflected back by the infant to the caregiver. They represent the barrage of sensory, affective, and cognitive experiences that characterize parent–infant interaction.

Other dimensions of a family's experience are not so brightly lit by our ways of looking, and may even be obscured by our focus on the parent–infant interaction, particularly if, for therapeutic reasons, our approach is strengths based.

> Perhaps most significantly, our "working model of therapy" holds that if we help ensure the bonds between (a mother) and her baby in the first days and weeks, we think the intruding ghosts will depart, as they do in most nurseries, when the child is protected by the magic circle of family." (Fraiberg et al., 1975, p. 421)

This belief can make it nearly impossible to even think, let alone mention, that, at its potential best, the relationship between a particular mother and her child is not always in either partner's best interest. Yet with a bit of time and space separating us from immediate engagement, that question does come to mind for every one of these six cases. As Stone eloquently stated in her discussion of Ruth's work with the Jones/Muhammad family:

> In strengths-based work, the therapist is often so enthusiastic to emphasize what can be done that no time is taken to mourn what may have been lost. Without acknowledgment of the gap between the longed for and the actual, the limitations that may be inherent in the difference between these two positions cannot be fully understood or worked with. Our failure to really explore this gap in work with families means the creative potential of "what is possible" will always be muted, filtered through what we have not acknowledged together. (p. 159)

We get so wrapped up in the hope and the possibility for a "new beginning" that little children inspire, that we often find it difficult to address the grief and tragedy that the birth of a child often entails. Whatever miraculous phoenix may rise from the ashes—and miracles do happen daily with babies—each one of these babies' births was also a tragedy. Perhaps it is only through being available to witness, feel, and honor the "mourning of what may have been lost" that we can find our way with such families.

## THE MOTHERHOOD CONSTELLATION REVISITED: TRANSFERENCE AND COUNTERTRANSFERENCE WITH TRAUMATIZED INFANTS AND FAMILIES

Typically, the therapeutic constellation in psychotherapeutic work with very young children and their families is thought of as a triangle, consisting of parent (usually mother), child, and therapist at each of the three poles. The emergent relationships and dynamics within such a triangle have been exquisitely described by Stern (1995). He posited a sort of "Indra's net" of cascading acts of reciprocal representation and mirroring. The mother initially may be unable to see her infant, or she may see him through the distorting lens of her own troubled childhood relationships with caregivers. In complementary fashion, she may see herself and her own mothering in a painful, distorted, and constricted way, perhaps as "bad," "perfect," "burdened," or "victimized" in relation to her infant. These distortions again reflect the dysfunctional relationships of her family of origin. The therapist, inviting and cultivating what Stern (1995, p. 186) called the *good grandmother transference*, offers her own consistent, benevolent, modulated, yet realistic capacity to see what is good, loving, and joyful in the mother, in the infant, and in their interactions and their developing relationship. Seen in this nurturing way, the mother and infant become increasingly able to *feel* and *act* in loving, joyful patterns of interaction, at first in the presence of the benevolent therapist and, over time, on their own. Jeree Pawl has repeatedly summarized this approach succinctly as "doing unto others what you would have others do unto others" (personal communication, November 5, 2007).

Heffron, Ivins, and Weston (2005) have offered a widely used conceptualization of *how* this trickle-down benevolence works, describing the therapist's use of self as a therapeutic technique. The therapist allows herself to share and to metabolize the emotional states of the dyad, thus mirroring them in a modulated fashion that renders them both thinkable and bearable. This process is described in the literature of object relations theory (Bion, 1979) as "containment." It echoes the kind of mirroring skilled parents do with infants (Fonagy, Gergely, Jurist, & Target, 2002) in that it is not literally mirroring or simply imitating or echoing the baby's communicative expression. Rather, such containing and mirroring processes and interprets the baby's expressive gesture and reflects a metabolized version that, first, helps the baby understand what she is experiencing and, second, gives the baby a soothing, calming experience of being held in another's mind. In infant–parent psychotherapy, it is thought that the therapist processes and interprets the communications of the dyad and reflects a metabolized version that, in similar fashion, fosters understanding and feeling understood.

Even for the many families who can use this kind of help, this model, like any model, entails certain risks—"side effects" if you will. There is perhaps a conflict or a contradiction inherent in trying simultaneously to contain emotional states (which invariably are both positive and negative, of varied intensity, etc.) and to identify and admire strengths. We may be at risk of being unable to see the cloud around the silver lining.

However, in our most difficult cases, and in each of the cases presented in the preceding chapters, this approach, combining use of self as a container for clients' difficult experiences, with a mandate to find and support clients' strengths, has real perils. First, the mental acrobatics required to look at these caregivers and children with hopeful admiration are nothing short of momentous. Second, true openness to the emotional chaos and trauma in which these clients live places the therapist at high risk for secondary traumatic stress. An intake worker assessing the caregivers in these families might well conclude that they were essentially untreatable as a result of varying combinations of

- Severe psychopathology;
- Overwhelming, chronic, and intransigent external stressors; and
- Lack of interest in, lack of belief in, resistance to, and hostility toward therapy that is based on exposing and understanding what has always had to be hidden and stifled.

Because we are not omniscient, our focusing on strengths, love, and joy inevitably results in some slighting of our attention to deficits, hatred, and wretchedness. In typical cases, this is not too much of a problem, and the therapist can fairly readily self-monitor and maintain a balance between hopefulness and realism.

The supportive, good grandmother paradigm becomes problematic when some combination of risk factors in the parent, the infant, and the network of supportive people and services prevents this warm "corrective attachment relationship" (Sklan, chapter 2) from forming.

As grandmothers around the world and through the ages tell us, in the absence of a good-enough parent, a "good grandmother" is less than a heartbeat away from becoming the de facto mother. Thus, a technique that asks us to provide a corrective emotional/attachment experience for infants in their caregiving environment, by genuinely caring for and loving what is good and hopeful in those systems, puts us at risk for developing a maternal countertransference characterized by an overwhelming and grandiose sense of responsibility, often accompanied by intense anxiety, feelings of isolation, and manic levels of activity. As Sklan wrote in her discussion of Heineman's case, the therapist feels a

> gravitational pull to both jump in and fill in the hole of overwhelming needs and also to feel pulled into a hole herself of overwhelming feelings in response to the overwhelming needs and feelings of the young child. (p. 247)

To some extent this happened to each of the therapist contributors to this volume, as they state in their own words:

- *Susan Sklan*: The absence was always present, and at times seemed shocking to me. I absorbed all of the pressures and responsibility of intervening in two vulnerable lives: an adolescent and her infant. I found myself wanting to cook her a meal and take care of Julia and her baby when the gaps felt difficult to bear. I procured a sling and later a stroller donation through my program so that Miguel could be safely transported and so Julia could better manage the logistics of going to day care on two buses and then school, twice a day. I tried to carefully time when to act and when to wait. I was constantly considering what Miguel needed at that moment, even if his young mother could not provide it. When can the infant or toddler wait and when is it critical that his needs take precedence? Miguel's dependency on such a young and at times so fragmented mother added to my sense of urgency and constant vigilance. I felt I had to keep them both in mind, and it made me anxious that no one else was doing so with a long-term commitment. (pp. 60–61)

- *Marian Birch*: The therapeutic role can easily become a venue for a field of dissociative responses on the part of the therapist who allows the observer to overpower the participant in the participant–observer role. Perhaps this is part of what happened to me with Ben. My continuing performance as the therapist became rigid and artificial as I ignored my inner reactions to feeling powerless to reach Ben. I was frightened and revolted by the cold violence of his scripts. Simply put, I kept acting "nice" and "helpful" when I felt neither. (p. 98)

- *Richard Ruth*: I felt grounded in my own sense of what therapy was, and grounded in a sense that I was holding important ambiguities, in more or less clear focus and at least much of the time. I kept asking myself whether these things were enough. I still ask myself, years later and after months of concentrated thinking. I kept thinking that, if we just had a little more time, things would work out. In parallel process, the same theme has gone through my mind as I have struggled to get what I think about this family and this therapy onto paper: It will all come clear if I just work on it a little more, but it never did. (p. 138)

- *Julie Stone*: What we had offered had been pushed aside, discarded, and reviled. This felt like the repetition of a destructive pattern we had not thought about clearly or fully enough in our work with Charlene and Jay. (p. 182)

- *Martin Maldonado-Durán*: Perhaps I was led by a "wish to cure" that in this case really was a misreading of the situation. The urgency to "cure" was more in the mind of the therapist than in the agenda of the family. Perhaps the complaints were taken too literally, and it might have been better to listen to more of the implications of the complaints, dealing empathically with them and to work harder first on establishing a true therapeutic alliance before intervening in any way. Without such an alliance, the interventions felt like an intrusion and alien to the family, who quickly discarded them.

  Another dynamic force is worth considering. I was "called in" to make some sort of "change" in this entrenched system. There was an internal pressure on the part of "the doctor" to make a difference when two other colleagues had felt "stuck." This led to a sort of messianic hope that somehow I—the doctor—would be able to offer something new. This was connected with the hope of finding some wonderful medication that might make things move along. Obviously, this was not the case. (p. 213)

- *Toni Vaughn Heineman*: Even though I knew better, when I could pull my rational self together, I felt as if we had been totally and completely abandoned—*forever*. My calls for help went unanswered. No one cared. No one even knew I needed help. . . . Indeed, during much of the time that I worked with Christina I alternated between feeling that there was no one to call and that I had to call everyone all of the time or all would be lost. . . . What made me want to cry? Everything about this child's life and our therapeutic life together. I had to take care of her, and I could not take care of her. . . . I wanted to cry because when Christina walked through my door, I instantly knew that there was no turning back, and that I had just put my sanity on the line. . . . I felt that on the most basic human level, I had no choice about resuming my therapeutic relationship with Christina. I had to see her. . . . I believe that my contribution to the crisis that we narrowly averted when Christina returned from the relatives who did not want her was my sense that I had to step into the parental void—not by adoption or becoming her foster parent—but by pulling all of the pieces and players together and holding them in mind for and with her. It was a job I had no hope of doing successfully and in the face of this formidable task, I felt hopeless and anxiously overwhelmed. Having psychically put myself into the center of the melee, everyone understandably looked to me to solve the problem. They themselves became anxious when they recognized that the limitations on my time, energy, and psychic space would make me fall short. (pp. 237–243)

## BACK FROM DESPAIR

The "perfect attunement" is not able to tolerate hate and rupture. It is a sign of the maturing in professional development in an individual therapist as well as the maturing of the field of infant mental health to be able to look at aspects of the work that feel unbearable. Just as the mother, as described by Winnicott (1947/1975), is able to walk the line of ambivalence of the love and the hate, the ability to contain the hate is the ability to acknowledge it. (Sklan, p. 252)

The fact that therapists are susceptible to such states of heightened anxiety, tunnel vision, and overwhelming sense of responsibility is not an indication that such therapy is wrongheaded. However, when therapists find themselves "blindsided" by such intense reactions to clients' predicaments, they need skills and support to enable them to use such feelings as information, rather than being sucked into a whirlwind of enactment as they try to single-handedly hold back the flood of disaster that threatens "their" baby.

In many of our cases, the therapist is trying harder and harder to present him- or herself as helpful and benevolent in the face of both direct and indirect messages from the family and system that he or she is experienced as neither. We are told in our training, as well as in our literature, of the importance of offering warmth, consistency, respect, and unwavering attention. We are taught less about the importance of tolerating, validating, and working with perceptions that we are uncaring, uncomprehending, unreliable, and dangerous. Our master clinicians have much to say about exploring the negative transference to the baby (in order to invalidate it), but far less to say about tolerating and exploring the negative transference to the therapist.

The discussion of the therapist's use of self in the literature tends to presume a degree of detachment and capacity for self-observation and restraint that, if it is possible, is certainly exceptional. There is a particular kind of counter-transference peril in work with infants that is related to the activation of the therapist's own attachment system.

To process and interpret and metabolize the unprocessed, unmetabolized expressions observed in the infant or client, the mother of the infant or the therapist of the dyad must first feel and experience them. When the care-giving parent or therapist is open to such raw feelings and experiences, her own earliest relational experiences, including her own states of mind with respect to relationship, are activated. This is not cognitive-behavioral or psychoeducational work; it is deep work and leaves the caregiving parent or therapist quite exposed and vulnerable to what is stirred by the baby or the client. Use of self is powerful, dangerous, and difficult. Like parenting, it cannot be done in isolation, without support, even by seasoned, gifted clinicians like those whose stories make up this book. Also, like parenting, it cannot, even at its best, compensate for deprivation and disrespect at a community, societal level.

Such countertransference responses are not a weakness or a failure in the therapist; they are inevitable consequences of this way of working. Metabolized and reflected on, they give us vital information about the extreme psychological danger in which a family dwells. Thus, regular consul-tation and working collaboratively with other services need to be require-ments for working with chronically traumatized and disorganized families, and not an optional choice. Consultation provides some containment for the therapist and increases the possibility of metabolizing such responses reflec-tively instead of acting them out. Collaboration with other kinds of services also provides support for a clearer definition of the therapist's role and its limitations.

We can also learn a great deal here from medicine, especially nursing, in developing intervention models that include the inevitability of failure, incurability, and psychological death. Sometimes our work is like the work of a pediatric oncology ward. Some families are very, very sick. Sometimes all our skill and caring fall short of what is needed. As Winnicott (1980) told us, there is no such thing as an infant without the caregiving environment, so we will fail to "save" many of the infants born into the kind of "perfect storm" of risk and deprivation described here.

We need to do better in our training programs to prepare practitioners for work with families that may have needs we cannot meet and that may defensively need to trash what we offer them.

We need to find greater professional clarity about the hospice-like palliative aspects of our work with severely impaired families so that we can continue to do it with a sense of being, in a humble way, useful.

Finally, we need to combine our intimate therapeutic engagement with individual families with a clear-eyed honesty with ourselves and with our clients about the limits of individual work and about the larger social issues that result in huge numbers of infants born into trauma and neglect throughout the world. As the saying goes, while we continue, as therapists, to "pull bodies out of the river," we must not lose sight of the fact that social forces upstream are throwing them in, and some will drown despite our best efforts.

## REFERENCES

Alvarez, A. (1999). Widening the bridge: Commentary on papers by Stephen Seligman and by Robin C. Silverman and Alicia F. Lieberman. *Psychoanalytic Dialogues*, 9(2), 205–217.

Beebe, B., & Lachmann, F. (2002). *Infant research and adult treatment: Co-constructing interactions.* Hillsdale, NJ: Analytic Press.

Bick, E. (2003). The experience of the skin in early object relations. In J. Rafael-Leff (Ed.), *Parent–infant psychodynamics: Wild things, mirrors and ghosts* (pp.74–82). London: Whurr Publishers. (Original work published 1968)

Bion, W. R. (1967). Notes on memory and desire. *Psychoanalytic Forum, 2,* 271–280.

Bion, W. R. (1979). *Elements of psychoanalysis*. Northvale, NJ: Jason Aronson.

Birch, M. (1994). Who's holding the environment? Issues of parents of traumatized children. *Section II Newsletter: Section on Childhood and Adolescence, Div. 39, American Psychological Association, 2*, 17–20.

Bromberg, P. (1998). *Standing in the spaces: Essays on clinical process, trauma and dissociation*. Hillsdale, NJ: Analytic Press.

Felitti, V. J., Anda, R. F., Nordenberg, D., Williamson, D. F., Spitz, A. M., Edwards, V., et al. (1998). Relationship of childhood abuse and household dysfunction to many of the leading causes of death in adults: The adverse childhood experiences (ACE) study. *American Journal of Preventive Medicine, 14*, 245–258.

Fonagy, P. (1998). Prevention, the appropriate target of infant psychotherapy. *Infant Mental Health Journal, 19*, 124–150.

Fonagy, P., Gergely, G., Jurist, E., & Target, M. (2002). *Affect regulation, mentalization and the development of the self*. New York: Other Press.

Fraiberg, S. (1980). *Clinical studies in infant mental health*. New York: Basic Books.

Fraiberg, S., Adelson, E., & Shapiro, V. (1975). Ghosts in the nursery: A psychoanalytic approach to impaired infant–mother relationships. *Journal of the American Academy of Child Psychiatry, 14*, 1387–1422.

Freud, S. (1955). The psychotherapy of hysteria. In J. Breuer & S. Freud, *Studies on hysteria* (pp. 1–305). J. Strachey (Ed. & Trans.), *Standard edition of collected works of Sigmund Freud* (Vol. 2). London: Hogarth.

Harris, W. W., Lieberman, A. F., & Marans, S. (2007). In the best interests of society. *Journal of Child Psychology and Psychiatry, 48*, 392–411.

Heffron, M. C., Ivins, B., & Weston, D. R. (2005). Finding an authentic voice-use of self: Essential learning processes for relationship-based work. *Infants and Young Children, 18*, 323–336.

Keats, J. (1970). *The letters of John Keats: A selection.* Oxford, England: Oxford University Press.

Lear, J. (2006). *Radical hope: Ethics in the face of cultural devastation.* Cambridge, MA: Harvard University Press.

Lieberman, A. F. (1993). *The emotional life of toddlers.* New York: Free Press.

Lieberman, A. F. (1997). Toddlers' internalization of maternal attributions as a factor in quality of attachment. In L. Atkinson & K. J. Zucker (Eds.), *Attachment and psychopathology* (pp. 277–291). New York: Guilford.

Lieberman, A. F., & Harris, W. W. (2006, April). *Still searching for the best interests of the child: Trauma treatment in infancy and early childhood.* Paper presented at the Albert J. Solnit Second Memorial Lecture, Yale University Child Study Center, New Haven, CT.

Lieberman, A. F., & Harris, W. W. (2007). Still searching for the best interests of the child: Trauma treatment in infancy and early childhood. *Psychoanalytic Study of the Child, 62,* 211–238.

Lieberman, A. F., Padron, E., Van Horn, P., & Harris, W. (2005). Angels in the nursery: The intergenerational transmission of benevolent parental influences. *Journal of Infant Mental Health, 26,* 504–520.

Lyons-Ruth, K. (1998). Implicit relational knowing: Its role in development and psychoanalytic treatment. *Infant Mental Health Journal, 19,* 282–289.

Lyons-Ruth, K., Bronfman, E., & Atwood, G. (1999). A relational diathesis model of hostile–helpless states of mind: Expressions in mother–infant interaction. In J. Solomon (Ed.), *Attachment disorganization* (pp. 33–70). New York: Guilford Press.

Lyons-Ruth, K., & Jacovitz, D. (1999). Attachment disorganization: Unresolved loss, relational violence, and lapses in behavioral and attention strategies. In J. Cassidy & P. Shaver (Eds.), *Handbook of attachment: Theory, research, and clinical applications* (pp. 520–554). New York: Guilford Press.

Main, M., & Hesse, E. (1990). Parents' unresolved traumatic experiences are related to infant disorganized attachment status: Is frightened and/or frightening parental behavior the linking mechanism? In M. Greenberg, D. Cicchetti, & E. M. Cummings (Eds.), *Attachment in the preschool years: Theory, research and intervention* (pp.161–184). Chicago: University of Chicago Press.

Mitchell, S. (2000). *Relationality: From attachment to intersubjectivity.* Hillsdale, NJ: Analytic Press.

Perry, B. D. (1997). Incubated in terror: Neurodevelopmental factors in the cycle of violence. In J. Osofsky (Ed.), *Children, youth and violence: The search for solutions* (pp. 124–149). New York: Guilford Press.

Schore, A. N. (2001a). Effects of a secure attachment relationship on right brain development, affect regulation, and infant mental health. *Infant Mental Health Journal, 22*(1–2), 7–66.

Schore, A. N. (2001b).The effects of early relational trauma on right brain development, affect regulation, and infant mental health. *Infant Mental Health Journal, 22*(1–2), 201–269.

Schore, A. N. (2004). *Affect regulation and the repair of the self.* New York: W. W. Norton.

Seligman, S., & Pawl, J. (1984). Impediments to the formation of the working alliance in infant–parent psychotherapy. In J. Call, E. Galenson, & R. Tyson (Eds.), *Frontiers of infant psychiatry* (Vol. 2, pp. 232–237). New York: Basic Books.

Siegel, D. (1999). Representations: Modes of processing and the construction of reality. In D. Siegel, *The developing mind: Toward a neurobiology of interpersonal experience* (pp. 160–207). New York: Guilford Press.

Siegel, D., & Hartzell, M. (2003). *Parenting with the brain in mind: How a deeper understanding can help you raise children who thrive.* New York: Jeremy Tarcher/Penguin.

Slade, A. (2007). Disorganized mother, disorganized child: The mentalization of affective regulation and therapeutic change. In D. Oppenheim & D. Goldsmith (Eds.), *Attachment theory in clinical work with children: Bridging the gap between research and practice* (pp. 226–250). New York: Guilford.

Sorce, J. F., Emde, R. N., Campos, J., & Klinnert, M. D. (1985). Maternal emotional signaling: Its effect on the visual cliff behavior of 1-year-olds. *Developmental Psychology, 21*(1), 195–200.

Sperling, M. B., & Berman, W. H. (1994). *Attachment in adults: Clinical and developmental perspectives.* New York: Guilford Press.

Stern, D. (1985). *The interpersonal world of the infant: A view from psychoanalysis and developmental psychology.* New York: Basic Books.

Stern, D. (1995). *The motherhood constellation: A unified view of parent–infant psychotherapy.* New York: Basic Books.

Trevarthen, C. (2001). Intrinsic motives for companionship in understanding: Their origin, development and significance for infant mental health. *Infant Mental Health Journal, 22,* 95–131.

Tronick, E. (1998). Dyadically expanded states of consciousness and the process of therapeutic change. *Infant Mental Health Journal, 19,* 290–299.

van der Kolk, B. (1994). *The body keeps the score: Memory and the evolving psychobiology of posttraumatic stress.* Boston, MA: Massachussetts General Hospital, Trauma Clinic, Harvard Medical School.

Winnicott, D. W. (1975). Hate in the countertransference. In D. W. Winnicott, *Through paediatrics to psychoanalysis* (pp. 194–203). New York: Basic Books. (Original work published 1947)

Winnicott, D. W. (1980). *The maturational process and the facilitating environment.* London: Karnac.

Winnicott, D. W. (1980). The theory of the parent-infant relationship. In D. W. Winnicott, *The maturational processes and the facilitating environment* (pp. 37–55). London: Karnac. (Original work published 1960)

Winnicott, D. W. (1989). Fear of breakdown. In C. Winnicott, R. Shepherd, & M. Davis (Eds.), *Psychoanalytic explorations* (pp. 87–95). Cambridge, MA: Harvard University Press. (Original work published 1963)

# INDEX

Adelson, E., 1–2. *See also* infant–parent psychotherapy, dominant model of intervention

adoption by therapists, 6, 7, 242

adoptive parents: awakened ghosts of, 81–82, 90, 96, 99, 281–282; effect of adopting a second child, 93–95, 279; fathers, 89–90, 262; parental attachment behavior in, 282. *See also* Birch's case (Ben and his adoptive family)

adults and therapy: and containment, 73–74; and language of countertransference, 309–310; recent insights into nature/vehicles of therapeutic change, 309–310

advocacy by therapists: Maldonado-Durán's discussion of Stone's case, 193–194; Ruth's case, 144–145

African American families and therapy: and contexts for experiencing denied promises of child welfare system, 141; office therapy and external constraints on, 124–128; reflections on blues music and African American experience, 117–118, 153–154; Ruth's case, 117–118, 119, 124–127, 141, 150, 153–155, 284–185; white/African American therapeutic couplings, 118, 119, 150, 284–285. *See also* race, class, and culture (issues of)

ages and symptoms of infants/children in case studies: Birch's case, 78–79, 280; distinctions between preventive work/reparative work, 265, 266–267; Heineman's case, 232–234, 238–239, 304; Maldonado-Durán's case, 298–299; Ruth's case, 118, 119, 134–135, 154, 159–160, 285; Sklan's case, 275; Stone's case, 168–169, 174, 292; treating older toddlers with relationship-independent symptoms, 256, 265–267

Alvarez, Anne, 165, 175

Amini, F., et al., 32, 49

angels, absence of (families lacking social support), 256, 260–263; absent and violent fathers, 261–262; Birch's case, 109–110, 279–280; community resources, 262–263; defining "angels," 260–261, 303; Heineman's case, 303; Maldonado-Durán's case, 297–298; Ruth's case, 284; Sklan's case, 274–275; Stone's case, 291

attachment-based intervention, 14–15; activation of parental attachment behavior, 7, 282; the "affective trio," 32; anxiously

attached infants as adult caregivers, 14, 84, 188; attachment disorders without reparative parental relationship in place, 250; Birch's case, 84, 85–86, 88–89, 93, 97–98, 282; and countertransference paradigm, 7, 321–322; defining, 14–15; disturbed attachment and inability to play, 85–86, 89, 97–98; disturbed attachment and predatory behavior, 85–86, 88–93; disturbed attachment behavior in traumatized children, 84, 85–86, 88–89, 92–93, 97–98, 282; Heineman's case, 250; implicit memories of early attachment relationships, 32; pondering the powerful attachment system and anxiety in children, 88–89; "right-brain-to-right brain" connections, 84; Sklan's case (attachment-based intervention), 31–32, 62, 68–69, 70, 273; traumatized infants' chronic fearful states of arousal, 83–84; unresolved trauma and disorganized attachment, 258–260; where a different approach might have succeeded, 68–69; and the working model of relationship, 84, 92–93

attunement/entrainment, 309

autism diagnoses, Stone's case and mother's pursuit of, 162–164, 172–173, 176, 181, 182–184, 191–193, 290, 292, 295; effects of hasty diagnoses on child's sense of self, 183–184, 192; the provisional diagnosis, 181, 182–184, 192; tension between assigning diagnosis/seeking understanding, 162–163; therapist recognition of autistic-like defenses and behavior, 174, 292; therapist's concern about the assessment, 182–183; what pediatric evaluations should ideally do, 183–184; what the autistic behaviors meant for mother, 292

autistic-like defenses/stereotypes, 98, 174, 180, 190, 291, 292

*The Baby as Subject* (Thomson-Salo and Paul), 164

Barnard, Kathryn, 3–4

Beebe, B., 309

Bion, W. R., 119, 269

Birch, Marian: comments on Sklan's case, 67–76; practice and professional background, 3–4, 10

Birch's case (Ben and his adoptive family), 10–11, 77–101, 103–115, 278–283;

140–141, 145, 155, 286, 288; Sklan's case, 30, 36, 37–38, 48, 58; therapies authorized/funded by, 269–270; withholding critical information from a therapist, 122–123, 129, 286. *See also* Child Protective Services (CPS); foster care system

choices about inclusion/exclusion, 256, 268–271; Birch's case, 79, 281–282; containment issues, 269–271; Heineman's case, 304–335; Maldonado-Durán's case, 212–216, 299–300; Ruth's case, 124, 126, 268–269, 286; Sklan's case, 37–38, 49, 58–59, 268, 276; Stone's case, 268–269, 293–294; and theoretical orientations of the therapists, 268–269

classical model of psychoanalytic practice: context of Fraiberg's modifications, 17–18; and discussions of treatment failures, viii–ix; historical adaptations of, 17–18; "interpretations of resistance" in, 20; and neutrality concept of, viii–ix, 106–109; the "superhuman" analyst and no countertransference, 21

class issues. *See* race, class, and culture (issues of)

Coltart, N., 156–157

community resources. *See* angels, absence of (families lacking social support)

containment: in adult therapy, 73–74; and choices about inclusion/exclusion, 269–271; containing without confronting, 270; and countertransference issues, 316–317; and dominant model of intervention in infant–parent psychotherapy, 16–17, 155–156; emotional side effects for the therapist, 135–136, 288–289, 316–317; and home visits, 32; and Kleinian notions of development and mental operations, 133; Maldonado-Durán's case, 299; metabolizing the experiences, 192–193, 299, 316–317; mirroring, 82–84, 288, 316–317; and object relations school, 269, 316; in play therapy, 99; Ruth's case, 133, 135–136, 145, 149–150, 155–156, 269, 288–289; Stone's case, 179–180, 269; and strengths-based therapy, 270–271; trickle-down benevolence, 20–21, 316–317; Winnicott's discussion of the "holding environment," 269

contributors and cases, 9–13; discussion of coauthors' case histories, 13; therapists' self-disclosure/courage to offer a problematic case, 9

cotherapy: and countertransference, 178–179, 295; Stone's case, 164, 166–168, 178–179, 193, 293, 295–296

countertransference and infant–parent psychotherapy, 6–7, 19–23, 21; acknowledging analysts' fallibility, 21; and ambivalence of therapeutic relationships (as professionals paid to care), 109–110, 249–250, 270–271; basic paradigm (activation of attachment systems), 7, 321–322; Birch's case, 98, 113, 282, 318; case management services obscuring the "play" of, 19; cases in which no "parental mind" is present, 250, 272–273; as central issue running through all cases, x, 13, 256, 308–313, 315–322; and challenges of effective intervention, 6–7, 21, 22–23; and classical model of psychoanalysis, 21; and cotherapy situations, 178–179, 295; disorganized transference-countertransference patterns, 257, 272–273, 308–310; and emotional availability of therapists to caregivers, 19; expansion of concept of, 21–22; finding the appropriate therapeutic stance, 22–23; and the good grandmother paradigm, 316, 317–318; and hate/love in therapeutic relationships, x, 22, 249; Heineman's case, 231, 235, 238, 239, 247–253, 305–306, 318, 319–320; home visits obscuring the "play" of, 19; and "hostile-helpless states of mind," 272; and impediments to the working alliance, 310–313; intensity of responses, 21–22; and isolation of therapist/necessity of collaboration, 267–268, 321; learning to understand/process responses and inevitability of failures, 310–13, 320–322; Maldonado-Durán's case, 213, 301–302, 319; "negative transference" (learning to accept), 311–313, 320–331; recent insights into nature/vehicles of therapeutic change in adults, 309–310; risks of therapist's use of self, 316–322; Ruth's case, 138, 287–289, 318–319; Sklan's case, 55–56, 60–62, 75, 277–278, 318; Stone's case, 178–179, 182, 295–296, 319; and strengths-based intervention, 20, 312–313; therapists' feelings of abandonment, 250; therapists' feelings of sadness, 7, 22–23, 175, 238, 239, 295; therapists' impulse to activity, 22, 59–61, 231, 252–253, 306, 319–320; therapists' intense feelings/thoughts, 7,